PHYSICIANS OF THE FUTURE

THE WILLIAM & BETTYE NOWLIN SERIES
in Art, History, and Culture of the Western Hemisphere

PHYSICIANS OF THE FUTURE

Doctor-Influencers, Patient-Consumers, and the Business of Functional Medicine

Rosalynn A. Vega

University of Texas Press

Austin

First edition, 2024

Requests for permission to reproduce material from this work should be sent to:
Permissions
University of Texas Press
P.O. Box 7819
Austin, TX 78713-7819
utpress.utexas.edu

♾ The paper used in this book meets the minimum requirements of ANSI/NISO Z39.48-1992 (R1997) (Permanence of Paper).

Library of Congress Cataloging-in-Publication Data

Names: Vega, Rosalynn A., author.
Title: Physicians of the future : doctor-influencers, patient-consumers, and the business of functional medicine / Rosalynn A. Vega.
Description: First edition. | Austin : University of Texas Press, 2024. | Includes bibliographical references and index.
Identifiers: LCCN 2023029872
ISBN 978-1-4773-2867-5 (hardcover)
ISBN 978-1-4773-2868-2 (paperback)
ISBN 978-1-4773-2869-9 (pdf)
ISBN 978-1-4773-2870-5 (epub)
Subjects: LCSH: Functional medicine—Social aspects. | Functional medicine—Administration. | Functional medicine—Costs. | Health services accessibility—Economic aspects. | Social media in medicine. | Traditional medicine—Social aspects. | Patient-centered health care. | Physician and patient.
Classification: LCC R733 .V445 2024 | DDC 610—dc23/eng/20230727
LC record available at https://lccn.loc.gov/2023029872

doi:10.7560/328675

For my mom, the woman who raised me to fight for social justice

為了我的波波。我想你，我愛你

CONTENTS

PHYSICIANS OF THE FUTURE

Prelude

TREAT THE PERSON, NOT THE DISEASE

The summer after my freshman year in Brown University's Program in Liberal Medical Education, I returned home to Sacramento, where I had lined up observerships in three different hospitals and enrolled in second-semester physics at UC Davis. One of the mentors I began observing was my own ob-gyn. It was exciting to see her work, and I pictured myself doing the different procedures and maneuvers she was demonstrating to me. Every consultation room was my classroom, and I was watching for technique.

On clinic days, my ob-gyn mentor consistently had an hour for lunch. One day she invited me to her home, explaining that she had purchased a house a few blocks from the hospital so she would waste no time commuting. The inside of her home was fairly bare; she had just finished paying it off. I walked around the living room and saw a photo of her with a man—someone I presumed was her boyfriend. I asked her about the picture, and she told me her boyfriend was a professional musician. Like her, he was raised in an Asian household where children were taught to play instruments like the violin or piano, and music became his profession. The two did not see each other much since he traveled with his symphony orchestra. The distance in their relationship was one of the many reasons it was important for her to own her own home.

Moments like these, visiting my doctor's home and learning about her love life, made me think of her less as a professional mentor and more as a "dee dee" (an older-sister figure). I could relate to her in so many ways—I had been brought up with a piano in my house and had started weekly lessons at age six. As a child and throughout my adolescence, whenever I had had any gift money—my Chinese family members had given me red "lucky money" envelopes instead of boxed gifts for Christmas, Chinese New Year, and my birthday—I had saved the money for my future house. (In my late twenties, I put that money toward the home I now own.) I could see myself in her, and I took all her advice to heart.

Three years later, I went into her office for a routine Pap smear. When I was in my late teens and early twenties, the guideline was to have a Pap smear annually. (Since then, the guideline has been changed to every three years in women with negative results.) I scheduled my Pap each summer like clockwork. Since it was a routine visit, I grabbed whatever appointment was available. This time, it was with her physician assistant. A week or two later, I received the result in my patient portal. The result read "POSITIVE." The test result included a note that biopsies of the abnormal tissue were required. For this procedure, I would not be observing over the ob-gyn's shoulder—I would be the biopsy patient.

My mother came with me. I told her I did not need her to come, but she insisted. Looking back, I know she was even more concerned than I was. She herself had had cervical dysplasia that required cryosurgery in her thirties. Furthermore, she had been indelibly affected by my grandmother's cervical cancer. She drove me to the hospital and waited with me in the waiting room. When I was called in to the procedure room, she joined me there too. My ob-gyn asked me if it was all right with me that my mom was there, and I responded that it was fine. I assumed she was referring to the possibility of my wanting privacy during a procedure that is rather intimate in nature.

I assumed wrong. As soon as I finished consenting to my mother's presence, my ob-gyn dove into a tongue lashing, implying I was now suffering the consequences of promiscuity. "HPV incidence increases with your number of sexual partners," she emphasized. I was caught off guard. I have never been promiscuous—I am a monogamous person by nature. She insisted, taking out a chart demonstrating the different degrees of cervical dysplasia, with the illustrated cells becoming more disfigured and sickly colored from one stage to the next. My Pap smear results were CIN-3, the highest level of dysplasia. She explained, "To get to CIN-3, this process had to have started at least ten years ago." I instantly did the math: in order for what she was saying to be correct, my cervical dysplasia needed to have begun when I was eleven, or even younger. Given my sexual history, I knew she was miles off the mark. However, if she had been correct, my ob-gyn should have been questioning whether I was the victim of childhood sexual abuse, not casting judgment.

My ob-gyn continued to tell me that cervical dysplasias are caused by HPV—the human papillomavirus—so I must have been infected by this sexually transmitted virus. I resisted her assertions as I had been inoculated against HPV as a teen. Could she test me? She responded, "It doesn't make any sense to test you because I already know you have it."

When she was finished berating me, she ordered me to lie on my back and place my feet in the stirrups. After snapping the speculum into place, she inserted a long metal tool that had a hole-punch-like mechanism on the end. She took six biopsy samples, punching into my cervix again and again. At the time I thought the procedure was always that awful. Now, having gone through the same procedure an additional seven times, I know she was lashing her judgment on my cervix. Looking back on this experience from the perspective of a medical anthropologist, I recognize that the way my ob-gyn shamed me was inappropriate and misplaced, and the way she performed the procedure could be considered violating.

If my ob-gyn had looked at my medical record more closely—in fact, if at all—she would have noticed that I had received annual Pap smears and I had never had a positive result. This immediately repudiated her assertion that my dysplasia was a decade or more in the making. As a detective, she should have questioned whether something other than what she was used to seeing was going on. If she had taken my word over her textbook definition of how cervical dysplasia unfolds, she would have been open to other etiologies. And she would have tested me for HPV, on the small chance that I did not have it.

This experience would also have been different if my ob-gyn had delved into my personal and family history. She might have understood how my living in Mexico for several years in a region with more than ten times the safe limit of arsenic in the water (see Golam Mostafa, Jahin Queen, and Cherry 2017; Alarcón-Herrera et al. 2020; Fisher et al. 2017; Galetovic Carabantes and de Fernicola 2003),[1] my lifetime of eating arsenic-contaminated rice (FDA 2016), my genetic predisposition (see Burk et al. 2017), and my weakened immune system (American Cancer Society 2020) had increased my risk of developing cervical cancer.

As an epidemiologist, I see clearly now that HPV is not the sole cause of cervical cancer (Mount Sinai Tisch Cancer Center n.d.). The virus is a component cause in many cases, but HPV alone is not sufficient to cause cervical cancer. If it were, all women who are infected with HPV at some point in their lives—about 80 percent of women—would go on to develop cervical cancer (Cleveland Clinic 2022). This certainly is not the case, so other factors must also come into play. That is, HPV, combined with specific other component causes, creates the proper circumstances in which cancer may develop. At the same time, other component causes, in the absence of HPV, may also lead to cancer (American Cancer Society 2020). However, doctors and public health officials have adopted a vaccine-oriented approach for preventing cervical cancer, and other potential causes (e.g., genetic predisposition, environmental exposures, gut dysbiosis, long-term use of birth control pills, etc.) have received meager attention (see Dyer 2002).

When my ob-gyn received the biopsy results, she suggested the loop electrosurgical excision procedure (LEEP) to remove the abnormal tissue, insisting the procedure was necessary since, per her explanation, when a dysplasia advances as far as mine had, there is no chance it will reverse on its own. CIN-3 dysplasias advance to cervical cancer, so I needed to surgically remove the dysplasia before the problem spread.

Two of the risks associated with the LEEP are an increased chance of preterm delivery and, in rare cases, a narrowing of the cervix resulting in infertility. Faced with these potential outcomes, I decided I could not risk affecting the success of my future pregnancies or, worse yet, losing the ability to become pregnant at all. Even though I was over a decade away from even considering having children, my future babies were already real in my mind. I fired my ob-gyn. I had grown up knowing her and had looked up to her as a role model, but the time had come for the relationship to end.

For my CIN-3 dysplasia to be correctly treated, I needed personalized medicine—not the standard protocol. Unfortunately, protocols define patient care in conventional medicine—especially in obstetrics and gynecology, where any deviation from the established protocols represents a personal risk for providers, who are already paying sky-high malpractice insurance premiums. Fortunately, I found another ob-gyn, and she was able to at least offer me more time while sticking to the conventional medical protocol.

During our initial visit, I immediately asked my new doctor to test me for HPV. She told me that while my prior ob-gyn was correct in asserting that most cases of cervical dysplasia are caused by HPV, a small percentage of cases are not. In those rare cases, the dysplasia may "spontaneously" resolve without surgical intervention, especially in women under twenty-five years old. She tested me for HPV and the results were negative. This ob-gyn performed another round of hole-punch biopsies—about six months after the first round—and determined my dysplasia at that point was CIN-2. Given these new findings, she decided it was permissible for me to wait until I turned twenty-five to take further action.

Thus began my first experience with cervical dysplasia. I went back for biopsies every six months for the next three years, for a total of forty-two hole-punch biopsies. I have always believed in "precision medicine." How could I make informed choices about my health if I did not make the most of existing technologies to understand what was going on in my body?

The three years during which I struggled with cervical dysplasia overlapped with the three years and seven months I spent in Mexico conducting research for my first book and teaching medical anthropology at the Autonomous National University of Mexico (UNAM). While I flew home to California for biopsies every six months, I otherwise did not have access to any medical care. Much of my research was conducted in rural settings with pirated electricity, corrugated metal roofs and dirt floors, no running water, and dilapidated, unmanned clinics. Although I did not yet have diagnoses for the web of chronic diseases I was struggling with, I could feel how fragile my body was—anyone with a cold seemed like a major threat as even common viruses could put me in bed for weeks or months. I was chronically fatigued, but I was committed to my research.

I turned to my upbringing with Traditional Chinese Medicine for ideas on recovering my health in this challenging time. For twenty-plus years, I had watched my maternal grandmother, Popo, plant, harvest, dry, store, and use her medicinal herbs. I created a tincture for cervical dysplasia and combined this with quality rest, diet, supplements, and other herbal remedies when needed. I had become my own doctor and herbalist, and I believed in my body's ability to heal itself. And I slowly got better. My dysplasia came down again, from CIN-2 to CIN-1, and finally to a negative result, just a couple of months before my twenty-fifth birthday.

I will forever be grateful to the gynecologist who entertained my decision to wait. My second ob-gyn offered me the LEEP each time I went in for biopsies, suggesting that having the procedure was actually the easier option. "If you ever get tired of this and you just want to have it out, we can just schedule you for the procedure and be done with it." Every time I responded the same way: I wanted to keep waiting. I turned down her offers with a lot of appreciation for how she was communicating with me but also with conviction in my decision. By not prioritizing her time over my choice, she gave me the gift of time. This was the best thing she could have given me since the medicine I truly needed was nowhere to be found—at least not to the knowledge of a twenty-one-year-old woman in the late 2000s.

I needed precise data collection to identify potential contributors to the worsening of my cervical dysplasia. This would have included an in-depth examination of my genome, not to grimly identify my genetic fate but to develop epigenetic tools for ridding my body of the dysplasia and preventing future disease. The ideal care would have used microbiome testing to evaluate how gut dysbiosis (an imbalance of intestinal flora) might be influencing my female hormones so I could precisely intervene where needed. It would have used nutritional testing to assess my absorption of important cancer-fighting nutrients. It would have tested for heavy metals to evaluate my toxic load and for viruses other than HPV to evaluate the state of my immune system. My dysplasia was particularly aggressive—in a matter of mere months it had progressed to a stage that, according to textbook explanations, requires many years. Nevertheless, the medicine I needed would have emphasized my body's capacity to heal itself if given the right support.

It was a full decade later when I discovered that the medicine I had needed at twenty-one was gaining a foothold in the American "healthscape" (see Pizzorno 2017).[2]

INTRODUCTION

This book interrogates the hidden logics of inclusion and exclusion in functional medicine, a holistic form of personalized medicine that targets chronic disease by focusing on nutrition and "lifestyle." Functional medicine traces its origins to 1990—the same year the Human Genome Project began. By positioning the genome as a "roadmap to function," functional medicine practitioners focus on the usefulness of genomic data for creating health instead of merely identifying disease risk. Using advanced diagnostic testing, these practitioners combine genomics with epigenomics (the effects of environmental inputs on gene expression) and metabolomics (the sum total of all the metabolic processes happening in the body in reaction to food, toxins, stress, and the outside environment) to create a telescopic understanding of what is occurring in the "bioindividual" patient at multiple levels, in real time. This "health-optimization medicine" has produced positive health outcomes for those who can afford it. In fact, a cohort study of 7,252 patients published in the *Journal of the American Medical Association* found that functional medicine patients exhibited significantly greater improvements than their conventional medicine counterparts (see Beidelschies et al. 2019).

Functional medicine is quickly becoming accepted as part of "mainstream" medicine. In 2021, the Institute for Functional Medicine received more than sixty-five thousand visits per month to its Find a Practitioner database and trained nearly ten thousand practitioners. Furthermore, the institute was awarded accreditation with commendation by the Accreditation Council for Continuing Medical Education for the third time in July 2022.[1] Meanwhile, large institutions such as the Department of Veterans Affairs and the Nebraska Methodist Hospital have adopted functional medicine to meet patient demand and treatment goals. According to the American College of Lifestyle Medicine's Health Systems Council, sixty health systems across the country are now providing "lifestyle medicine."[2] Furthermore, functional medicine interlocutors are reaching an international audience, as evidenced by some of the presentations at the June 2022 Integrative & Personalised Medicine Congress in London.

Some conventionally trained doctors have turned to functional medicine after struggling with chronic disease themselves or caring for a close family member with chronic disease. In either instance, these "wounded healers" discovered they did not possess the tools to cure the problem and felt betrayed by their conventional medical training. Their personal experience of illness and recovery, which often involved poor treatment or stigmatization within the conventional medicine paradigm, led them to embrace practicing functional medicine as the final destination of their "hero's journey."

Power and authority operate differently in functional medicine than in conventional medicine—perhaps due to the personal experiences of functional medicine practitioners but also largely because functional medicine services are paid for out of pocket by socioeconomically privileged "clients." Functional medicine interlocutors such as Sachin Patel, a best-selling author and founder of the Living Proof Institute, position the patients of functional medicine as "the doctors of the future," meaning they take a leadership role in medical decision-making regarding their own bodies—as will be the way of the future—while the provider takes on the role of guide or health coach. In this book, I make the following three interventions.

First, I argue that multiple relational shifts, including those in emergent forms of biosociality, are occurring in the functional medicine realm. Biosociality, a concept first introduced by Paul Rabinow in 1992, explores how people with shared biological conditions form social networks. A narrow approach to this concept analyzes how people diagnosed with a disease or condition form a new identity based on their diagnosis. A broader interpretation of biosociality examines how the social status of humans relates to their biological status. I extend the concept of biosociality to ask how, as wounded healers, functional medicine practitioners relate to one another as former chronic-disease sufferers, thus reconfiguring their illness narratives as a form of social capital. And, as the doctors of the future, functional medicine clients lay claim to expert insight through their embodied knowledge, a shift away from the traditional patient-doctor relationship. However, this relational shift is not accessible to everyone since out-of-pocket expenses for functional medicine are prohibitive for many. Online support groups have emerged to provide those struggling with similar diagnoses and interested in a functional approach with peer-to-peer guidance, thus critiquing the high hourly rates charged by some functional medicine practitioners. Based on advice and feedback from these groups, some less privileged individuals have been able to implement functional medicine protocols on their own—turning to the group instead of the "guru" for support.

Second, I analyze the social underpinnings of functional medicine entrepreneurship. Functional medicine practitioners have needed to learn entrepreneurial skills to be successful in private practice. Many have enrolled in the same coaching programs and thus have developed strikingly homogeneous entrepreneurial strategies. These include positioning themselves as "doctor-influencers" by harnessing the power of social media to engage potential consumers. Functional medicine entrepreneurs further participate in community-based marketing, thus reinforcing the biosociality among practitioners. I argue that entrepreneurship in functional medicine inadvertently reinscribes racialized inequality when it romanticizes the "ancient healing traditions" of far-flung cultures while excluding racialized "Others" from profit streams. Thus, functional medicine entrepreneurship is premised on an "us"/"them" binary that unwittingly glorifies poverty and fails to defend the intellectual property rights of the originators of traditional knowledge.

Third, I open up avenues for possibility in functional medicine. Functional medicine practitioners critique the existing health care system and argue that the pharmaceutical and insurance industries have placed companies' profits over lasting wellness for patients. In this context, functional medicine practitioners and advocates have aimed to develop strategies for the "mainstreaming" of their approach, for example, by offering group-delivered care. While I acknowledge the benefits of group visits, I simultaneously argue that functional medicine delivery models have inadvertently been steeped in neoliberal ideology. Functional medicine's emphasis on (bio)individuality places the responsibility for healing on the individual and often sidesteps important issues of "racial" and socioeconomic inequality. Given disparate COVID-19 outcomes based on "race,"[3] combined with the 2020 resurgence of the Black Lives Matter movement, functional medicine interlocutors are beginning to wrestle with their responsibility for making functional medicine accessible to all. I argue that, through a commitment to community (a key theme in functional medicine), functional medicine practitioners can position themselves as champions for "health justice."

METHODS

Through discussion of my twenty-seven months of in-depth digital, traditional, and autoethnographic research from 2019 to 2022, I illuminate multiple perspectives regarding functional medicine, relational shifts, and access to recovery. My digital autoethnographic approach gives new meaning to "multisited ethnography." I create a cartography of functional medicine in the United States, thus identifying different "windows" through which chronic-disease reversal and issues of inequality can be examined (see Marcus 1995; Menéndez 1996; Rapp 2000; Wilson 2004). To accomplish this task, I weave together the stories of myself and others as they unfold across multiple physical and digital spaces, thus analyzing social life in its multiple contemporary forms (see Kent 2021). As a whole, this "braided tale" (Lester 2019) tells an important story about unequal access to health. It emphasizes that recovery is possible but that in our society, healing is facilitated by privilege.

Over the course of my ethnographic research, I observed hundreds of functional medicine practitioners and proponents, as indicated in table 1. Readers will find in the appendix a list of the sources from which each functional medicine interlocutor is referenced or quoted. I also endeavor to list in the appendix the training and professional background of each of the individuals discussed in this book. I have intentionally avoided cherry-picking the voices featured in this text—instead, I present the functional medicine network exactly as I encountered it during my ethnographic research. Using social-network data, I was able to map the saturation and cohesion of the functional medicine community (see figures 0.1 and 0.2). Although this study does not encompass every individual who practices or advocates for functional medicine, my methodology helps confirm that the individuals included in it are representative of the functional medicine community at large.

I culled the majority of my data from "public" online spaces (e.g., conferences, summits, docuseries, blogs, podcasts, YouTube videos, TED talks, etc.) where functional medicine biosociality can be observed and discourse unfolds, as indicated in table 2. Over the course of my ethnographic fieldwork, I recognized that the individuals I was observing form a cohesive community whose discourse revolves around common themes. I became digitally familiar with almost all the functional medicine practitioners who have a significant online presence, and I listened to virtually every aspect of their discourse. In the following subsections, I provide further detail regarding the process of digital ethnography, participant observation, and illness autoethnography.

Table 1. Research Subjects

Profession/role	**Number of individuals included in this ethnographic research project**
Medical doctors (MD)	77
Health and science doctorates (PhD, DHSc)	63
Entrepreneurs, health advocates, and consultants	39
Patients	28
Nutrition experts (PhD, CCN, CN, FACN, DACBN, MS)	26
Health coaches and educators	18
Chiropractors (DC)	15
Naturopathic doctors (ND)	13
Filmmakers and show hosts	10
Health science journalists, editors, and authors	9
Administrators of functional and integrative medicine clinics and organizations	6
Osteopaths (DO)	6
Nurses (RN, CNS)	6
Acupuncturists	6
Politicians	5
Oriental medicine practitioners (DOM, MSOM/MSAOM)	4
Dieticians (RD, RDN)	3
Pharmacists (PharmD, RPh)	3
Food activists	2
Ayurvedic doctor (AD)	1
Institute for Functional Medicine Certified Practitioner (IFMCP)	1
Other allied health professionals	6

Note: *I include here only the number of individuals whom I quote or refer to directly in this book or in* Nested Ecologies *(2023). I refer to most of these individuals in both books. I do not include the hundreds of thousandsof other individuals who participated in online summits and conferences, appeared on YouTube channels and podcasts, belonged to Facebook groups, were featured in docuseries, attended continuing medical education courses, or delivered presentations on online health education platforms but are not directly referred to in my work.*

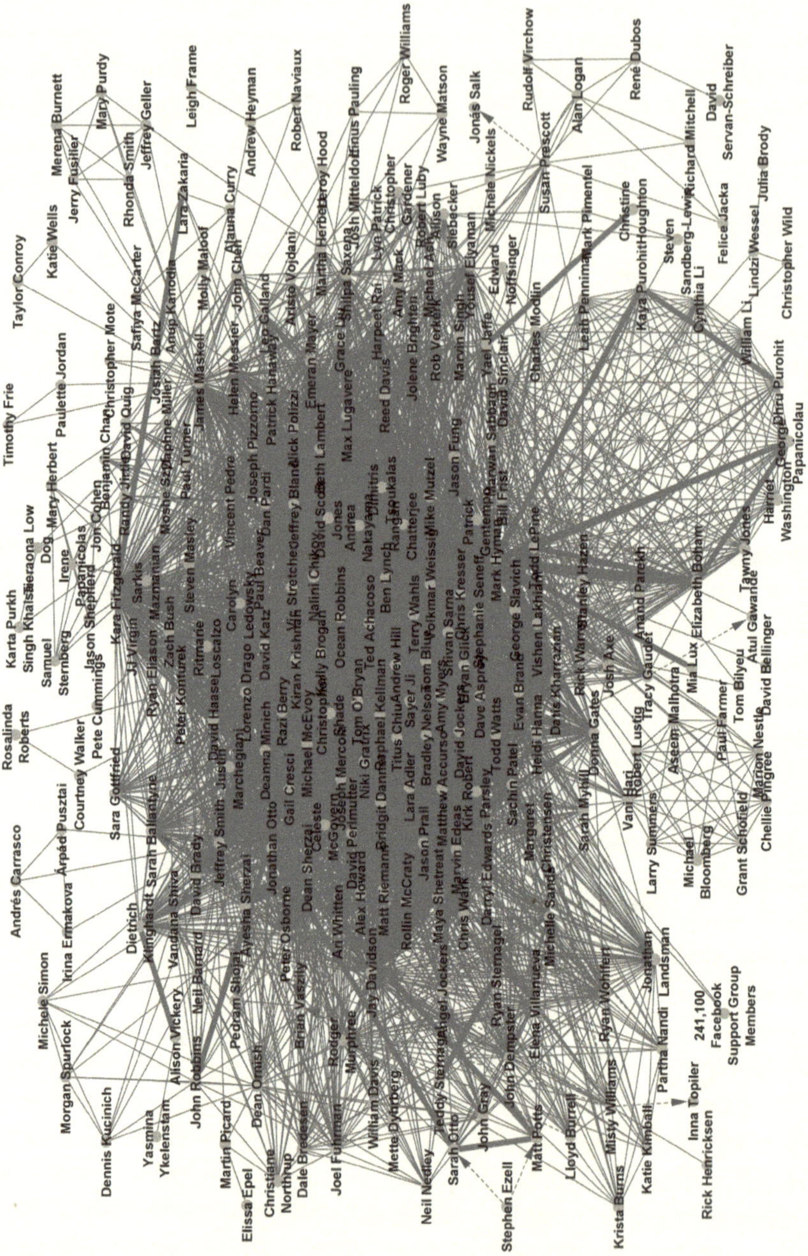

Figure 0.1. People-centric social network. This social network map demonstrates how different interlocutors are connected to one another. Bold lines represent "real-life" connections (e.g., individuals who are coworkers, siblings, or spouses). Dashed lines indicate when an individual referenced another individual. Credit: Jason Vega. Full-color image hosted at https://tinyurl.com/Physicians-of-the-Future.

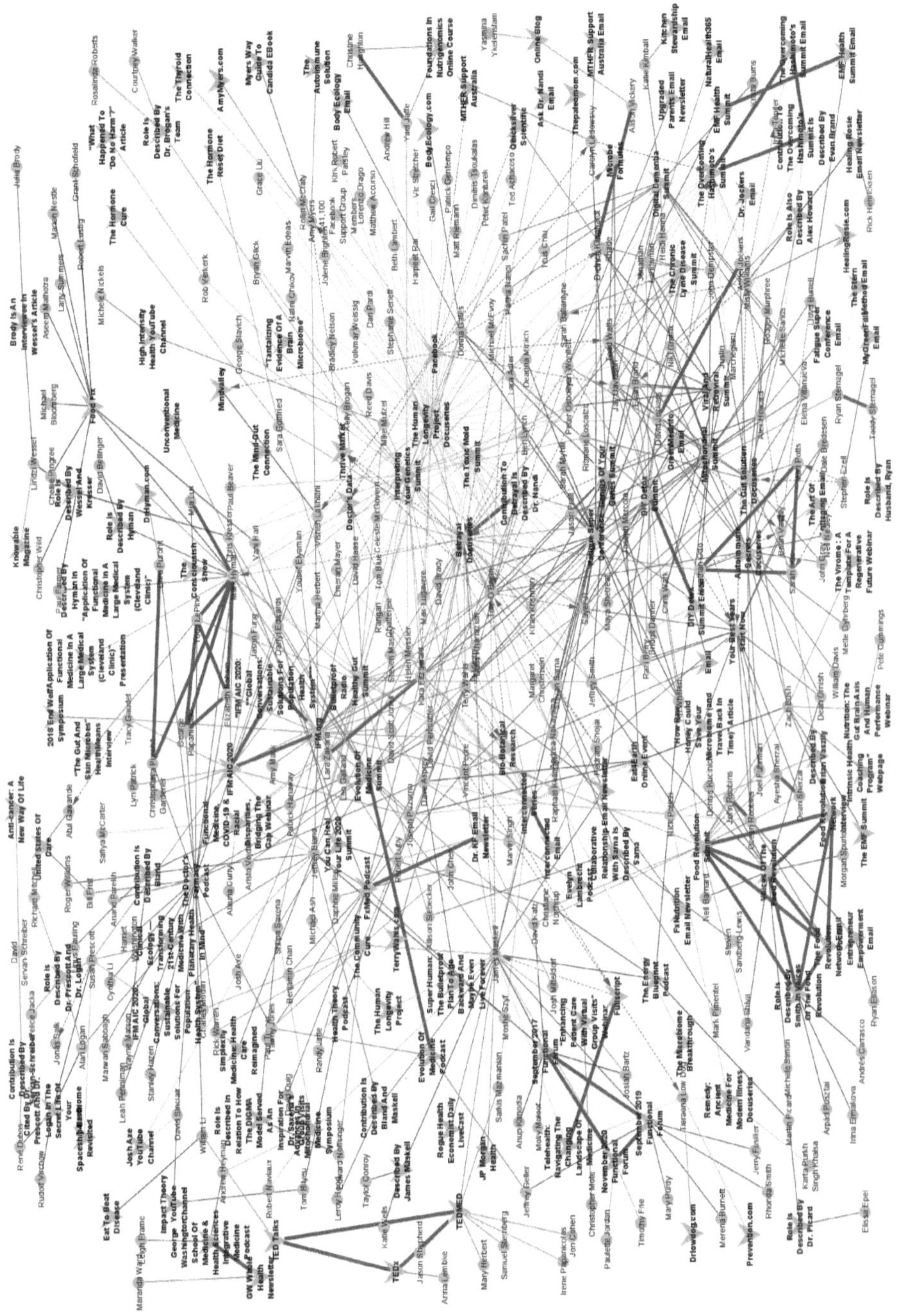

Figure 0.2. Source-centric social network. This social network indicates how individuals are connected to one another through their participation in different sources (e.g., podcasts, webinars, or summits). Bold lines represent "real-life" connections (e.g., individuals who are coworkers, siblings, or spouses). Dashed lines are indicative of "promotional relationships" (individuals or platforms that promoted the products or services of companies or of other individuals). Credit: Jason Vega. Full-color image hosted at https://tinyurl.com/Physicians-of-the-Future.

Table 2. Data Sources

Data source type	Number incorporated into this ethnographic research project
Hours of online coursework in nutrigenetics and nutrigenomics	60
Continuing medical education credits	52
Functional medicine interlocutors' newsletters	29
Books intended for a wide audience	19
Webinars, eCourses, and master classes	19
Online summits and conferences	18
Company newsletters	16
YouTube channels	11
Facebook groups (totaling 241,100+ online members in December 2020)	9
Docuseries	6
Podcasts	6
Blogs	4
Magazine and newspaper subscriptions	3
Online health education platforms	2

Digital Ethnography

My first pieces of ethnographic data emerged when I was searching for answers regarding my own health issues. My search led me to the web pages of individuals who had launched careers as health coaches after struggling with similar issues, seeking additional training, and interviewing leading medical experts. As I delved deeper into the topics presented in these health coaches' blogs, I encountered multiple conventionally trained doctors who had transitioned to practicing functional medicine. These doctors had struggled with chronic disease themselves or had witnessed a close family member's experience of chronic disease. In the process, they discovered that while their conventional medical training provided them with tools for managing chronic disease, they were ill equipped to address root causes and restore themselves and their loved ones to health. My early research into functional medicine led me to HealthMeans and DrTalks, web platforms that host online summits and conferences on different functional medicine topics. I listened to numerous conferences and summits, thus gaining up-to-the-moment insights from dozens of functional medicine practitioners on a wide variety of health-related topics. My attendance at these events exposed me to how functional medicine discourse unfolds among large groups of colleagues.

Following my participation in many online events on different platforms, I began receiving email newsletters from numerous functional medicine practitioners and their allies. These emails often included links to podcasts and blogs and offers of free registration for webinars and eCourses. Thus, while the HealthMeans and DrTalks platforms brought numerous functional medicine practitioners together for each online event, webinars and eCourses were usually delivered by either a single functional medicine practitioner or a small group of functional medicine colleagues. Often, this format exposed me to individual practitioners' illness narratives. As I became more interested in the perspectives of particular functional medicine practitioners, I began looking for them in increasingly public digital spaces such as YouTube and TED talks. The videos I watched were often extensions of functional medicine practitioners' audio podcasts.

At times, I found that email newsletters promoted online docuseries in which functional medicine practitioners were featured. These docuseries were oriented around specific topics—for example, reversing autoimmunity, improving gut health, using stem cell therapy, increasing longevity, and so forth. The different series, generally lasting a week or so, were delivered in daily episodes that were only available through purchase after the event "expired." They were created by filmmakers who either suffered from the disease being investigated or had a family member who had suffered from it. After personally experiencing the effectiveness of functional medicine for reversing chronic disease and promoting health, these filmmakers used their skills to conduct in-depth interviews with different functional medicine practitioners, and sometimes recovered patients, on the topic.

The email newsletters from functional medicine practitioners also promoted products, thus blurring the line between health professional and health "influencer." Initially, I ignored promotional emails, sifting through the daily mountain of inbox items for useful information. At a certain point, however, I recognized that promotional emails were in fact a valuable source of ethnographic data. Clicking on products promoted by health "influencers" connected me to different companies' commercial listservs and, in one case, resulted in a monthly magazine being delivered to my house. These marketing materials exposed me to functional medicine entrepreneurs' multiple strategies for attracting consumers.

While I considered many more sources of ethnographic data—especially webinars, eCourses, master classes, summits, and docuseries—I stopped when I felt my data had reached "saturation"; that is, I concluded my research when additional online events no longer exposed me to new faces or ideas.

Participant Observation

My observations of online meetings, blogs, docuseries, videos, and talks provided me with a clear picture of how functional medicine practitioners engage one another before a virtual public audience. However, I felt the need to also observe biosocial interactions among these practitioners as colleagues and wounded healers in person. Thus, I conducted participant observation and earned continuing medical education credits from the American Medical Association while attending the Advances in Mitochondrial Medicine Symposium in Dallas in 2019. This in-person participant observation provided me with the opportunity to connect with numerous functional medicine practitioners in a face-to-face setting.

I likewise felt the need to observe biosocial interactions among functional medicine patients. Some of the functional medicine practitioners in my study created online Facebook groups as a platform for directly engaging patients, followers, and the public. As I began exploring these groups, Facebook suggested related groups to me. I joined nine Facebook support groups for topics related to my own healing journey. These groups' membership totaled approximately 241,100. Interacting with these group members via Facebook provided me with insight into how patients actively use functional medicine techniques to tackle their chronic health conditions. I participated in and observed the constant mutual support these digital communities provide. As someone suffering from chronic disease, I empathized with fellow patients. I both sought and offered encouraging feedback within online support groups at different points in my healing journey. I took note of how, in a matter of months, every group I joined grew by one to six thousand members.

I use pseudonyms for fellow members in closed Facebook groups. This decision was informed by the original purpose of the data source. While docuseries were created to spread the word about functional medicine, the content of closed Facebook groups is made accessible only to the groups' members in an effort to keep sensitive health information private. With the goal of respecting the wishes of these group members, I have also omitted dates, photos, and any other identifiable information. Given that the membership of these groups totals nearly a quarter million people, I believe this form of anonymization is effective for concealing the identity of individual group members.

Illness Autoethnography

In addition to digital ethnography and participant observation, I have incorporated in this book my personal experiences as someone who has struggled with, and recovered from, chronic disease. In so doing, I hope to render visible the process of participant observation that informs this book, thus actively resisting the notion that the researcher is absent or neutral (Hertz 2006). My training in the ethnographic method provided me with the necessary skills for finding answers regarding how to reverse my chronic health problems. Autoethnography underscores the usefulness of ethnography for everyday life.

I am building upon a rich tradition of illness autoethnography in medical anthropology and medical sociology. Autoethnography provides a "thick description" of multiple layers of consciousness. As a form of emotional and vulnerable postmodern witnessing, autoethnographies "give voice to the structured silence of embodied illness experiences" (Ettorre 2006, 156). Autoethnography demonstrates how the emotions of anxiety, despair, agony, disgust, triumph, hope, joy, and pleasure are refracted through the body to create the intricate texture of illness.

Autoethnography connects the personal to the cultural and societal (Ettorre 2005, 2006). Although ethnographic writing has been viewed as too emotional and personal to be academic (Atkinson 1997), it allows researchers to situate themselves in a larger context and document the details of their lived experience (Ellis and Bochner 2000). In this way, autoethnography problematizes the binary splits between self and society, between subjective and objective, and between medical understandings of disease and perception of illness as embodied experience (Reed-Danahay 1997).

While the point of this book is not to describe my own experiences, autoethnography does appear here in the form of a prelude and three interludes between chapters to demonstrate what is at stake for individual patients. Autoethnography renders the person suffering with chronic illness visible without portraying her as other. Medical narratives are often dominated by the voice of a distant expert, and while people suffering from chronic illness are frequently the subjects of research, their personhood tends to be obscured (Richards 2008). In contrast, autoethnography makes it difficult to read the narrative as a story of disease instead of a story about "the impact of an illness on a person's life" (Sullivan 1986, 332). Embodiment and emotionality gain legitimacy as mediums of lived experience, and bodily dysfunctions are imbued with value when the body is connected to the self (see Bochner 2001). Autoethnography may raise awareness and provoke change by offering a theorized and politicized yet intensely individual and subjective point of view (Garro 1992; Kleinman 1992; Marks 1999).

By including my experiences in brief interludes, I am furthermore able to include raw ethnographic data that demonstrate emerging forms of biosociality in functional medicine. To provide the reader with access to my lived experience, and with the intent of demonstrating relational shifts in action, I have decided to share in this book my email correspondence with two practitioners on my functional medicine team. I then submit these emails to the same critical analysis I apply to all the discourse in this ethnographic study.

Discourse—the circulation of concepts and ideas—takes on a unique shape and is carried on through distinctive means within the functional medicine realm. In particular, functional medicine practitioners encourage each other to share their personal stories of illness and recovery among themselves and with their patients. The "illness narrative" (Kleinman [1988] 2020) of "wounded healers" was a discursive form I came across time and time again when conducting research for this book. In fact, sharing the details of how they personally reversed chronic disease is a common way functional medicine practitioners introduce themselves during podcasts and online webinars.

By sharing my own illness narrative, I hope to both *describe* the ethnographic phenomena I observed as an anthropologist and *demonstrate*, through my own story, how functional medicine is experienced by individuals. This allows me to simultaneously engage in two types of discourse. I extend anthropological discourse when describing what I experienced as a participant observer of functional medicine. And by writing in a way that incorporates the unique style of functional medicine discourse, I simultaneously enact how this discourse unfolds among functional medicine practitioners and patients. While preparing to write this book, I reproduced the form and format of illness narratives among functional medicine interlocutors when I described my healing journey in a forty-five-minute interview for KSDT radio in San Diego. This double engagement—both analytical and illustrative—with functional medicine's discursive forms is a key feature of this book since the culture of functional medicine comes to life through the particular types of knowledge that are circulated and made known (see Strathern 1994, 347).

It is important to note that while I am incorporating the discursive forms of the people I studied and observed, the respective goals of our communication—that is, functional medicine practitioners sharing their illness narratives with colleagues and patients, and my doing so with readers—are distinct. While the illness narrative is a *prescriptive* discursive form among functional medicine practitioners, my aim is *descriptive and analytical.* That is, functional medicine practitioners share their stories when explaining how to reverse disease. In certain cases, the protocols that functional practitioners have developed are outgrowths of the strategies they used to heal themselves. By sharing their stories, these practitioners are instructing their colleagues and patients on how to identify root causes and reach lasting wellness. In contrast, I am not holding myself out to be a medical expert by any means. The goal of sharing my story is not to teach others specific healing strategies. Instead, I adopt the illness narrative as a discursive form to help readers think critically about their own lives and their relationships to health and disease. In essence, I hope to stimulate "the dialectic of revelation" in which the autoethnographic writer and reader co-create or (re) negotiate an interpretation of the topic at hand (see Warren et al. 2000).

By combining digital autoethnography and engagement with the existing literature, I aim to write in a way that engages multiple audiences (social scientists, health care providers, patients and their families, policymakers, etc.). By revealing the lived experience of illness, this reflexive approach may prompt readers from diverse backgrounds to question their attitudes about health, illness, and disease, and to (re)negotiate their beliefs (Richards 2008).

WHAT IS TO COME

Chapter 1 sets the stage for the rest of the book by examining functional medicine in the context of the current state of technoscience and medical practice. I address the question of whether functional medicine is a pseudoscience by exploring the varying qualifications of its practitioners, its (lack of) conformity to existing scientific research methods, the (absence of) uniformity in its application, its potential for offering false hope, and its links to complementary and alternative medicines. I argue that while functional medicine resists most of the defining characteristics of pseudoscience, some features of it unfold in the area between science and pseudoscience. Turning to the literature on boundary work—a term that refers to how boundaries between fields of knowledge are continually created, reinforced, challenged, and dismantled—I suggest that functional medicine interlocutors engage in "inclusionary" boundary work when they aim to expand the limits of conventional medicine.

The next three chapters explore different relational shifts (e.g., emerging forms of biosociality) at play in functional medicine. Through a reconfiguration of the body, functional medicine opens up new possibilities for relationships between providers and patients, among providers, and among patients. Chapter 2 analyzes shifts in provider-provider relationships. I explore the illness narratives of functional medicine practitioners as a particular discursive form that reconfigures understandings of health, disease, vulnerability, and recovery. "Wounded healers" are doctors who have transitioned to functional medicine after experiencing chronic disease close up and realizing their conventional medical training has not equipped them to cure the problem. I argue that functional medicine providers' illness narratives take on the form of a "hero's journey" since, through their narratives, these providers shed their façade of impenetrability, reveal their former health struggles, explain how they were "betrayed" by the conventional paradigm, describe experiments in which their own health was at stake, and challenge biomedical hegemony in order to champion the functional medicine model. I interrogate how, in so doing, functional medicine practitioners must resist the stigmatization of disease—a tendency that would threaten their authority as health care providers within the conventional paradigm.[4] Ultimately, the recounting of illness narratives establishes a sense of commonality among practitioners while instilling them with a sense of purpose. I thus extend biosociality to provider-provider relationships—a type of relationship that has been underappreciated and underexamined in medical anthropology.

Chapter 3 explores how, while in conventional medicine the medical practitioner is the sole authority, the functional medicine model represents a shift in hierarchical power. Through enthusiastic engagement of disruptive technologies (e.g., wearable devices, apps, and at-home tests), functional medicine repositions the patient as the doctor of the future. In the process, the role of the provider is rescripted to that of a coach or guide rather than an authority to whom "compliance" is owed. These relational shifts are buttressed by individuals' ability to shape their biology through marketplace alternatives. Since functional medicine patients are paying "clients," their embodied knowledge demands legitimacy, thus decentering the authoritative knowledge embedded in conventional medicine (Jordan 1992). These patient-consumers tend to be socioeconomically privileged, thus evincing the relationship between capital and power.

Using the information and understanding I gained during my participant observation in Facebook support groups, I explore in chapter 4 emerging forms of digitized biosociality among functional medicine patients (Rabinow 1996; Gibbon and Novas 2007). In the digital age, the majority of patient-patient interaction unfolds online. While in-person groups tend to unite people who share the same locality and some degree of socioeconomic similarity, online biosociality spans geographic distance and economic difference in ways that are made possible only by digital means, thus rendering stark socioeconomic inequalities visible to participants. During my ethnographic research, I observed and interacted with functional medicine patients of diverse socioeconomic means from Australia, Austria, Belgium, Canada, Costa Rica, Czech Republic, Denmark, England, France, Germany, Hungary, Iceland, Mexico, the Netherlands, New Zealand, Norway, Portugal, Scotland, Serbia, South Africa, Spain, and Wales.

I analyze how online functional medicine communities are sometimes monetized and framed as commodities. Given this context, members of Facebook support groups that are open to the public and free of charge often critique the limited affordability of functional medicine protocols; these groups are valuable information resources for less privileged individuals who are unable to afford out-of-pocket care from a functional medicine provider. In these online spaces, members describe shared experiences and develop mutual understandings of disease etiologies. When individual members seek guidance, the group's "hive mind" produces suggestions for diets, supplementation, and lab testing. At the same time, economic capital sometimes facilitates social capital. In functional medicine circles, self-knowledge costs money (through expensive lab tests, functional medicine care, etc.) and (self-)knowledge (knowledge learned on one's own path toward healing that is later shared with others) becomes social capital.

Digitized relationships among patients simultaneously critique and set the stage for consumption; meanwhile, biosociality among practitioners creates the conditions for functional medicine entrepreneurship. Chapters 5 and 6 explore consumption-based inclusion and exclusion in functional medicine. Chapter 5 turns to how, as functional medicine practitioners have sought creative ways to practice outside of the insurance model, their activities have become increasingly entrepreneurial. I track the multiple strategies functional medicine entrepreneurs employ when interpellating health seekers as consumers. Functional medicine entrepreneurs participate in "community-based marketing"—multiple members of the community market products and services to the mutual benefit of these multiple members, thus constituting and reinforcing relational ties. Furthermore, functional medicine practitioners and health educators turn to social media, corporate sponsors, and online stores to create a (false?) sense of familiarity with potential consumers, build their brands, and earn income as "health and wellness influencers."

The products sold in the functional medicine realm are often said to be inspired by "ancient healing traditions." In chapter 6, I describe how functional medicine entrepreneurs suppress or exalt different ethnic identities for financial profit, thus inadvertently commodifying non-American cultures and reconfiguring traditional healing methods from other societies for mass consumption. Functional medicine discourse romanticizes the ancient healing traditions of "other cultures." At the same time, it describes cultural "Others" (i.e., "non-Westerners") as frozen in an idealized past and does not equitably include them in functional medicine discourse or profit streams. In the process, I contend, functional medicine discourse inadvertently glorifies poverty and reinscribes political, economic, and "racial" inequality. I argue instead for multilateral discourse. This would require functional medicine interlocutors to resist otherization, to view ethnic heritage as a legitimate source of expertise, and to defend the intellectual property rights of the people from whom knowledge originates. In the absence of these elements, functional medicine entrepreneurship runs the risk of venturing into the territory of biopiracy.

The final two chapters turn to systemic shifts that I argue will be required to ensure equitable access to strategies and techniques that create health and reverse chronic disease. Chapter 7 emphasizes the importance of switching to value-based care—that is, paying doctors based on positive patient outcomes rather than the number of services they provide. Functional medicine providers and health educators point to the health care system's inherent conflict of interest: by operating through a fee-for-service model, providers are incentivized to manage but not to heal chronic disease. I furthermore argue, along with many functional medicine practitioners, that incentives preconfigure outcomes and that the neoliberal incentives of "Big Pharma" have led to a system that profits from ill health. I identify both challenges and opportunities for the change these practitioners propose. To achieve meaningful change in the health care system, the funding structures for academic research and, indeed, our very understanding of what constitutes legitimate science must also undergo change. If this change is accomplished, incentives will shift from managing disease to creating health. This chapter provides context for functional medicine practitioners' emerging strategy for "mainstreaming" their therapeutic approach.

Since the 1990s, functional medicine mavericks have turned to private practice to use their expanded skill set in patient care. Acknowledging that this model is inaccessible to many Americans because it is not covered by health insurance, functional medicine proponents have recently argued for "bringing functional medicine to the masses" (i.e., via group medicine). In chapter 8, I argue that despite efforts to make functional medicine more readily accessible, the strategy of group visits is unwittingly steeped in neoliberal ideology. Functional medicine practitioners have used group visits as a savvy solution to their problem of not having enough time and needing to see too many patients. At the same time, this business strategy allows functional medicine practitioners to earn a large income while seeing patients who have limited economic resources. By positioning functional medicine practitioners as entrepreneurs and patients as consumers, functional medicine inadvertently perpetuates neoliberal notions of good citizenship, casts health as a consumer item for purchase in private markets, and promotes individual responsibility at the expense of true social solidarity. I argue that through a commitment to community, functional medicine can begin to decenter neoliberal ideology and its individualistic underpinnings, thus championing health as a matter of social justice.

Finally, in the conclusion, I argue that health is a matter of social justice, and thus I call for a health system that not only is effective at preventing and reversing chronic disease but also responds to "racial" and economic disparities. Functional medicine discourse has often avoided the concept of "race," thus ignoring the question of how functional medicine practitioners can ensure that their approach is adapted to and equitably reaches people of all "racial" and ethnic backgrounds. The Black Lives Matter resurgence in 2020, paired with obvious "racial" disparities in COVID-19 deaths, has brought the topic of "race" and health equity to the fore among functional medicine interlocutors—leading to increased attention to how intersecting "race-" and class-based inequalities structure what is possible for individuals, including recovery from chronic disease. I argue for "health justice"—the removal of racism, exploitation, and oppression in the health care system and the establishment of equitable access to health-promoting resources. In so doing, I point to untapped opportunities for challenging the neoliberal mindset, for unseating the very logics that sustain unequal health care in the United States, and for engaging both providers and patients in a politicized struggle for health justice. Ultimately, I critique the concept of health as a consumer item and argue for health as a citizenship-based right.

While I point to a few prominent advocates for equitable access to functional medicine techniques and approaches, these individuals are—so far—exceptions among the functional medicine community. At present, functional medicine is a path toward healing for a rapidly growing number of people, but since functional medicine is now almost exclusively available to patients through out-of-pocket services, those people tend to represent the socioeconomic elite. By critiquing the current inaccessibility of functional medicine, I am not discounting the value of functional medicine. Rather, I am highlighting, along with certain prominent members of the functional medicine community, the need for a more equitable future. Since I have benefited from functional medicine myself, my hope for writing this book is that reversal of chronic disease will become possible for all.

CHAPTER 1

IS FUNCTIONAL MEDICINE PSEUDOSCIENCE?

In this chapter, I attempt to locate functional medicine in the contemporary technoscientific and medical landscape and ask, Is functional medicine science or pseudoscience? To answer this question, I hold functional medicine to criteria laid out by Karl Popper, an early twentieth-century philosopher of science, and by current scholars Sven Ove Hansson, Barry L. Beyerstein, and Massimo Pigliucci and Maarten Boudry. I argue that while functional medicine resists most of the characteristics Hansson (2013, 2017) and Beyerstein (1996) describe when defining pseudoscience, some features of functional medicine suggest that it unfolds in an area between science and pseudoscience. I analyze this in-between area vis-à-vis existing literature on boundary work. Ultimately, I argue that, by aiming to expand the limits of conventional medicine, functional medicine interlocutors are engaged in "inclusionary" boundary work.[1]

In addressing this chapter's question, I explore five characteristics of functional medicine that may indicate it is pseudoscience. First, functional medicine practitioners possess a wide range of educational backgrounds, potentially signaling a lack of appropriate credentials among them. Second, the functional medicine approach resists conformity to existing scientific research methods (e.g., the randomized control trial design), with implications for patient care. Third, the functional medicine pursuit of "P4" medicine (medicine that is predictive, precise, personalized, and participatory)[2] results in an absence of uniformity in application. When exploring functional medicine's efforts to predict disease for individual patients, I contextualize the decision to seek functional medicine therapeutics within broader anxieties among the privileged. Fourth, functional medicine may offer false hope and simultaneously inadvertently blame victims when it focuses on the body's natural healing capacity and neglects structural factors. Finally, functional medicine providers use health-promoting compounds that are linked to complementary and alternative medicines.

INTERROGATING FUNCTIONAL MEDICINE

In 1934, Popper asked what distinguishes science from nonscience and pseudoscience ([1934] 1959). He termed this question the "demarcation problem." Popper believed he had solved the demarcation problem by offering the criterion of falsifiability. According to his logic of discovery, scientific theories begin with hypotheses that are tested until they are falsified, and if they cannot be falsified, they are deemed scientifically valid.[3]

Philosophers of science are reexamining the demarcation problem by developing what they call the "philosophy of pseudoscience." Hansson (2013) suggests that pseudoscience is characterized not only by not being science but also by failing one important quality criterion of science: reliability. Reliability signals genuine knowledge. That is, for a statement to be reliable, it should be correct or come as close to correctness as can currently be achieved. He furthermore presents science denialism as a form of pseudoscience (2017). He points to three prominent areas of science denialism—relativity theory denialism, evolution denialism, and climate science denialism—and suggests that science denialism and other forms of pseudoscience are characterized by the fabrication of fake controversies, extraordinary male dominance among their activists, and a strong connection to right-wing politics.

Others consider the question differently. Functional medicine may be considered by some to fall into what Pigliucci and Boudry call "borderline cases [that] are hotly disputed among scientists and philosophers" (2013, 2) or what Beyerstein deems a "gray area"—that is, the borderland between science and pseudoscience—neither generally accepted nor total quackery (1996, 11). This perception of functional medicine as a "borderline case" can be attributed to the lack of credentials among a minority of its practitioners, its nonconformity with the randomized control trial study design, the absence of uniformity in its application, its potential for offering false hope and blame for patients, and its use of health-promoting compounds linked to complementary and alternative medicines. I will explore each of these issues in turn.

(Lack of?) Credentials

The individuals I observed generally fell into three groups. Only a subset of them hold themselves out to be functional medicine practitioners. These individuals are licensed health care professionals, many of whom have been certified as functional medicine practitioners by the Institute for Functional Medicine.[4] Approximately 70 percent of the people in my study who identify as functional medicine practitioners are MDs. Others identify themselves as allied health professionals who support functional medicine practitioners, including nutrition coaches and dieticians; health coaches and educators; nurses; and clinic administrators. A final subset of individuals are not involved with the provision of functional medicine in any capacity; they advocate for functional medicine from a range of positionalities—as entrepreneurs, consultants, filmmakers, journalists, food activists, etc. I observed how a few uncredentialed hangers-on from this final group threaten the validity of functional medicine as a whole when they (loosely, tangentially, and even inaccurately) parrot the principles and findings of functional medicine, often venturing into the territory of pseudoscience, for personal financial gain.

Nonconformity with Randomized Control Trial Study Design (and Implications for Patient Care)

Functional medicine occupies the borderland between what is considered science and pseudoscience with regard to research methods. As in conventional medicine, functional medicine practitioners value empirical observation, experimentation, reproducible findings, debate, and intellectual fermentation. The field embraces falsifiability and is therefore self-correcting. At the same time, functional medicine proponents hope to broaden what are considered valid scientific research methods.

Randomized control trials—currently the gold standard for conventional clinical research—assume comparability among people, except for the therapeutic factor being examined. These trials often compare two groups of people, one group while taking an experimental drug and the second group while taking a placebo. All individuals in such a study share a common denominator: they suffer from the same disease. Functional medicine interlocutors question the value of randomized control trials since the individuals enrolled in the trials are, from a functional medicine standpoint, not comparable.[5] They consider it misleading to compare cases on the basis of one mutual diagnosis because this obscures from view the rest of each individual's unique biology and circumstances. Thus, trials inspired by functional medicine are not limited to studying one compound in isolation but, rather, are based on studying the effects of a multipronged, lifestyle-based protocol. Since functional medicine relies so heavily on dynamic interventions and coaching relationships, trial designs cannot be double-blind and the potential for the placebo effect cannot be eliminated (see Sforzo et al. 2017).

Functional medicine's assertions about what forms of data are important and how this data must be analyzed are reminiscent of some of Charles Ragin's arguments in *The Comparative Method: Moving beyond Qualitative and Quantitative Strategies* ([1987] 2014). Ragin is critical of multivariate statistical techniques because, he argues, these methods encourage investigators to skirt issues of comparability. He points to a "bias" that discourages investigators from examining historically, culturally, or geographically defined social phenomena. These statistical methods (and their emphasis on increasing sample size) cause researchers to reformulate their questions so that they apply to wider categories, and they separate a cause from its context, assessing a cause's influence across a variety of settings (vii). By arguing for "case-oriented methods," Ragin points to the relevant social bases and origins of phenomena and the importance of preserving complexity and historical specificity (x).

Functional medicine interlocutors similarly advocate for deep, individualized data analysis instead of broad, "high-powered" studies based on the false premise of comparability. Referring to the contemporary era of Big Data, Dr. Kara Fitzgerald, a functional naturopath, host of the podcast *FxMed*, and clinical director of her functional medicine and nutrition clinic in Newtown, CT, notes, "We're . . . moving away from the double-blind, placebo-controlled trial and really attempting to measure, observe, and see what's happening in real time." That is, using laboratory testing, functional medicine practitioners attempt to capture what is occurring within individual patients at molecular, genomic, and metabolomic levels in the moment. This individualized data is what functional medicine practitioners consider the gold standard for scientific evidence.

However, existing study designs inform population-based guidelines. Dr. Fitzgerald distributed an email newsletter with a leading question in the subject line: "Are population-based guidelines obsolete?" She expanded in the newsletter, "As the US Dietary Guidelines Committee gets ready to release its 2020–2025 updates, we pose the question: Do population-based guidelines even work?" She then answered her own question, stating, "While the guidelines aim to be evidence-based, science now clearly demonstrates that nutritional guidelines cannot be one-size-fits-all." A myriad of interindividual differences shape responses to dietary inputs, including genomics, metabolism, microbiome, and nutrient status. Dr. Fitzgerald argued that since six out of ten American adults have one or more chronic diseases, the same statistic the Centers for Disease Control and Prevention gives on its website (CDC 2022), generalized dietary advice has been proven ineffective and individualized interventions must be initiated at scale.

The individualized nutrition plans that functional medicine practitioners envision hark back to the question of what counts as valid scientific evidence. Dr. Fitzgerald asked Dr. Mark Hyman, a functional medicine physician, eleven-time best-selling author, founder and medical director of the UltraWellness Center, and host of the podcast *The Doctor's Farmacy*, how he decides what to advise individual patients regarding their personalized diets. Dr. Hyman responded by saying each person is truly a study of an *n* of 1. Instead of collecting data on one factor across *n* number of people and assuming that all else is equal, from the perspective of personalized medicine, each person, with all their individual intricacies, is their own study. Providers then consider each patient's improvement or decline to be valid scientific evidence.

Functional medicine practitioners incorporate this concept of bioindividuality into their clinical practices in different ways. Nutrition counselor and holistic health coach Andrea Nakayama analyzes bioindividuality within the context of each person's life and ancestry. According to Nakayama, the current evidence-based approach in medicine is focused on factors external to the individual. For her, uncovering the "truth of the individual" includes really connecting with the person to understand their situation in life, their ancestry, and their reactions to foods and environmental factors—all of which are elements that fall outside the purview of conventional "evidence."

Functional medicine explicitly challenges what counts as "evidence" by validating, and even prioritizing, embodied knowledge as scientific data.[6] In Nakayama's view, for example, the patient's experience contains more evidence than anything the provider could read on paper. She explains, "In the process of relying so much on evidence-based medicine, we are missing what I like to call clinical intuition." In contrast, by treating patients in a way that is "evidence-informed," Nakayama hopes to avoid rote implementation of protocol. Furthermore, she argues that if it works in clinic, and if patient after patient improves, those experiences of healing and recovery are a legitimate validation of efficacy.

Nakayama takes a functional medicine approach that focuses on "the truth of the individual"; similarly, medical anthropologists critically analyze how social, cultural, and political factors affect individual bodies using in-depth interviews and participant observation. In their seminal article "The Mindful Body: A Prolegomenon to Future Work in Medical Anthropology," Nancy Scheper-Hughes and Margaret M. Lock (1987) critique how assumptions about the body affect research paradigms and health care planning and delivery. They propose a tripartite model that adds layers of complexity to biologized understandings of the body: "The body may be viewed: (1) as a phenomenally experienced individual body-self; (2) as a social body, a natural symbol for thinking about relationships among nature, society, and culture; and (3) as a body politic, an artifact of social and political control" (6). Over the course of my ethnographic research, I observed how functional medicine proponents prioritize patients' individual experience and discuss relationships between their unique bodies and their natural, social, and cultural factors; however, functional medicine proponents were not very attentive to the body politic.

Instead, functional medicine proponents focus their critique of randomized control trials on their limited degrees of validity given varying external factors in real-world settings (see Horn and Gassaway 2007). For example, Dr. Jeffrey Bland, a biochemist and clinical nutritionist who is regarded as the founding father of functional medicine, critiques how health care providers assume that simultaneously inoculating individuals with multiple vaccines is safe because each individual vaccine has been proven safe in clinical trials. These providers do not consider how trials have confirmed the safety of individual vaccines only when administered in isolation. Bland likens this approach to conducting a study on the patient without sufficient data since the effects to the patient's long-term health are unknown. Furthermore, regarding vaccination the effects cannot be known since it is nearly impossible to prove that downstream consequences were caused by (poly)vaccination, and even if a patient were able to produce evidence, "no vaccine manufacturer shall be liable in a civil action for damages arising from a vaccine-related injury or death associated with the administration of a vaccine," according to federal law.[7]

Functional medicine proponents with a research background similarly critique the process of determining prescription pharmaceuticals' safety. Dr. Datis Kharrazian, a clinical research scientist, professor, and functional medicine provider, emphasizes that researchers "never look at polypharmacy, or how these medications all interact with each other." Furthermore, clinical trials do not consider how drugs affect different genotypes—different genetic constitutions of individual organisms. Dr. Kharrazian explains that pharmaco-genotype interactions can result in a completely different response from one person to the next. Thus, real-life polypharmacy results in diverse impacts to individuals' receptor-site responses, brains, and microbiomes in ways that are still unknown. Despite the fact that clinical trials do not document the effects of drugs under real-life conditions, these trials are legitimized as evidence-based research.

In addition to critiquing existing research methods, functional medicine practitioners also critique the time it takes for emerging findings from medical research to make their way into medical school curricula and for a whole new generation of doctors to complete their training and begin putting those findings into practice. This time lag between when research findings emerge and when they are reflected in clinical protocols is referred to as the "translational gap." Zoë Slote Morris, Steven Wooding, and Jonathan Grant (2011, 510) determined that the translational gap in medicine is seventeen years. The Institute for Functional Medicine's strategic advisor for industry, Tom Blue, reacts to this gap, exclaiming, "Where else in our entire economy would you find the breakthrough thing taking seventeen years to make it into your household, your new smart phone, your computer, or whatever?" From a functional medicine perspective, the translational gap is both "insane" and "tragic," Blue says.

However, functional medicine practitioners do not attribute the translational gap to doctors' indolence. Given the enormous number of new scientific papers published each year—approximately two and a half million (Boon 2017)—doctors are forced to read primarily within their specialties. Nonetheless, as Dr. Hyman asserts in the docuseries *The Human Longevity Project*, "There's enormous amounts of information that we're not able to assimilate and use." Dr. Fitzgerald describes how she browses her inbox for articles that directly shape clinical practice, writing, "I am most likely to open and read (i.e., actually click on) those heavy on the science, especially featuring new research." Doctors must develop effective methods for determining which studies to read.

Since pharmaceuticals are not functional medicine practitioners' primary resource for treating disease, the papers of most interest to them focus on topics such as systems biology, lifestyle interventions, environmental toxins, epigenetics, the microbiome, diet, food, and nutrition. While the number of papers that interest functional medicine practitioners are a small subset of the total being published, they also address a wider array of topics than would generally be of interest to most specialists. Furthermore, the mode of discourse that functional medicine practitioners use to communicate emerging scientific discoveries extends far beyond papers published in scientific journals.

As I have already mentioned, the ideas rapidly circulating and evolving in the functional medicine community take on a vibrant social life in digital spaces—through webinars, master classes, podcasts, YouTube episodes, online summits, email newsletters, listservs, etc. These digital spaces are often open to the public. In the case of Facebook groups, sometimes hosted by a functional medicine practitioner, the aim is to bring patients into the digital-social discourse. When functional medicine researchers do publish their findings, they often choose to do so in books written for public audiences over scientific papers that may be read by only a few colleagues in their areas of expertise. Dr. David Sinclair, a professor who researches aging and epigenetics at Harvard Medical School, indicates, "I've been so busy, I haven't written a lot of these ideas down in scientific publications. I've been working on the book. So it could be that the world will be able to read about all this science before scientists do." This emphasis on publishing for the public signals how functional medicine has reconfigured the role of the patient-consumer.

Functional medicine practitioners also make it a priority to close the translational gap by introducing new therapeutic techniques into their clinical practice "in real time." Blue indicates, "What functional medicine is accomplishing is an acceleration of the application of modern science in the day-to-day practice of medicine rather than a divergence." He also explains that many conventionally trained doctors invest additional time and money to become functional medicine doctors so they can implement interventions in their practices as soon as there is enough literature to support clinical efficacy for reversing chronic disease.

Over the course of my ethnographic research, functional medicine proponents shared with me their personal experiences of seeking out further education to understand the root causes of disease. Dr. Volkmar Weissig learned about mitochondrial DNA diseases by attending lectures offered by specialists and basic scientists at United Mitochondrial Disease Foundation meetings. As a professor to future doctors of pharmacy, he noted that "mitochondrial diseases are not yet in the curriculum." Dr. Ted Achacoso, medical director of the BioBalance Institute and a specialist in antiaging and nutritional medicine, confirmed that "metabolomics, epigenetics, bioenergetics dealing with mitochondria, the gut immune system being the gut microbiota, [and] exposomics" are not presently taught in medical schools. In the absence of change to medical and pharmacy school curricula, doctors become personally responsible for seeking out further knowledge and training.

While this self-led training allows functional medicine practitioners to expand their tool kits and use advanced diagnostics, it also results in significant shortcomings and concerns. Dr. Andrew Heyman, a conventionally trained doctor turned researcher in the field of integrative and functional medicine, explains, "This is the promise and peril of integrative medicine, which is, by definition, we integrate: diet, and exercise, and stress management, sometimes meds, and botanicals, and supplements, and acupuncture needles." This process of integration often produces positive outcomes, but even so, functional medicine providers cannot be sure which elements have contributed the most to a patient's improvement. Nonetheless, these practitioners attempt to close the translational gap in medical research by, in Dr. Heyman's words, exercising a practical willingness to "do whatever it takes" to help the patient improve, including "suspending their own disbelief" when trying new methods.

Functional medicine practitioners describe how, by engaging in functional medicine, they began to practice "outside of the box." Dr. Fitzgerald describes this as "an open-mindedness and a willingness to jump in and try something out." On his podcast *The Doctor's Farmacy*, Dr. Hyman recounts how he began instructing patients to do things that were beyond what he had learned in medical school—for example, dietary changes. He explains, "It really took me years and years to expect that people would get better. . . . People just recovered. It was just amazing to me!" When patients reported improvement, he says, his thought process was immediate disbelief, followed by reluctant acceptance, and, finally, commitment to the functional medicine model.

Functional medicine practitioners' dismissal of discrete treatment paths (i.e., protocols) introduces both disadvantages and advantages. On the one hand, Dr. Heyman notes, there is evidence to support each of his clinical decisions. On the other hand, he admits, "I'm not always certain which were the steps that were the most responsible for improvement. And it might be different in different patients. So you do feel like it's a little bit of a kitchen sink approach." Meanwhile, Dr. Robert Luby, a board-certified family physician who was in the first class of Institute for Functional Medicine certified practitioners, in 2013, expresses his fear that, in the absence of functional medicine training in medical school curricula, mavericks with insufficient training will practice beyond the scope of their licensure, especially as more diagnostic and therapeutic products become publicly available. Both doctors advocate for the incorporation of functional medicine into medical education.

In sum, attempts in functional medicine to redefine what counts as valid science present both strengths and weaknesses. Functional medicine proponents uncover how the nature of statistical methods tends to discourage awareness of the assumptions required by these methods (see Ragin [1987] 2014). They critique how the framing of individuals as exchangeable units in randomized control trials belies the relevance of contextual factors. However, while functional medicine's individualized approach attempts to sidestep this pitfall, functional medicine proponents often fail to interrogate the political and economic factors shaping individual health. Similarly, functional medicine practitioners' tendency to eschew standardized protocols creates an opportunity for the tailoring of predictive, precise, personalized, and participatory (P4) interventions; however, this tendency also opens the door to the practice of pseudoscience under the flag of functional medicine. I will explore functional medicine's commitment to P4 medicine in the next section.

Absence of Uniformity in Application (P4 Medicine)

In functional medicine, protocols shown to produce beneficial results through clinical trials, such as those conducted and published by Dr. Terry Wahls and colleagues for multiple sclerosis (Wahls, Chenard, and Snetselaar 2019; see also Bisht et al. 2014), Dr. Fitzgerald and colleagues for DNA methylation (Fitzgerald et al. 2021), and Dr. Dale Bredesen for Alzheimer's (2014), are reproduced and applied to large cohorts of patients. However, their application differs from conventional trial methods in that functional medicine practitioners hold space for the tailoring of protocols to individual patients. That is, clinically validated protocols are not applied in a one-size-fits-all approach; rather, they are viewed as guiding insights for P4 medicine. I will explore each *P* in turn.

PREDICTION

Functional medicine practitioners aim to achieve targeted prevention through prediction of specific risks for individual patients. Likewise, functional medicine patient-clients proactively seek preventive strategies to allay their concerns about chronic diseases they could potentially develop in the future. Their concerns are fueled, at least in part, by increases in chronic-disease prevalence (see Terzic and Waldman 2011). Ruth Q. Wolever et al. (2013) observe, "Global rates of preventable chronic disease have reached epidemic proportions" (38). In functional medicine, prediction is an integral component of personalized medicine since risks are always unique to the individual.

Researchers in functional medicine are developing further predictive tools with direct application for clinical care. For example, Dr. Marvin Edeas describes how his current research aims to identify specific metabolites in the gut microbiome, thus providing critical information for the prediction and prevention of chronic disease. The spectrum of diseases that can be prevented by maintaining a healthy gut microbiota includes neurodegenerative disease, kidney disease, liver disease, and metabolic syndrome, to name a few. In essence, the goals of this type of functional medicine research are to use metabolomics and microbiome data to predict personalized risk for disease and to effectively prevent future suffering before it even occurs by using pharmaceuticals, probiotics, prebiotics, diet, or a mixture of these. This approach turns "reactive disease care" on its head.[8]

Prevention through prediction also differs from the way the public health sector aims to blunt population-level crises through preparedness. While public health hopes to be prepared for unknowable population health risks such as pandemics, functional medicine seeks to predict health risks for individual people. To clarify the difference between preparedness and prediction, I will turn to the work of medical anthropologist Andrew Lakoff.

Lakoff (2012) describes how in 1976, the possibility of vaccinating the entire population to a sudden new strain of influenza became feasible for the first time. In 2005, the combination of urgency and uncertainty surrounding avian flu led US health officials and politicians alike to conjecture about when the next pandemic would occur. In November of that year, the White House unveiled a $7.1 billion pandemic preparedness strategy—the most robust public health proposal up to that time. This plan included funds for disease surveillance, stockpiling medicine, and developing new methods of vaccine production. The proposal was criticized for overemphasizing pharmaceutical interventions, but the consensus was that pandemic planning for present and future threats was of urgent concern and the nation was currently not prepared.

Lakoff suggests that in this way, the avian flu became a vehicle for a form of planning that is oriented toward a variety of dangerous events. The norm of preparedness came to structure thought about threats to public health. The need to be prepared generates an effect of urgency among officials in the absence of the event itself and knowledge about vulnerabilities in response capability. In essence, Lakoff is pointing to how imagined futures (and so-called anticipatory knowledge) shape political actions in the present. This was certainly true during the Obama presidency, when a pandemic preparedness infrastructure was set into place. This infrastructure was largely dismantled during the Trump presidency, leaving the nation vulnerable to disease threats and biological incidents.

At issue is Niklas Luhmann's 1998 question "In what form does the future manifest itself in the present?" (401). Critiquing fear-based responses to unknown risks, entrepreneur and functional medicine advocate James Maskell asks, "Prevention is such a weird concept because, how do you know what you prevented? You don't!" Dr. Bland echoes this critique when he points to unknowable risks and indicates that it is impossible to know what you have prevented. Despite the significant shortcoming Maskell and Dr. Bland signal, preparedness continues to shape public health.

The primacy of preparedness came to the fore at the outset of the COVID-19 pandemic in 2020. While many individuals and families were isolated in their homes, they were bombarded with media messages about the deadly consequences of being unprepared. In making this observation, I do not mean to underplay the devastating death toll wrought by COVID-19; rather, I aim to note that mass media contributes to a profitable, ideology-driven "fear machine" that produces feelings of risk and danger (see Altheide 1997). In this context, functional medicine interlocutors emphasized—via webinar, online summits, YouTube videos, podcasts, and other virtual platforms—that COVID-19 mortalities were usually occurring in individuals with comorbidities. They argued that by eliminating metabolic disease and increasing resilience (for example, by consuming a nutritionally complete diet), individuals could prevent the most serious consequences of COVID-19 infection.

In my view, both prediction and preparedness have a role to play in prevention. Using precise laboratory testing to predict future disease and prevent it before it happens could potentially revolutionize medicine—although Maskell's critique also applies here since, in most cases, it is impossible to know for sure what outcomes have been prevented. At the same time, this approach requires financial investments. Since the current health care system is primarily set up to treat disease, not to prevent it, prevention through prediction currently takes place through neoliberal consumption. On the other hand, as the COVID-19 pandemic has proved, preparedness at the population level is essential. However, since it is impossible to adequately prepare pharmaceuticals for viruses that have yet to exist, the focus of preparedness should be geared toward creating the infrastructure for immediate response (for example, laboratories and machinery to develop and produce vaccines when they are needed, trained research and hospital personnel, sufficient hospital beds and physical infrastructure for quarantining infectious patients, stockpiles of masks and gloves, etc.) and planning for the equitable provision of resources across gendered, racialized, and socioeconomic groups.

With regard to the functional medicine approach to individualized prediction, I argue that patient-clients' striving to prevent disease is shaped by the aura of knowability in our postgenomic era. Due to functional medicine's use of genomic testing, future-facing concerns regarding chronic disease are often highly specific. While Peter N. Stearns (2006, 100) writes, "Threats to health, though objectively reduced from the past, shifted toward less familiar sources such as cancer or hypertension," I suggest that genomic testing has rendered chronic-disease threats anticipatable and, from a functional medicine perspective, preventable. Functional medicine interlocutors argue that, with the exception of congenital diseases, our genes merely indicate predispositions, not future manifestations. Seen through this lens, the results of genetic testing can serve as a roadmap for averting disease.

Furthermore, I situate the desire to predict within broader anxieties among the privileged. Although many middle- and upper-class Americans have experienced increasing anxiety across multiple areas of life (see De Courville Nicol 2021; Jetten, Mols, and Healy 2017),[9] health is a particularly strong area of concern for the wealthy. My ethnographic observations of functional medicine patient-clients support the sociologist Nikolas Rose's arguments that ever-increasing rates of anxiety result from "reshaping discontents" (2008, 46) and that humans increasingly make sense of their own suffering through somatic processes (2007a, 2008). I apply Rose's approach to contemporary notions of prevention and preparedness, and meritocracy and aspirations, to historicize privileged individuals' concerns about future health.

In essence, prevention through prediction is a form of capital within an ethico-moral meritocracy. According to Alain de Botton (2004), a meritocratic outlook produces status anxiety among relatively prosperous Americans, whose quest for betterment generates feelings of insecurity and relative deprivation. Rose suggests that by acting upon their bodies, people strive not just to make themselves better physically but also to make themselves better persons (Rose 2007a, 2008). Participation in functional medicine is a specific form of health consumerism that constitutes social capital among aspirationals (see Vega 2018, 20, 25, 73, 74, 83, 86).

PRECISION

Functional medicine is characterized as "precision medicine" because of its reliance on advanced diagnostic tools. Functional medicine practitioners often express how much they "love data" and are unable to create a personalized treatment protocol for a patient without knowing exactly what processes are occurring in that patient. Dr. Fitzgerald's website instructs new patients to "send at least one year of medical records, including most recent laboratory data" in preparation for their first visit. For patients who have records dating back further than one year, the website continues, "Err on the side of sending more, rather than less, of your records." Copious data collection on the individual person is the hallmark of "precision medicine," and this element of the P4 approach enhances "personalized medicine."

Personalization is achieved through precision in clinical diagnosis. Dr. Marwan Sabbagh, a geriatric neurologist, research professor of neurology at the University of Arizona College of Medicine–Phoenix, and director of the Alzheimer's Disease and Memory Disorders Division at the Barrow Neurological Institute, notes, "We are not all the same. We can now, using molecular diagnostics, determine the differences between [our patients]." For example, Dr. Chilkov describes a situation where she was approached by a woman who had a mass in her breast. The patient asked, "Can you treat me?" Dr. Chilkov responded, "Treat what? There are breast *cancers*. If I don't know what kind of cells are there, I can't put a plan together for you.'" The patient agreed to a biopsy, allowing Dr. Chilkov to put together a personalized treatment plan. Thus, while functional medicine may seem "anti-medicine" to outsiders who observe its resistance to long-term pharmaceutical use, functional medicine practitioners are not opposed to using medical procedures and medical technology for precise diagnosis.

In fact, functional medicine practitioners are often enthusiastic about automated informational biology data analysis because they consider the human body to be an organism beyond human comprehension. Dr. Dale Bredesen, an expert on neurodegenerative diseases such as Alzheimer's, opines that while doctors attempt to keep up with the rapid speed of scientific discovery by obtaining continued medical education, their efforts will never be enough, indicating, "You can't cram all the [continuing medical education] in the world into one lifetime." Furthermore, as science progresses, clinical considerations become more nuanced and complicated.

Functional medicine practitioners need "support from a Silicon Valley approach," Dr. Bredesen says. The emphasis on precision within personalized medicine relies heavily on increased incorporation of artificial intelligence into health care delivery. Many functional medicine practitioners characterize artificial intelligence as an indispensable tool that augments their clinical decision-making process. Moving forward, Dr. Bredesen indicates, "What would be very, very helpful with these larger data sets would be to have an assistant that would be an expert system." Essentially, the "assistant" he describes is data-analysis software that can flag a patient's health problems, identify contributing factors, and propose an initial plan. Dr. Bredesen anthropomorphizes the software and describes it as saying, "I've gone through the entire genome for you. I've gone through the metabolome, the lipidome, and the proteome, and so on, and I can generate for you an initial idea." Artificial intelligence can analyze enormous amounts of data, thus potentiating informational biology beyond its current applications. However, it would ultimately be up to the patient and the physician to "fine tune" these recommendations and make therapeutic decisions.

The incorporation of artificial intelligence into clinical care is predicated on the merging of two previously distinct industries. Dr. Bland explains that this transition will be led by individuals at major health care innovation companies like Google, Apple, Microsoft, and Cisco—"people that were previously not even considered part of the health care community." Dr. Bland argues that, due to the expansive size of data sets exploring interactions between genes and the environment, technology companies will play a primary role in aggregating information using machine learning and complex informatics. Stated simply, the involvement of these companies will shape medical knowledge (both *what* is known and *how* it is known) in the future.

Health care and tech industry cross-pollination is already underway. Dr. Bland describes his work with Dr. Leroy Hood, a leader in the field of systems biology, at the Institute for Systems Biology in what they call the Pioneer One Hundred Project. At the time of his presentation, Dr. Bland had collected over three million data points for the project. These data points are inserted into an informatics system to evaluate trends. The first paper resulting from this project was published in *Nature Biotechnology*, titled, "A Wellness Study of 108 Individuals Using Personal, Dense, Dynamic Data Clouds" (Price et al. 2017). Dr. Bland's work with Dr. Hood highlights the new methods of proof in the age of complex lifestyle disease and "multiscale biology."

Ragin's proposal of considering individual cases as whole entities and comparing these entities in a data matrix is useful for understanding the future of precision medicine ([1987] 2014, xiv). While multivariate statistical analysis breaks cases into parts (variables) that are difficult to reassemble into wholes, Ragin explains that "case-oriented methods" treat cases as whole entities and not as collections of parts (ix). In his view, relations between parts of a whole are understood within the context of the whole (i.e., the person), not within the context of general patterns of covariation among members of a population of "comparable units" (xiv). In essence, Ragin's method allows for the comparison of full persons as "constellations, configurations, and conjectures" (x).

Ragin develops an algebraic technique of qualitative comparison that uses Boolean algebra to simplify complex data structures (using set theory and producing something similar to a data matrix), thus transitioning to a case-oriented (as opposed to variable-oriented) and historical (as opposed to abstractly causal) approach. When employing this technique, "causation is understood conjuncturally. Outcomes are analyzed in terms of intersections of conditions" (Ragin [1987] 2014, x). Multiple combinations of conditions may produce the same outcome, thereby adding complexity to existing notions of cause and effect.

While functional medicine similarly resists comparing patients based on diagnosis—arguing that similar etiologies can lead to multiple disease outcomes and that a single outcome can be traced back to divergent etiologies—it has tended to focus primarily on the genome when considering each patient's bioindividuality. This tendency is linked to the history of complex informatics in functional medicine. As Dr. Bland describes it, emerging technologies for data management were first used to understand interactions between genes and the environment. Dr. Hyman offers this critique of how precision medicine has been realized thus far: "It is often just about pharmacogenomics—which is important but is really not sufficient. It's really more about all the variables." He lists the microbiome, environmental toxins, and nutritional status as some of the necessary variables to include. At present, functional medicine practitioners are arguing for the expansion of these technologies.

From this perspective, Ragin's matrix approach for managing and evaluating data would preserve the holism of each person as a unique data set and then use informatics to identify trends among a number of data sets. Dr. Hyman elaborates, "With the advent of big data, and with artificial intelligence, we'll be able to make more sense of what's happening. Integrate faster. And build training models that will actually allow doctors to do this." The hope of functional medicine providers is that this precise, data-rich approach will allow them to treat patients in a radically holistic way.

Precision medicine is firmly rooted in genomic science and "Big Data" informatics. Although these connections to advances in biology and technology are not suggestive of pseudoscience, precision medicine can nonetheless result in inadvertent harm to patients through what Sara Degli-Esposti refers to as "dataveillance" (2014), or surveillance and potential use of personal data by third parties. I will explore the "dark side" of dataveillance in chapter 3. For now, I turn to prediction—an extension of precision medicine since it relies on advanced laboratory testing to determine personalized risks.

PERSONALIZATION

Each person represents a unique genome, set of environmental factors (including social relationships, stress level, etc.), habits and behaviors, and life history. Compiling both quantitative and qualitative data for each individual patient allows functional medicine practitioners to tailor their recommendations to each individual's unique biology. Dr. Hyman refers to a common single nucleotide polymorphism—MTHFR—and indicates how knowing patients' MTHFR status provides insight into how they will metabolize folate: "Some people might need 400 micrograms of folate, which you can buy over the counter, and some people might need 5 milligrams of methyl folate—a special kind because they have this unique gene." The goals of functional medicine's personalized approach to data analysis are to identify the individual patient's unique needs, optimize their treatment plan, and create the conditions for both healing and maintaining wellness.

According to Dr. Bland, the personalization of medicine rests on Roger Williams's (1998) concept of biochemical individuality and Linus Pauling's (Pauling et al. 1949) concept of molecular medicine. Through the practice of functional medicine, these concepts manifest into unique therapeutics based on each individual's situation. In Dr. Bland's words, "The health of the world is really a result of the health of each individual, one at a time. So if you want to get the world to be healthy, you need a bunch of healthy individuals." Each individual, of course, is a bioindividual whose genome will respond uniquely to environmental inputs. Thus, Dr. Todd LePine, a board-certified internal medicine and functional medicine physician, notes, "I've never treated two patients the same way from a functional approach. . . . The person comes in with their own genetic uniqueness, their own personality, makeup, their own story." Dr. Hyman concurs with Dr. LePine: "In functional medicine, there is no recipe, there is actually having to think every time you see a patient." This principle of uniqueness is what many functional medicine practitioners consider the most fascinating part of their work.

The personalization of medicine harks back to how functional medicine practitioners are trained to listen to their patients' illness narratives and take thorough histories.[10] Without these skills, providers can misdiagnose and mistreat problems. Dr. Nalini Chilkov, a doctor of Oriental medicine and licensed acupuncturist, provides the example of one of her patients, a breast cancer survivor. While Dr. Chilkov's patient had had successful treatment ten or fifteen years earlier, she was still struggling with fatigue—a long-term sequela from the chemotherapy treatment. Her primary doctor, not knowing she had had chemotherapy, worked her up for hypothyroidism. Had her primary doctor taken a complete history instead of focusing on fatigue as an isolated symptom, they may also have screened her for early signs of a cancer recurrence.

Dr. Chilkov went on to explain her unique role in bringing a functional approach to oncology. "It is my job to make sure that we have highly individualized therapy—which is not the usual approach in conventional oncology." Furthermore, Dr. Chilkov aims to ensure that each patient's treatment plan "optimizes the therapeutic effects and minimizes the adverse or negative effects." Since Dr. Chilkov is not an oncologist herself, her role often involves pointing out overlooked features of the patient's history to the oncologist and providing additional support to the patient (through recommendations for diet, supplements, etc.) to offset some of the side effects of chemotherapy. In so doing, Dr. Chilkov works collaboratively with oncologists to augment the effectiveness of her patients' therapy.

Personalization of medicine is appealing but time intensive for providers and expensive for patients. While functional medicine can be combined with conventional medicine, as Dr. Chilkov describes, only conventional interventions are covered by insurance. I am wary of how personalized medicine is synonymous with medicine for the privileged. Furthermore, personalized medicine must be situated within a larger tendency toward personalization in our neoliberal economy. That is, personalization appeals to upper- and upper-middle-class sensibilities because it is a status marker of privilege.

PARTICIPATION

From a functional medicine perspective, the reversal of chronic disease is possible, and individual patients have a primary role to play in their healing processes. Using cancer as an example, Sachin Patel, author and founder of the Living Proof Institute, explains that he intentionally avoids saying that a patient "got" a disease because while it effectively releases the patient from personal responsibility for the outcome, it simultaneously disempowers them by obscuring their proactive role in healing. Patel opines that by describing disease as largely unfolding at the intersection of choice and environment—not merely genetics—he empowers them to act. He adds, "When there's no hope, there's absolutely no healing." From a functional medicine perspective, whether an individual feels a sense of empowerment is of great consequence since it can determine that person's outcome.

The perspective of one cancer survivor may shed light on Patel's argument. Chris Wark was diagnosed with stage 3 colon cancer at age twenty-six. Wark felt powerless after being diagnosed. He describes a common experience for cancer patients undergoing treatment: when the patient asks his doctor why he developed cancer, his doctor replies that it is either bad luck or genetics, saying something along the lines of, "It's nothing you did. You just go home and eat whatever you want, and don't change anything about your life and you let us take care of it." While the intention of the doctor that Wark describes is to release the patient from potential feelings of guilt, this approach has another, inadvertent effect: it places the patient in a position of powerlessness. Wark explains, "What that does is [it] takes the power away from the patient. They believe that nothing they did contributed to their cancer, and nothing they can do will help them." Pushing back against powerlessness, Wark says, "I did everything I could find and afford to help my body heal, and it did heal." He received surgery to remove the cancer but refused chemotherapy, and he is now a cancer survivor and health coach.

Dr. David Servan-Schreiber—a neuroscientist who survived brain cancer twice before finally succumbing to the disease—also adds nuance to Patel's perspective on the role of mindset in medicine when he describes the concrete ways mindset shapes cancer treatment in his book *Anticancer: A New Way of Life*. Like Wark, he recounts an exchange he had with his oncologist, a colleague he refers to as a "leading light in modern medicine," when seeking advice about how to lead a healthy life and avoid a relapse:

> ONCOLOGIST: There is nothing special to do. Lead your life normally. We'll do MRI scans at regular intervals and if your tumor comes back, we'll detect it early.
> DR. SERVAN-SCHREIBER: But aren't there exercises I could do, a diet to follow or to avoid? Shouldn't I be working on my mental outlook?
> ONCOLOGIST: In this domain, do what you like. It can't do any harm. But we don't have any scientific evidence that any of these approaches can prevent relapse. (Servan-Schreiber 2009, 11)

Ultimately, Dr. Servan-Schreiber critiques how, by failing to acknowledge environmental effects, conventional oncology inadvertently robs cancer patients of their agency. He indicates, "In reality, what my doctor meant was that . . . as for more theoretical mind-body or nutritional approaches, he clearly lacked the time or interest to explore these avenues" (2009, 7). In contrast, Dr. Hyman indicates that in functional medicine, "If someone gets diagnosed with cancer, you don't just say, 'Come back every six months or year for a scan.' You go, 'Wait a minute. There is a lot of stuff that can be addressed.'" By exploring the patient's nutrient status, insulin resistance score, hormone metabolism, toxic load, gut microbiome, etc., functional medicine practitioners interpellate cancer patients as proactive participants in their healing journeys.

In essence, conventionally trained functional medicine doctors reveal that their medical school education did not prepare them to pursue "lifestyle"- and "mindset"-based strategies. For example, physician and researcher Dr. William Li describes a memory from his time working as a doctor at the Veterans Hospital. After delivering very bad diagnoses to veterans, he would answer their initial questions regarding the treatment process. His patients would listen to his explanations and begin heading out the door to leave, but then, in many instances, they would turn to him and ask one final question: "Hey, doc. What can I do for myself? What can I eat?" Dr. Li acknowledges, "I didn't have the answer because I wasn't taught. We weren't taught to give that answer. And I thought that was wrong" (Li 2019, xix). Over the course of my ethnographic research, I heard and read about many conventionally trained functional medicine doctors who likewise described turning to functional medicine when they became frustrated with their clinical capabilities.

While interpellating patients as agentive actors in their own healing journeys may lead to empowerment, it can also inadvertently bolster inattention to structural inequality and lead to blaming the victim. That is, the framing of healing as something that should be actively pursued by patients may unwittingly create a meritocracy in which patients' "failure" to heal is attributed to their not having done the right things. In reality, patients' well-being is also dependent on larger issues such as the food system and the environment. In addition, disadvantaged populations often lack the material resources needed for healing, "lifestyle changes" may be insufficient to reverse advanced disease and some diseases may simply be irreversible, and functional medicine's healing promise may give some false hope.

False Hope(lessness?)

The vast majority of functional medicine patients have already exhausted conventional treatment options before turning to functional medicine. Responding to critics who disregard functional medicine as "resort medicine," Dr. LePine points out that for patients of his who have already been to the Mayo Clinic or Massachusetts General Hospital and have tried everything conventional medicine has to offer, to no avail, functional medicine is "actually the medicine of *last* resort." Likewise, Dr. Heyman elicited confirmation from his audience—individuals seeking continuing medical education in functional medicine—that they frequently treat chronically ill patients who have nowhere else to turn.

Despite their patients' dire circumstances, functional medicine practitioners are remarkably optimistic. Dr. Heyman pauses, and, after a few moments, in a heartfelt tone, says to his audience at the Advances in Mitochondrial Medicine Symposium, "I know we see miracles in what we do, and we keep going as a result." In a similar vein, Dr. Kelly Brogan, a holistic psychiatrist and best-selling author, signals, "You see healing that makes no sense." She describes how, after many years of taking multiple medications, her patients not only improve but "achieve states of being that they never even knew were possible." Given these experiences, functional medicine practitioners aim to inspire hope in the patients they treat.

Hope is vital for healing from a functional medicine perspective. Dr. LePine explains that he often asks patients if they think they are going to get better, since how patients think about their future plays a determining role in their health outcomes. "If I have a patient who thinks they are going to get better, then together, we are going to get better. But if I have a patient that doesn't think they are going to get better, then I try to change their mindset." This is fundamental to his practice of functional medicine, which aims to support the body's amazing "intelligence" with regard to self-healing.

By counseling patients to truly believe they are going to get better, functional medicine providers are pushing back against what Dr. Servan-Schreiber calls a "culture of false hopelessness." When acknowledging that diet- and mindset-based approaches might be critiqued for arousing "false hope," Dr. Servan-Schreiber emphasizes the participatory nature of lifestyle medicine, writing, "I have learned this when I faced my own cancer—that such thinking robs patients of their power to act; and I mean this in terms of real power, not some illusion" (2009, 5). He goes on to argue that promoting a mindset of helplessness is not just psychologically demeaning but is also medically dangerous and unscientific, and he points to prodigious advances in science that have demonstrated individuals' abilities to protect themselves from cancer and to contribute to their own means of healing it. Dr. Susan Prescott, a pediatrician, immunologist, artist, and award-winning author, extends Dr. Servan-Schreiber's comments when she argues that despair and hopelessness lead to disengagement; meanwhile, positive emotions produce lifelong implications for health behaviors.

These perspectives hint at a foundational premise of functional medicine: healing is only possible because of the patient's natural capacity for healing. Citing the fact that the body is constantly producing new cells—to the extent that we have a "new" body every seven years—chiropractor and autoimmune expert Dr. Tom O'Bryan indicates, "The really good news is that the body always wants to be healthy." According to the functional medicine paradigm, the body will return to health if given the right conditions. Regarding the body as self-healing is simple yet radical, since it challenges the existing paradigm in conventional medicine and is a core tenet within functional medicine.[11]

This concept calls to mind the remarks of Dr. René Dubos, professor of microbiology at Rockefeller University, discoverer of the first antibiotic in clinical use (in 1939), and founder of the first Earth Summit of the United Nations (in 1972). Dr. Dubos opined, "I have always felt that the only trouble with scientific medicine is that it is not scientific enough. Modern medicine will become really scientific only when physicians and their patients have learned to manage the forces of the body and the mind that operate via *vis medicatrix naturae* (the healing power of nature)" (as cited by Servan-Schreiber 2009, 215–216). Dr. Dubos's perspective is revered by many functional medicine practitioners today since it perfectly encapsulates the goal of functional medicine to harness cutting-edge science while also incorporating the wisdom of ancient healing systems and trusting in the body's ability to heal itself.

The true ability of *vis medicatrix naturae* within functional medicine circles is increasingly substantiated by scientific evidence and acknowledged by the media. A 2019 research article in *Science Advances* confirmed the innate tissue-repair capacity in human lower-limb cartilages (Hsueh et al. 2019). CNN correspondent Jessie Yeung described the conclusions of the study authors thus: "Humans have a 'salamander-like' ability to regrow cartilage" (Yeung 2019). The findings of this study—in particular, the expression of limb-regenerative microRNAs—disprove former notions that cumulative damage to adult cartilage is irreversible. Thus, at the same time that laboratory testing is allowing for functional medicine physicians to examine increasingly intricate details about the body's inner workings, the emphasis on trusting the body's innate capacity to heal is becoming more pronounced.

According to functional medicine, patients are empowered to heal themselves from chronic disease—including those affecting the mind—when they learn to trust their bodies' natural ability to heal. Patel tells a patient simply, "You have to trust this body." Echoing these sentiments, neonatologist Dr. Mary Newport says, "We've healed ourselves because we are born with that ability. That is how we are made." Extending Dr. Newport's perspective, Dr. Martin Picard, a neurology researcher at Columbia University, insists that the "real way forward for health care" is "to help people develop and harness their own resilience and ability to heal and recover." Thus, an invaluable part of the functional medicine practitioner's role is to teach patients to trust in their own, innate capacity for healing.

Functional medicine interlocutors emphasize how important it is that patients acknowledge that their biologies are working in their best interests and that they resist conventional messages that can place them and their bodies in opposition. For example, Jason Prall, a filmmaker and health-optimization practitioner, contends, "We are too afraid of our own bodies. 'My thyroid is attacking me. My microbiota are giving me gut problems.' We are anti–our body. We are trying to overcome it and conquer it." Instead, functional medicine teaches patients that by protecting, honoring, and trusting their bodies, they create the conditions of possibility for lasting wellness.

Entrepreneur and health consultant Matthew Accurso describes functional medicine's radical trust in the human body as a "vitalistic approach." Accurso explains that this approach communicates to the patient, "Hey, you don't need to go outside of yourself to find the answers. The answers are already inside your body. You've been made like that." His comments are echoed by Dr. Rob Verkerk, executive and scientific director of the Alliance for Natural Health International, who, in his article "What Happened to 'Do No Harm'?," emphasizes, "It's time to radically rethink how we practice medicine to unlock our full healing potential. We need to unlock that extraordinary internal pharmacy of ours to promote self-healing" (2019). Together with Accurso's, Dr. Verkerk's comments underline how functional medicine's trust in the human body again places the patient at the center.

Functional medicine interlocutors position the patient as "the doctor of the future," emphasizing that it is the patient's body that heals itself,[12] when they explain the relationship between mindset and healing. Patel compares the body to a car—an analogy common among functional medicine practitioners. In this analogy, the body is the machinery, nutrients and other health-promoting compounds are the fuel, and the mind is the steering wheel. Patel explains, "If we know where we want to go, we've got to steer our thoughts and our mind in the right direction, and that sends this machinery the right instruction set so we can get us where we want to go." Viewing the mind in this way places the patient, not the provider, in the driver's seat. While the provider may guide the driver toward the right "fuel," it is the patient who must drive the car to health and well-being.

In this view, both thoughts and the actions they produce directly impact health. Functional diagnostic nutritionist Reed Davis explains that an attitude of gratitude motivates individuals to take care of themselves to the best of their ability: "If you get up every day and you're thankful, and you count your blessings, and [you] acknowledge that you're so lucky to be here, you probably have a better chance of being healthy." This emphasis on perception is rooted in biology—functional medicine practitioners are acutely aware of the specific mechanisms by which thoughts shape human physiology, often citing how meditation can reverse the corrosion of telomeres, a measure of aging.

Thoughts also shape the physical structure of our brains. Speaking on a topic that has been extensively researched and eloquently explained by medical anthropologist Tobias Rees in his ethnography *Plastic Reason: An Anthropology of Brain Science in Embryogenetic Terms* (2016), Dr. Titus Chiu, a functional neurologist and best-selling author, asserts, "Neuroplasticity, simply put, is our brain's ability to literally change its physical structure based on our experiences." Dr. Chiu clarifies that "experiences" include the thoughts that we (choose to) think. He has coined the term "sensory genomics" to encompass the potential of neuroplasticity, the power of epigenetics, and the influence of our five basic senses. He indicates, "Using the five common senses to activate genetic responses in our brain . . . we can exercise specific areas of our brain that actually light our nervous system." From a functional medicine perspective, our senses can play a role in reversing some of the mental decline associated with aging.

Vishen Lakhiani, founder and CEO of Mindvalley, describes how his elderly father relied on "neurological strength"—not rapid muscle growth—to create a "massive reversal" in his loss of physical strength. Lakhiani furthermore asserts that this shift in self-perception will have a positive effect on his father's overall health, stating, "Now he knows he's going to live beyond five years and he knows that he can take control of his health." This comment reiterates a common perspective among functional medicine interlocutors: patients are empowered to play a proactive role in their healing when they view their health as something that is under their control, not something that is merely happening to them.

I take seriously the power of the mind in shaping health outcomes; at the same time, this mindset-based approach to healing presents two flaws. First, I must flag the dangerous potential slippage embedded in arguments that link healing to an individual's thought processes, specifically hope. An inordinate focus on a hopeful outlook can lapse into noxious assumptions that biological outcomes are fully dependent on the patient's "mental strength." This, in turn, can create a meritocracy in which those exhibiting the most "mental strength" achieve the greatest healing. In contrast, "failure" to heal could be pinned on a lack of hope or insufficient "mental strength." In essence, this slippage would result in blaming the victim—the poor outcomes of those who continue to suffer from chronic disease would be attributed to their "mindset."

Second, the "mindset" approach to healing is effective only *when other health-creating resources are also in place*. "Mindset" goes hand in hand with "empowerment," and in our contemporary neoliberal world system, one's degree of "empowerment" is correlated with one's degree of *purchasing power*. That is, individuals' ability to feel and believe that they, as opposed to external forces, have control over the outcomes in their lives is instantiated by having at least the minimum requirements for survival and is potentiated by increasing capital. Privileged individuals with greater access to economic and material resources are better positioned to "empower" themselves. Functional medicine patients tend to be relatively privileged and are thus in the socioeconomic position to experience "mindset as medicine." The perspective that empowered patient-consumers—those with the right mindset—routinely achieve disease reversal is doubly rooted in the privilege of both functional medicine providers and their patient-consumers.

That is, functional medicine practitioners exhibit what I call structural myopia—a term I have used to describe how their socioeconomic privilege allows for a type of "nearsightedness" that obscures the struggles of the disadvantaged—when they underscore the power of mindset instead of the necessity to change the real conditions in which people live (Vega 2023, 147–150, 243). Functional medicine experts, focused on the positive effects of hope, may inadvertently disregard structural inequality because they are shielded from the effects of disadvantage in their practices, where patient-consumers primarily pay for healing out of pocket. This inattention to inequality unwittingly suggests that those suffering from chronic illness should shoulder the burden of intersecting inequalities while "thinking their way" to good health. While individuals can change their thoughts, there are limits to the benefits these changes can provide in the absence of social justice, especially with regard to access to quality health care. If someone has developed cancer and faces financial barriers to obtaining the chemotherapy treatment they need, no amount of positive thinking will heal them. Thus, I suggest that functional medicine practitioners themselves should harness the power of mindset while also championing for social justice.

Use of Health-Promoting Compounds

Functional medicine incorporates "salugens"—a term coined by Dr. Robert Naviaux, a mitochondrial medicine expert, to describe health-promoting compounds such as herbs and supplements that, at first glance, may seem to be associated with complementary and alternative medicines; however, functional medicine practitioners turn to laboratory science when deciding what compounds are valuable for clinical use. For example, Traditional Chinese Medicine may employ herbs based on their effects on "vital energies" and "meridians," while functional medicine practitioners rely on published studies that measure and validate the effects of herbal compounds using conventional scientific methods when incorporating these compounds into their practices.

However, as more and more salugens emerge, doctors will have to pay careful attention not to lapse into medicine's current reductionistic model wherein each symptom is isolated and treated using a non–systems biology, one-to-one approach.[13] Accurso explains why supplements—even when they are considered salugens—can lose their health-promoting potential if they are not prescribed as part of a systems biology approach (i.e., viewing the body as an integrated system that must be treated as a unified whole). "We know that there are supplements out there that are wonderful. . . . But the fact is that if I'm addressing the body mechanistically, then it's a glorified drug," he says. A whole-person approach is needed.

Functional medicine's embrace of salugens can be viewed as opening new avenues for patient care; on the other hand, since the supplement industry is largely unregulated, salugens can also be flagged as a potential danger or a waste of money. In 2015, an investigation led by New York Attorney General Eric Schneiderman focusing on a variety of herbal supplements from four major retailers (GNC, Target, Walmart, and Walgreens) determined that only 21 percent of the products contained DNA from the plants listed on their labels (CBS News 2015). Functional medicine practitioners have attempted to sidestep this hazard by creating their own "doctor's brand" supplements.[14] While this may sometimes ensure the safety of the supplements being recommended, doctor's brand supplements are often not third-party tested and tend to be more expensive than generic versions available on the market. Functional medicine patients may turn to cheaper alternatives and risk consuming fake or poor-quality supplements. Additionally, the effects and proper dosing of salugens are not always known due to insufficient research. Over the course of my ethnographic research, I found countless practitioners pointing to empirical evidence supporting the use of salugens and numerous patients recounting their positive outcomes; nonetheless, salugens must be used with caution given the lack of regulation and gaps in existing research.

Functional medicine resists most of the characteristics Beyerstein (1996) and Hansson (2013, 2017) describe when defining pseudoscience. Most functional medicine practitioners are trained scientists who employ methods based on scientific evidence, not on a mystical worldview or magical beliefs, when making clinical decisions. Far from touting arcane skills, religious dogma, or proprietary secrets, functional medicine practitioners aim to close the clinical translational gap by applying the latest scientific discoveries in clinical care (see Vega 2023, 57–60). The functional medicine approach does not contradict or deny well-established scientific knowledge such as relativity theory, evolution, climate science, the inverse square law, laws of thermodynamics, injunctions against reverse causality, C. D. Broad's basic limiting principles, or laws of conservation of energy, momentum, etc. The healing it offers is not spontaneous—rather, it is produced through the effort of the patient and the close, personalized care of the practitioner.

At the same time, some features of functional medicine suggest that it unfolds in the gray area between science and pseudoscience. I have observed how a small number of uncredentialed functional medicine interlocutors threaten the legitimacy of functional medicine as a whole. In an effort to redefine what counts as legitimate science, functional medicine critiques and resists the randomized controlled trial design—the existing gold standard for clinical research. Functional medicine exhibits a lack of uniformity in its application due to the pursuit of P4 medicine. Through this pursuit it delivers medicine that is inaccessible to many and must be situated within the broader anxieties of the privileged. Given functional medicine's focus on hope and the body's natural capacity to heal, it may inadvertently offer false hope or lead to victim blaming. Lastly, functional medicine relies on herbs and supplements that are often unregulated and may pose a danger to patients. If functional medicine is to prosper in mainstream medicine, its practitioners and proponents must explicitly address these potential shortcomings with their conventional medicine counterparts and the public at large.

BOUNDARY WORK

For now, functional medicine sits uncomfortably at the fringe of conventional medicine. It is not a pseudoscience and yet it is not mainstream. While functional medicine offers a series of deviations from "normal science" (see Kuhn 1962), its practitioners readily acknowledge how indispensable existing conventional medical therapies and interventions are in some cases.[15] At the same time, they hope to decenter pharmaceutical management of chronic disease and in its place designate personalization, prediction, precision, and participation as primary goals of medicine. I turn to scholarship on boundary work by Thomas F. Gieryn; Davina Allen; Steven P. Wainwright et al.; and Regula Valérie Burri to explore how functional medicine practitioners aim to incorporate new tools into existing medical practice.

Functional medicine proponents perform boundary work—pushing against the edges of what is currently accepted in mainstream medicine—in their quest to stimulate a transformative *expansion* of the current paradigm. Maskell explains, "Our work has been able to sort of, shift the medical system to understand these new truths and help medicine adapt to its new environment." Maskell indicates that the project of health creation requires functional medicine advocates to "rejig the medical system." At the same time, functional medicine doctors consider the work they do as functional practitioners to be an *extension* of what they were taught in medical school—they are "insiders" engaged in a struggle to renegotiate what constitutes medicine from within the discipline. Before I explore this argument further, I will describe how the term "boundary work" has been deployed in the existing literature.

In his seminal piece "Boundary-Work and the Demarcation of Science from Non-Science" (1983), Thomas F. Gieryn defines boundary work as attempts by scientists to create a favorable public image for science by contrasting it with nonscientific activities. He argues that scientists do boundary work as part of the pursuit of professional goals—for example, to acquire intellectual authority and career opportunities, to deny these resources to "pseudoscientists," and to protect their research from political interference.

Ultimately, Gieryn concludes that the boundaries of science are drawn and redrawn in flexible, historically changing, and often ambiguous ways.

More recently, scholars have used ethnography to observe boundary work in clinical and laboratory settings, sometimes building upon the original conceptualization of boundary work to adequately explain their ethnographic observations. For example, Davina Allen (2000) aims to understand the microsociological processes that constitute occupational jurisdictions and the practical accomplishment of the hospital division of labor. Steven P. Wainwright et al. (2006) explore what they call "ethical boundary-work" in the embryonic stem cell laboratory when they study scientists' perspectives on regulatory frameworks in stem cell research and what scientists consider to be ethical sources of human embryos and stem cells. Regula Valérie Burri uses the lens of visualization technologies such as magnetic resonance imaging (MRI) in radiology to merge Gieryn's concept of boundary work with Pierre Bourdieu's (1984) theory of distinction. She argues that the introduction of novel imaging practices forced radiologists to renegotiate visual expertise and reconstitute their disciplinary identity by regaining authority and accumulating symbolic capital within the professional field.

In Gieryn's original conceptualization, scientists perform *exclusionary* boundary work to distinguish science from nonscience and pseudoscience. This work often involves differentiating people: scientists from nonscientists, experts from nonexperts, etc. In contrast, functional medicine practitioners do not aim to invalidate the work of conventional medicine practitioners. In fact, the functional medicine proponents I observed repeatedly acknowledged the valuable role conventional medicine has played in treating acute conditions with anesthesia and surgical interventions, virtually eradicating many debilitating and life-threatening viruses with vaccines, fighting infection with the appropriate use of antibiotics, and partnering with public-health apparatuses to provide clean drinking water and sanitation (see Vega 2023).

Thus, conventional medicine and functional medicine are not necessarily incommensurable models—instead, the conventional model and the functional model can be combined to create a more diverse tool kit. Furthermore, "disease care" and "health-optimization medicine" may be complementarily combined to the benefit of certain patients. Speaking about cancer treatment, Dr. Chilkov opines, "You need a disease expert who understands what tools can go after the tumor, and you need a health expert to say, 'How do we actually orchestrate this so that we have the best outcome possible, not just cell kill?'" Many functional medicine doctors, agreeing with Dr. Chilkov, support teamwork with conventional medicine counterparts in order to de-normalize illness and create the conditions for patients to experience resilient health.

In essence, the boundary work of functional medicine practitioners is *inclusionary* and unfolds on a *paradigmatic* plane. Their goal is not to draw a boundary but to shift and expand the existing boundary to address the root causes of chronic disease. While functional medicine practitioners often work in conjunction with nutritionists and other allied health professionals, their struggle is not primarily about what categories of health professionals do legitimate work but, rather, the very goals of medicine. They argue that while the existing medical system is poised to treat acute disease, the goals of medicine should extend to the ongoing creation of health and the prevention of chronic disease through lifestyle interventions.

This inclusionary, paradigmatic boundary work has epistemic and material consequences. Many of the functional medicine doctors I observed had sought further training in functional medicine in order to include additional microbiological, nutritional, metabolic, and genomic tools in their medical tool kits. For example, while the average medical school student receives a mere nineteen total hours of training in nutrition (Li 2019, xviii), functional medicine practitioners invest time and resources to obtain additional training in nutrition from metabolic and genomic standpoints. They then use advanced laboratory testing to observe individual patients' metabolic processes and to tailor personalized nutraceutical interventions.

Furthermore, while the scientists engaged in exclusionary boundary work hope to protect their work from political interference, functional medicine advocates are fighting for political recognition and reimbursement for services through health insurance.[16] Using peer-reviewed research like the 2019 study published by Michelle Beidelschies et al. in the *Journal of the American Medical Association*, functional medicine practitioners argue for inclusion within existing health insurance structures. Their work aims to extend the existing boundary surrounding medical care to imbue reimbursable value to lifestyle interventions and prevention in addition to treatment of existing disease. In so doing, these advocates hope to renegotiate the hospital division of labor and place prevention at the forefront of primary care.

Interlude

MAPPING OUT MY SYSTEMS BIOLOGY

Throughout my healing journey, as a dining room table "provider" with a patient list of one, I was determined to understand the interconnections among my different ailments. With no artificial intelligence to aid me, I drew out a rudimentary concept map to depict how my different health issues were related to one another—updating the map each time I came across further relevant information (figure 1.1). While this depiction is limited by its two-dimensional quality, the reader can imagine the map as a sphere that can be rotated and spun. No one particular data point is the center of this "data universe." All the points manifest in constant relation to each other.[1] Ragin's data matrix, along with Dr. Bland and Dr. Hood's "dynamic data clouds" (Price et al. 2017), analyzes how spheres like mine—each representing a "data universe"—relate to those of hundreds of other individuals, each with their unique biology.

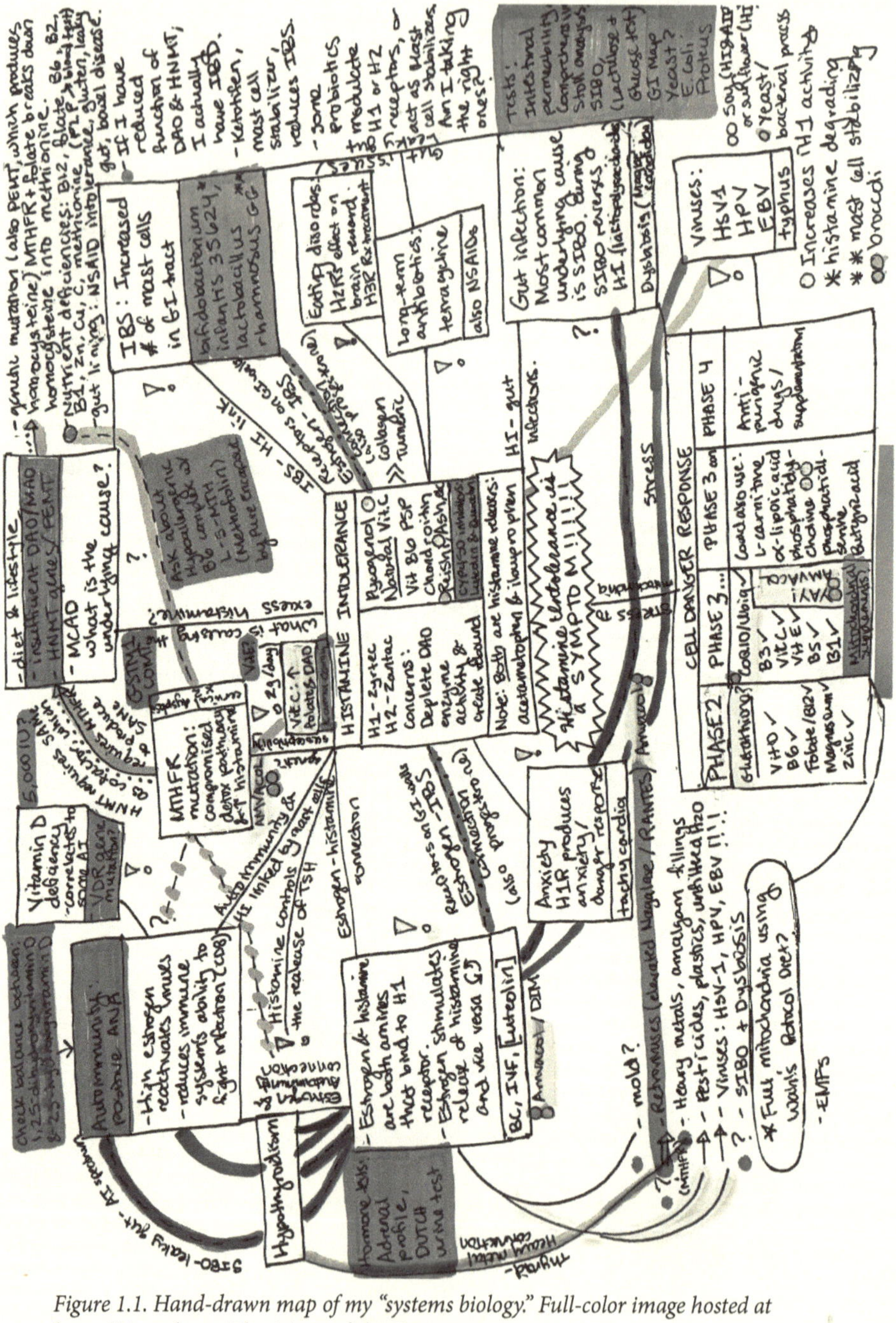

Figure 1.1. Hand-drawn map of my "systems biology." Full-color image hosted at https://tinyurl.com/Physicians-of-the-Future.

CHAPTER 2

WOUNDED HEALERS

"Wounded healers" nearly always share their personal histories of struggling with and triumphing over disease. Why, and in what context, do functional medicine practitioners recount their stories of illness and recovery? The functional medicine matrix—a tool for understanding the antecedents, triggering events, and mediators that have contributed to and perpetuated an illness—elicits narratives that strive to explain how the onset of illness was contingent on underlying factors. In addition, functional medicine practitioners use illness narratives to describe the experiences that impel them to create change in health care provisioning. These practitioners also rely on illness narratives as a form of social capital. In all these cases, functional medicine practitioners reconstruct their personal identities in terms of their *recovery* from illness. Thus, while illness narratives generally lack an "ending" (see Good 1994, 157), the illness narratives of functional medicine practitioners follow a moral arc that ultimately results in triumph.

A primary theme in providers' illness narratives is feeling betrayed by conventional medicine. Wounded healers describe turning to integrative therapies after discovering that the conventional methods they learned in medical school are insufficient for healing their own disease or that of a loved one. In this chapter, I include multiple examples of how functional medicine experts discovered such inadequacies in their training. As a result of these experiences, the illness narratives of wounded healers are firsthand accounts of the noxious effects of medicalization.

I analyze how, through telling their illness narratives, wounded healers describe their "felt experience of dissonance"—in the words of Dr. Kelly Brogan—and critique medical hegemony. These practitioners explain how their transition to functional medicine required "reschooling." Scholars have discussed how illness narratives resemble stories of religious conversion, and, with a similar outcome, functional medicine practitioners describe how their successful recovery from chronic disease gave them a sense of purpose—which can even be described as zealotry—with regard to health coaching and education. They suggest that without these personal experiences of illness, they would not have been sufficiently impelled to challenge the limits of conventional medicine.

Furthermore, providers' dissatisfaction with their personal experiences as patients—including being ridiculed and dismissed by colleagues—has fomented an increased capacity for empathy in them. In conventional medicine, doctors' suffering is usually rendered invisible. Suffering is framed as part of the medical school experience, and from the time of their initiation into medical school, future doctors are not shown empathy—not even when they become patients. However, my research confirms observations by Sayantani DasGupta and Rita Charon (2004) regarding the utility of eliciting the illness narratives of providers to teach fellow doctors empathy and create therapeutic connections. Functional medicine practitioners' empathetic approach to patients relocates the locus of their authority from their technical expertise to their shared experience of suffering.

In turn, this relocation of authority supports the creation of dialectical relationships between functional medicine patients and providers. Providers often come to acknowledge their own illnesses through treating patients whose cases resemble their own. By the same token, functional medicine practitioners locate answers for patients when attempting to locate answers for themselves. Their personal experiences of suffering inspire their clinical approach, which includes "slow medicine"—a meaning-centered approach that acknowledges and affirms the patient's and family's experiences of suffering (see Kleinman [1988] 2020, 3)—and the moral act of caregiving. The shared experience of suffering realigns the doctor-patient relationship, making the patients' speech acts more valuable. While functional medicine providers position themselves as "health care heroes" vis-à-vis their illness narratives, they simultaneously position patients as heroes of their own journeys.

Ultimately, I analyze how illness narratives are relationally constructed through interaction between the narrator and the listener. Identifying oneself as a wounded healer sets the stage for novel types of relationships and creates a sense of unity among functional medicine practitioners. Biosociality among wounded healers is sustained and evidenced by unifying speech acts. The illness narratives of wounded healers collectivize their experiences as both providers and sufferers, and they use them as a strategic device to achieve social effects.

I have opted to refer to functional medicine doctors by their titles and surnames in other chapters of this book, thus indicating their positionality vis-à-vis functional medicine. In contrast, I refer to practitioners in this chapter by their first names after using their full names on first mention, signaling how in the process of telling their illness narratives, functional medicine providers shed some of the power and mystique of the white coat and reveal themselves to be just as human, and just as vulnerable to disease, as their patients.

I now turn to the illness narratives of Terry Wahls, Amy Myers, and Andrea Nakayama—three prominent examples of functional medicine providers who lead with their illness narratives when introducing themselves in emails, books, and online events.

ILLNESS NARRATIVES AMONG FUNCTIONAL MEDICINE PRACTITIONERS

> *Terry Wahls was initially diagnosed with relapsing remitting multiple sclerosis (MS) on the basis of a history of optic neuritis and weakness in her left leg.*[1] *She had a variety of tests done, including spinal taps, MRIs, blood and vision tests, etc. She wanted to treat her disease as aggressively as possible, so she sought out the people doing the latest research and prescribing the newest drugs. She saw specialists at Marshall Health (recognized as the first Center for Comprehensive Multiple Sclerosis Care in West Virginia), the University of Iowa Hospitals and Clinics, and the Cleveland Clinic. Despite receiving the most recent treatments, her well-being went steadily downhill.*
>
> *Within three years Terry needed a reclining wheelchair. Her disease was reclassified as secondary progressive MS. Her doctors told her that once she lost physical functions they would never come back. Hearing this, she was on board with taking more and more aggressive drugs because she did not want to become permanently disabled. However, despite her aggressive treatments, "nothing seemed to stop this relentless march toward being bedridden and possibly demented." At the same time, she was struggling with worsening pain and realizing that on top of being bedridden, having uncontrolled pain was an additional prospect.*
>
> *She began reading basic science studies related to her condition and looking for drug trials. Then she had an "Aha!" moment: it occurred to her to look at the mechanism of the disease rather than the drugs that had been tried to treat it. She decided to transition to focusing on studies using animal models to test the effects of specific nutrients for improving disease states involving shrinking brains—diseases such as amyotrophic*

lateral sclerosis, Parkinson's, and Huntington's. She found that diminished mitochondrial function was a hallmark of all those diseases. Even though no one was writing about the relationship between mitochondria and MS at the time, she hypothesized that disordered mitochondria were a big driver of MS. Based on existing scientific studies using animal models, Terry decided to create a supplement protocol for her mitochondria. This step helped build her energy and alleviate her fatigue.

However, Terry continued losing muscle function until she needed to be in a zero-gravity wheelchair. At that point, she was assigned job duties she knew she physically could not do. It was the VA's way of saying, "We are done redesigning your position. You are going to have to take medical disability." The following month, she discovered the Institute for Functional Medicine and enrolled in its course on neurological protection. Taking the course was a struggle since she was in the midst of brain fog, but she slogged through it and came out with a longer list of vitamins and supplements. Then she had another very fortuitous "Aha!" moment: she realized that the nutrients she needed might be more effective if they came from diet.

Terry decided to start with her now even longer list of supplements and research how she could get the same mitochondria-supporting nutrients through diet. She restructured her paleo diet to make it more nutrient dense for the mitochondria and the brain. Within a month, she started a new role at work that she had initially assumed she could not do, but as it turned out, she could do it. Her brain fog was clearing and her energy was improving. After one more month, she was walking with a cane throughout the hospital. In a couple more months, she was walking without a cane in the hospital. In six months, she was biking around the neighborhood. She describes these moments of progress, saying, "I was crying, my wife was crying, and my kids were crying." In a year, she was able to do a twenty-mile bike ride.

Terry's experience changed how she thinks about disease. She shares how before her experience of recovery, she was very skeptical of supplements and complementary and alternative medicines. She thought people were "wasting a lot of money and time." However, given her amazing chronic-disease reversal using functional medicine techniques, she acknowledges, "God works in mysterious ways."

Terry's experience also restructured how she practices medicine. Initially, her director at the University of Iowa Hospitals and Clinics told her to write up her own experience as a case report. Her first step was to reflect on herself as an "n *of 1." Subsequently she received a small grant* *for a slightly larger study. Her chief of medicine told her to change her entire research agenda to using diet and lifestyle to treat MS and other complex chronic diseases. In August 2018, the National MS Society awarded Terry over $1 million to conduct a clinical trial comparing the effect of the Wahls diet with that of a low-saturated-fat diet on MS outcomes. In this clinical trial, the Wahls diet produced better outcomes.*[2] *Terry explains, tongue in cheek, that the biggest side effect of her dietary protocol is rapid weight loss, "but not too much—once patients reach a healthy weight, they stabilize." The second biggest side effect is mood regulation.*

In 2019, Terry and her team received a $2 million gift from Dr. Howard Urnovitz to support the Wahls Therapeutic Lifestyle Fund. The gift money is to be used for Terry's current study comparing dietary and lifestyle changes without drugs to the standard of care in MS treatment. The lifestyle changes that she includes are meditation and exercise.

Terry used multiple methods, including her email listserv, to recruit potential study subjects. In an automated email titled "Research opportunities for you!" Terry wrote, "Rosalynn, As I've mentioned before, it's been a busy and exciting year for research! . . . The sooner I have the data that shows the protocol works, the sooner we can influence clinical practice around the world." Terry's mission is to create an "epidemic of health."

While Terry's illness narrative is exemplary, it also possesses many elements that are representative of most illness narratives among functional medicine practitioners. Her narrative emphasizes the height of the struggle: she discusses her experience of losing physical function to multiple sclerosis and worrying that she would end up "demented" and in uncontrollable pain. As a conventionally trained physician, she first turned to the most aggressive and cutting-edge therapies in conventional medicine to treat her disease. However, as her symptoms progressed and she began losing more and more physical function, Terry became desperate. She embarked on a personal quest involving an investigation of basic science literature and experimentation with supplementation and dietary protocols she created. This self-designed alternative approach produced unexpected, positive results. Terry is one of the most well-known and well-regarded practitioners in the functional medicine community due to her astounding disease reversal and her translation of that reversal into clinical practice and medical research. Her own healing journey fuels her sense of purpose as a functional medicine physician.

Amy Myers's struggle began when she was in her second year of medical school and she started experiencing the "nightmarish symptoms" of hyperthyroidism.[3] *For the first time in her life, Amy was seized by panic attacks. Within a few months, she dropped from a size 4 to a size 0, despite barely exercising and eating massive amounts of pizza and oatmeal cookies. Her heart and mind were constantly racing and she was always in a mild sweat. She began to have uncontrollable tremors. At night, she was tormented by insomnia, and she began spiraling into a pattern of anxiety, dizziness, and fatigue. "I couldn't believe this was happening to me," Amy writes in* The Autoimmune Solution. *"Awful as the symptoms were, the helplessness was worse—the feeling that my life was no longer my own."*

When Amy's tremors became impossible to conceal, her friends urged her to see a doctor, but when she did, the doctor dismissed her symptoms as stress and told her, "I wouldn't worry about it." This doctor's visit served as a painful lesson for Amy to listen to her own patients and tell them, "You know your own body better than I do."

Amy demanded a full workup, and her lab results provided a diagnosis: Graves's disease, an autoimmune condition of the thyroid gland. "Finally, my misery had a name," she writes. Unfortunately, conventional medical treatments for Graves's disease are either procedures to destroy or to remove the thyroid or medication with a long list of serious side effects. Amy confides, "Despite my enrollment in a conventional medical school, I believed there were other roads to health besides medications and surgery."

Reflecting on her family life in her childhood, Amy explains that her mother prepared "1970s health food" from scratch. However, when she discovered functional medicine, Amy realized that the "healthy" family diet—predominantly whole-wheat bread, grains, and legumes—could have "actually been poisoning us all." Her mother developed pancreatic cancer at age fifty-nine, and her father has struggled with worsening polymyositis—an autoimmune disease characterized by joint pain and muscle weakness.

Conventional medicine's only approach to her mother's cancer was chemotherapy. When she asked her mother's doctor about nutritional interventions, the doctor scoffed, saying, "Your mom could put a watermelon in her ear and jump up and down on one foot, and that might help too, but it probably won't." Amy concludes, "My mother died less than five months after she was diagnosed. I entered medical school the following year—and one year later I was suffering from Graves'."

Amy faced terrible options for treating her Graves's disease with conventional medicine, but as far as she knew, there was no other way. It was the year 2000, and functional medicine was in its infancy. Initially, she opted for the medication route, but this caused disastrous side effects—the prescription drug began destroying her liver and caused toxic hepatitis. Thus, Amy explains, "I chose ablation and said goodbye to my thyroid, a choice I regret to this day." Since she no longer has a thyroid, Amy is reliant on synthetic hormones. She tells readers that if she had known about functional medicine at the time, she might be living symptom-free today, with her body intact.

Although her major health issues nearly forced her to drop out of medical school, she persevered, graduated, and became an emergency room physician. While in this role, she was proud of being able to save trauma patients, but she also became increasingly aware of how little she could do for her chronic-disease patients. Meanwhile, her own health problems persisted. She developed irritable bowel syndrome (IBS). She never really felt healthy—the best she could feel was "not sick." Then, finally, she found functional medicine.

As a spokesperson for functional medicine, Amy aims to address some of the fifty million Americans suffering from an autoimmune disease, as well as their parents, spouses, siblings, friends, and children. Furthermore, she hopes her message reaches some of the hundreds of millions of people struggling with inflammatory conditions that put them at risk for developing an autoimmune disease. In her book, Amy indicates she will show readers how to use a healthy diet, high-quality supplements, and lifestyle to eliminate symptoms and get off of medications. Amy's goal is to help readers take charge of their health, reduce their toxic burdens, heal their infections, reduce their stress, and make choices that support their bodies. She asks, "Why do I sound so confident? Because over the years, I've treated thousands of patients with this approach—and I've also treated myself. . . . If you give me just thirty days, I can help you take back your life too."

Like Terry's narrative, Amy's provides a rich description of how she felt at the height of the struggle, emphasizing her helplessness. Amy reveals her anxiety and fear as she struggled to complete medical school shortly after her mother died and while experiencing both the symptoms of Graves's disease and the side effects from conventional treatment. Despite her conventional training, she felt intuitively that there must be an alternative to surgery or medication. Amy describes how her efforts to advocate for herself and her mother were dismissed and ridiculed by doctors. As a medical student suffering from an autoimmune disease, and as the daughter of parents who were succumbing to cancer and autoimmunity, Amy was not shown empathy by medical providers. These experiences inform how she practices functional medicine, including how she intentionally listens to patients, resists the normalization of feeling unwell, and aims to use diet, supplements, and lifestyle to liberate patients from chronic disease. Her work as a functional medicine doctor pushes back against medicalization and pharmaceuticalization.

Andrea Nakayama begins her story, "Many of us have these life events—either health circumstances that happen to ourselves or a loved one—that change everything from that point forward. In functional medicine, we might call that a trigger."[4] *While the terminology of a "trigger" is usually applied to a life event that spurs the onset of symptoms, Andrea uses this terminology to describe the way many practitioners are called to do the work of functional medicine.*

Turning to her own story, Andrea explains that her husband was diagnosed with a very aggressive brain tumor in April 2000, when she was seven weeks pregnant. His doctors told him he had six months to live and he would not see the birth of their child. Andrea and her husband did everything they could to shift his prognosis. They took a "yes and" approach to combine allopathic treatments with nonconventional medical approaches. Andrea explains, "He, in fact, lived for two and a half years. . . . He died when our son was 19 months old."

When she reflected on the experience, it did not make sense to Andrea that her husband's doctors treated him as a diagnosis instead of a whole person. "Here I had the man who was my soulmate and my partner . . . who was about to be a father and [was] a husband, and a son, and a brother, and a worker, and he was treated like a dead man walking." Andrea acknowledges that while those experiences occurred many years earlier, she characterizes them as "a huge life-changing event." As a result, when she eventually found functional medicine, its holistic approach made extraordinary sense to her.

Andrea has also had her own journey with disease—in her case, with the chronic autoimmune disease Hashimoto's thyroiditis. She began experiencing symptoms after her husband died. "Certainly, pregnancy is a trigger for autoimmunity. . . . And the stress that my body was under during pregnancy was profound—not just the regular hormonal changes you go through [during] pregnancy, but a whole lot of added

> *stress on top of that," she says. Additionally, she had inherited the genetic predisposition for Hashimoto's from her mother. Understanding how her genetic propensities had been triggered by life events was integral to Andrea's healing journey.*
>
> *Andrea's painful experiences of disease and loss led to her becoming a functional medicine nutritionist. When interacting with patients and colleagues, Andrea introduces herself by explaining how these life events have framed her work. For example, in an automated email titled "Welcome, Rosalynn! I can't wait to meet you," Andrea wrote, "Hi Rosalynn, The hardest thing I've said to my husband Isamu was that it was OK to die." The email included three photos—the first is of Andrea and her husband on their wedding day in 1998; the second is of the couple and their young son while Isamu was in hospice in 2002; and the third is of Andrea and her son, Gilbert, at the farmer's market in 2011. Andrea continued, "The pictures above give you a little glimpse into my journey with my husband's illness and death, becoming a Functional Medicine Nutritionist, raising a son as a single mom, and building an online school for people like you."*

In the same vein as both Terry's and Amy's illness narratives, Andrea's likewise points to a defining moment in her journey—what I have referred to as "the height of struggle" and what Andrea refers to as a "life event." She describes the acute stress of learning that her husband was terminally ill while she was pregnant with their child and the deep pain that followed when her husband passed and she was left to rear their son. Like Amy, Terry describes how a loved one, her husband, was treated poorly by medical personnel. While Amy alludes to how her mother's death just one year prior to her onset of Graves' disease was a contributing factor in her own illness experience, Andrea explicitly explains how the acute stress of her husband's terminal illness, combined with hormonal changes during pregnancy and an underlying disposition for Hashimoto's, triggered her autoimmunity. These experiences impelled Andrea to become a functional medicine nutritionist and to create an online school for functional medicine nutrition. When interpellating others as future students in her school, Andrea shares deeply intimate details and photos of her experiences of suffering and loss. In this way, she turns to her illness narrative as a medium for potential connection with other wounded healers.

Terry's, Amy's, and Andrea's stories contain common themes, exemplify how sufferers reconstruct their personal identities and life histories in terms of an illness, point to how illness narratives become a powerful discursive form among wounded healers, and demonstrate how illness narratives are told in social contexts that are unique to the functional medicine community. Lars-Christer Hydén (1997) identifies three different social contexts in which illness narratives often unfold: people tell others about their illnesses in everyday contexts; interview subjects deliver illness narratives to researchers in elicited contexts; and patients tell their doctors or therapists about their symptoms when they seek help in the institutional context. The three social contexts Hydén identifies are insufficient for capturing the full utility of wounded healers' illness narratives since, in the functional medicine realm, these narratives often unfold in entrepreneurial contexts, where they are leveraged as a form of biosocial currency.

On their way to constructing biosocially relevant and entrepreneurially profitable illness narratives, however, functional medicine providers transitionally construct "contingent" narratives. Contingent narratives address the origins of a disease, the causes of illness episodes, and the effects of illness on everyday life. Illness narratives are a medium for discussing possible explanations for an illness and to help others relating to the illness (Hydén 1997). Functional medicine practitioners-in-training, at once patients and providers, are taught to seek and deliver contingent illness narratives when learning about the functional medicine matrix—a tool for understanding the antecedents, triggering events, and mediators that contribute to and perpetuate illness.

Functional medicine providers generally commit to functional medicine after personally experiencing recovery or witnessing the recovery of others; in the process, their contingent narratives begin to morph into moral narratives. Moral narratives constitute changes between the person, the illness, and their social identity, thus (re)establishing the moral status of the individual and maintaining social distance. The articulation of illness narratives allows sufferers to attribute meaning to their symptoms within the context of their lives (Hydén 1997). By reframing their illness narratives as moral narratives, functional medicine practitioners explain what impels them to create change in health care provisioning. In turn, their narratives become biosocially relevant and entrepreneurially profitable when functional medicine practitioners embed their sense of purpose into their personal experiences of illness and subsequent recovery.

While the social context in which the illness narratives of wounded healers are told—the underlying purpose for their retelling—is unique to the functional medicine community, the arcs of these narratives also differ from narratives told in other contexts. Outside of the functional medicine realm, illness narratives are considered incomplete. According to Byron J. Good (1994, 157), an illness narrative lacks an "ending" since, after a person falls ill, it is unknown how the situation will develop. The suffering could lead to death, slow deterioration, or eventual recovery. Without an ending, Hydén notes, it is difficult to make sense of illness symptoms because "there is no temporal horizon to give them meaning" (1997, 61). As a result, Good (1994, 157) argues, illness narratives undergo continual negotiation—they are always ambiguous and forever in search of meaning. During this process, J. Wiltshire (1994, 211) says, the narrator's voice is routed through the doctor, and may switch between the voice of the "ill" and the voice of the "healthy." That is, narrators toggle between the vantage points of ongoing suffering and of illness as something that invaded one's life at an earlier time. This code switching can be seen as the narrator's struggle to define the end of their illness narrative.

In contrast, functional medicine interlocutors consider the illness narratives of wounded healers to be complete. Their stories end with triumph over disease—reversal of symptoms and recovery from illness. Thus, while patients elsewhere tend to reconfigure their identities in terms of the illness when telling their illness narratives, wounded healers reconfigure their identities—and particularly their drive to help others—in terms of their recovery.

In the next section, I turn to where the illness narratives of wounded healers begin: when the practitioner or scientist discovers that their existing knowledge is insufficient to heal their own disease or that of a loved one.[5] This defining feature of wounded healers' illness narratives results in an agentive search for knowledge beyond the scope of their training. Wounded healers later apply the lessons they have learned as patients and family members of patients to their patient care. The dissonance between functional medicine providers' conventional medical training and their personal experiences of suffering fuels their desire to create change in health care provisioning.

BETRAYAL: FELT DISSONANCE AND THE DESIRE TO CREATE CHANGE

Kelly Brogan, a holistic psychiatrist, "awoke to the possibility of putting a chronic autoimmune disease into remission" when she began to have her own emergent symptoms. Kelly was diagnosed with Hashimoto's disease postpartum, nine months after the birth of her second child. She engaged with her own health crisis by "hitting the books" and asking,

"Well, is this evidence based? Putting an autoimmune disease into complete and total remission?" She found decades of reports documenting total remission in patients; however, were it not for her personal experience, she confesses, "I would have dismissed it out of hand." She reversed her Hashimoto's by following functional medicine principles: eliminating food sensitivities, taking supplements, and recommitting to exercise.

David Servan-Schreiber, a neurologist, describes how he discovered from his own brain-scanning experiment that he had brain cancer. David writes, "No longer wrapped in the comfortable mantle of physician and scientist, I had become a cancer patient" (2009, 1). He used his skills as a physician-scientist to delve into the medical literature, in search of complementary approaches to help him "change the odds." The integrated techniques David discovered were often criticized and dismissed by his conventional medicine colleagues. David's experience sheds light on how alternatives are rendered thinkable only when scientists are seeking answers for their own healing—not in their day-to-day patient care.

Elizabeth Boham describes how, as a woman who studied nutritional biochemistry at Cornell University, became board certified in family medicine by Albany Medical School, and completed further graduate training to become a registered dietician at Columbia University, she seemed like an unlikely candidate for breast cancer. However, learning about functional medicine helped Elizabeth to realize that eating well and exercising were insufficient for preventing cancer in her case. She explains, "For some people [those are] really important area[s to] focus on in terms of prevention of cancer—but for me . . . I needed to focus on managing my stress better, or helping my body detoxify." Elizabeth's specialization in functional medicine prompted her to develop an amplified perspective of health and thus helped her put her breast cancer into remission.

At other times, practitioners' narratives do not describe their personal experience of illness. Rather, these narratives describe the illness experiences of close kin—usually a parent or child. Tom O'Bryan, a chiropractor and autoimmune expert, tells the story of his father's death, saying, "When my father died suddenly, the pathologist called me and said, 'I don't know why your father died.' I said, 'What do you mean?'" The pathologist went on to explain that while Tom's father died of a heart attack, the autopsy did not reveal any of the underlying etiologies that are known to cause a heart attack. These results sent Tom on a hunt for answers. After lots of research, he realized that his father had had an undiagnosed gluten intolerance that led to inflammation and vitamin B deficiency, which, in turn, led to elevated homocysteine and, ultimately, vasospasm. Elevated homocysteine does not cause any apparent symptoms and is thus referred to as "the silent killer." Tom immediately began checking himself and his family members. As it turns out, he, his brother, his sister, and nineteen of his twenty-one first cousins have elevated homocysteine—a problem that is reversible in just three weeks by taking B vitamins. Tom's experience demonstrates how many functional medicine practitioners arrive at a deeper understanding of biology through the biology of a loved one.

In the same vein, Rangan Chatterjee, a physician and star of the hit BBC One series Doctor in the House, *explains, "For me, the big moment was my son. When my son was six months old, he nearly died. He had a convulsion. . . . It was a really, really scary time." On a quest to help his son, Rangan learned more about science, nutrition, and the immune system. The experience caused him to open his mind to all the possibilities for healing.*

Similarly, physician and researcher William Li's commitment to "food as medicine" is based on results he has personally witnessed. William's mother had metastatic endometrial cancer for which she received immunotherapy. On the podcast The Doctor's Farmacy, *William noted that only about 20 percent of people respond strongly to immunotherapy—those with a certain gut bacteria. Knowing this, William guided his mother toward a diet that would enhance her microbiome. Within thirty days, his mother was cancer-free.*

For his part, acupuncturist and health coach Chris Kresser witnessed through a family member how medicalization can have negative effects. Chris attributes his grandfather's death to the inappropriate treatments offered by conventional medicine. He states that his grandfather's death "was totally unnecessary," going on to assert that surgery "basically killed him. He didn't die right away, but he just kind of withered away after that." In Chris's view, his grandfather was medicalized, and subsequently perished, due to a "faulty paradigm."

Like their MD counterparts, many functional medicine educators have also suffered from disease and have also played the role of protagonist in their recovery. For example, Matt Riemann, an author and educator on personalized health and the prevention of chronic pain, describes the moment he realized he needed to find the answers for himself, explaining, "One day, about ten years ago, I woke up in excruciating pain. I couldn't breathe. I couldn't move. I actually thought I was having a heart attack." Matt sought care from the leading specialists around the world and was diagnosed with a terminal illness—a TTI genetic mutation. Needing to find out how to "switch his gene off," he began exploring the existing literature on epigenetics.[6] Matt possesses a master's degree in applied human sciences. While he is not an MD, his scientific literacy and experience identifying the data he needed to heal himself resemble that of many functional medicine practitioners.

Functional health educator Dr. Sarah Ballantyne similarly describes how she relied on her academic training while recovering from multiple overlapping autoimmune diseases. Sarah indicates she initially dismissed the functional medicine approach only to then get "hooked" on the science. She explains, "I dove into PubMed. . . . And, it all started to make sense." She quickly identified gaps in her existing perspective—although she had conducted extensive medical research on the immune system and the gut barrier, her research background was focused on basic science and drug development.[7] She continues, "I needed to teach myself nutritional sciences. Fortunately, I had experience switching scientific fields, so teaching myself a new branch of science was something I had the skills to do." Like Matt, she used her scientific agility to research and reverse her own health conditions. Sarah and Matt are not MDs—thus, they do not offer patient care—but they are considered functional medicine experts and are included in online summits and conferences alongside providers.

In their illness narratives, these wounded healers describe a certain sense of betrayal by conventional medicine. In Terry's case, she was already working as an internal medicine physician when she began losing motor functions. Her doctors told her that there was no hope for remission from her MS. Realizing that her training in conventional medicine did not equip her with the knowledge needed to combat her declining health, Terry sought out education in functional medicine and set out to design her own dietary protocol. Amy was undergoing training as a conventional medical doctor when, in her words, the conventional medicine system "failed her." She was presented with terrible options to treat her Graves' disease—each of which presented awful side effects or long-term consequences. Kelly successfully placed her Hashimoto's into remission after "hitting the books" and studying documented cases of remission. She learned strategies she would have immediately dismissed based on her medical school training alone. David was told by his oncologist that there was nothing he could do as far as diet or lifestyle to improve his outcome; however, despite being critiqued and dismissed by his colleagues, he decided to embrace integrative methods to shift the odds in his favor when battling brain cancer. Elizabeth was doing everything "right" according to her training—she was eating nutritious food and doing plenty of exercise—however, she needed to learn the functional medicine approach to stress management and detoxification to put her breast cancer into remission. After his father's death, Tom learned that a blood test that is not usually ordered by conventional medicine physicians would have revealed a vitamin B deficiency. Knowing this sooner would have saved his father's life. He used this information to alert his siblings and cousins and help twenty-one of them prevent a fate similar to his father's. When his son had a convulsion, Rangan sought out scientific studies regarding nutrition and the immune system since his medical school training provided him with little knowledge that would help his son. William recognized that the prognosis for individuals with metastatic endometrial cancer is bleak when treated with immunotherapy alone. In a successful attempt to ensure the best possible outcome for his mother, he turned to the most recent microbiome research and helped her adjust her diet. These narratives are representative of those of the many functional medicine practitioners who switch to functional medicine after they or someone they love struggles with health problems and the practitioners realize that their conventional medical training does not provide them with the necessary tools for healing.

The transition to functional medicine requires thorough reschooling—practitioners must embrace fresh knowledge and develop a systems-based view of the body. Rangan describes the experience of conducting extensive research for healing his son as "basically getting another degree." Cynthia Li, a doctor and author whose work focused on public health in underserved populations before she transitioned to integrative and functional medicine, explains to Mark Hyman how, after being told by her endocrinologist that her hypothyroidism is "genetic" and there was nothing she could do to improve her thyroid function, she decided to find answers that would help her heal herself. In the process, she learned to understand the body as a system. Cynthia indicates, "When my thyroid was out of whack, it wasn't just my thyroid. It was my whole hormone system, which is tied then to the digestive system, which is tied to the immune system." This process of initiation leads functional medicine practitioners to realize just how little they know.[8]

In essence, conventionally trained doctors "cross over" to functional medicine after a "felt experience of dissonance" with what they learned in their training. Kelly indicates that doctors go "rogue" after an "experience of awakening" that shows them "a greater version of the truth than what they were exposed to through their pharma-funded education." During this process, their sustained commitment to emerging science trumps their allegiance to the current paradigm.

When wounded healers share their illness narratives, they challenge existing structures in conventional medicine, an idea that returns us to how illness narratives were originally seen by Arthur Kleinman and pointing to the underlying utility of this discursive form. In 1988, Kleinman, a physician and medical anthropologist, wrote *The Illness Narratives: Suffering, Healing, and the Human Condition* as a guide for altering medical education; he published a new edition in 2020.[9] Kleinman argues that interpreting narratives of illness experience is a core task of doctoring, but the skill has atrophied in biomedical training. While he admires many aspects of biomedicine, he asserts that the medical care system diverts the practitioner's attention away from the illness experience. As a result, he characterizes chronic-disease care as a failure of contemporary medicine (Kleinman [1988] 2020). While Kleinman's conception of illness narratives positions patients as narrators and providers as interpreters of illness narratives, wounded healers are at once patients and providers, narrators and interpreters. Being multiply positioned allows wounded healers to interpret and prioritize their patients' illness experiences while working to reverse the "epidemic" of chronic disease (see Terzic and Waldman 2011).

Wounded healers often frame their illness narratives as a critique of conventional medicine and the care they offer as a corrective to underlying structural issues in the health care system. Similarly, in the preface to the 2020 edition of *The Illness Narratives*, Kleinman reflects on bureaucratic, commercial, and governmental influences in medicine, arguing, "Professional practitioners have been proletarianized as workers in large-scale institutions [and] patients and families feel powerless in the face of the dominance of health care as big business and big government" (iii). In his view, both patient mistrust and physician burnout are evidence of a health care system in disarray and in need of moral reform. The "meaning-centered slow medicine" approach of functional medicine practitioners resembles the "cult resistance that will lead to reform through moral acts of caregiving (witnessing, acknowledging, affirming)" (3) that Kleinman hopes his work will inspire.

As functional medicine practitioners experience and witness reversal of chronic disease, they are instilled with a strong sense of purpose. For Sarah, her successful chronic-disease reversal inspired what she calls "zealotry." Her IBS and gastroesophageal reflux disease (GERD) completely disappeared, her anxiety attacks stopped, her aches and pains greatly diminished, she no longer required daily medications to control her asthma, her weird allergies (e.g., breaking out into a rash every time she touched cardboard) vanished, her eczema and acne cleared, and she was able to lose weight after plateauing for months. As a result of all these positive outcomes, Sarah explains, "I became a zealot. I was all in. Like, 'Let's start a blog as an outlet for my enthusiasm' level." Sarah's description exemplifies what scholars have identified as a Christian narrative pattern in illness narratives.

Anne Hunsaker Hawkins (1990) indicates that many illness narratives constitute a separate genre, which she calls "pathographies." These pathographies detail patients' illnesses, their struggles to overcome them, and the process of regeneration. Hunsaker Hawkins argues that pathographies have replaced religious conversion stories depicting how a "sinner" has become a follower of God. Pathographies are thus an extension of an ancient Christian narrative genre involving a sinful life, the realization of sinfulness, the experience of regret, and the turn to a new life (see also Freccero 1986).

Like Sarah, many other functional medicine interlocutors funnel their newfound sense of purpose into health coaching and health education. Chiropractor Dr. Ryan Wohlfert recalls, "I don't like to talk about it, but I battled brain fog and fatigue, migraines, and poor focus. My wife . . . she struggled with tiredness and exhaustion. And I've seen sickness and disease repeatedly in my family." For twenty years, Ryan also witnessed these symptoms in his patients. He indicates, "That's exactly why I created a one-on-one coaching program that reveals the causes of fatigue, brain fog, poor focus, exhaustion, and tiredness." In the same vein, Jonathan Landsman, a holistic oral health expert, explains that his wife struggled with mercury poisoning. After his wife recovered, Jonathan felt impelled to educate others so they could also protect their health. In essence, personal experiences give many functional medicine interlocutors, MDs and non-MDs alike, a strong sense of purpose with regard to health education.

Without personal experiences of recovery, many would-be functional medicine interlocutors may not feel sufficiently motivated to engage in boundary work and expand the current paradigm. Lloyd Burrell, creator of the EMF Health Summit and best-selling author, explains, "You need to be so committed, and have so much belief in it, and the only way you are going to get that is if you have actually directly experienced the problem—the pain—or someone really close to you has." Lloyd identifies this shared experience of pain as a unifying factor among the guests on his summit. Speaking to Lloyd's point, chiropractor and integrative health coach Elena

Villanueva explains that having been "really sick once," she has "a passion [for getting] the education out there" and for encouraging people to "take massive action." Elena's commitment to getting the word out about functional medicine demonstrates how experiences of personal healing, and the resulting passion for bringing functional medicine to others, propel the functional medicine movement forward.

PROVIDERS' SUFFERING POTENTIATES EMPATHETIC THERAPEUTIC CONNECTIONS

In illness narratives, providers position themselves as wounded healers. This seemingly paradoxical role emphasizes that functional medicine providers have also suffered from chronic diseases and thus possess intimate insight into their patients' perspectives. These narratives, furthermore, point to dissatisfaction with (mis)treatment by biomedical professionals. Here I am using a parenthetical reference to signal the dual meaning of the word "treatment"—the manner in which providers behave toward patients and also the medications and interventions they recommend. Amy describes both how her Graves' symptoms were dismissed as stress and how her mother's doctor mocked Amy's comments regarding the healing potential of diet. Andrea recounts how her husband was treated like a "dead man walking" instead of a man who was still alive and needed to be engaged as a person, not a disease. In all these examples, providers and their family members were treated poorly by medical personnel and were offered inadequate treatment—thus motivating their subsequent turn to diet and lifestyle interventions.

Over the course of my ethnographic research, I observed how wounded healers told of how experiences of being ridiculed, dismissed, and disregarded had impelled them to practice functional medicine with empathy and with respect for patients' embodied knowledge. Sarah explains, "My passion for helping others was ignited by decades of seeking help from medical professionals and being figuratively patted on the head and told that I was just a stressed student who needed Prozac and to count my calories and exercise." Having similarly faced degrading treatment from a medical authority and having her questions dismissed out of hand, Amy intentionally listens to patients and reassures them they are the primary authority with regard to their body. Andrea likewise strives to understand not just the patient's biology but also all the life events and triggers that led to the onset of their disease. After experiencing (mis)treatment by providers, these wounded healers describe their commitment to behaving compassionately and diligently toward the patients they serve.

Why is conventional medicine providers' suffering so infrequently cited as a source of compassion for patients? It is not that conventional doctors do not suffer; rather, they conceal their suffering from peers and patients to avoid potential stigma. According to Cynthia, conventional medicine lacks empathy toward its own practitioners since there is "this taboo about doctors not disclosing their health problems." Mark links this lack of empathy to what he characterizes as "the hazing of medical school." During medical school, many future doctors become "unwell," and this experience is normalized. As if participating in this conversation, Dr. Kirk Robert Parsley, a medical doctor, former Navy SEAL, and CEO of Doc Parsley Sleep Remedy, elaborates on how hazing occurs: "It took a threat of congressional action just to get a training doctor's work week down to one hundred hours or less." Pointing to how this situation is detrimental to the health of both doctors and patients, Cynthia comments, "It's a kind of trauma and we pass it on to our patients inadvertently." Kirk links this normalization of suffering to the production of biomedicine's authoritative knowledge and notes, "Doctors are sort of this upper echelon of admired professions—for whatever reason, I have no idea." Comments from these functional medicine practitioners, all of whom are trained in conventional medicine, support Kirk's conclusion that his peers are "by and large a pretty miserable group."

While functional medicine practitioners argue that medical schools normalize the physical, mental, and emotional burdens of their students—thus making it more difficult for them to demonstrate empathy for their patients moving forward—published research suggests that the illness narratives of providers can be used to teach empathy. DasGupta and Charon (2004), both physician researchers, argue that medical training creates a dichotomy that identifies patients by their bodies and physicians by their minds. As a result, physicians dedicate their time to examining, diagnosing, and treating the bodies of others but are afforded little opportunity to deal with their own illness experiences or those of their loved ones. After administering a reflective writing exercise to second-year medical students and then asking them to evaluate the exercise, DasGupta and Charon conclude that eliciting the personal illness narratives of physicians may counteract the conventional distancing of physicians' minds from their bodies and lead to more empathetic practice. This possibility comes to fruition within the realm of functional medicine.

Having learned through personal experience to identify with patients, wounded healers engage with this empathy to create therapeutic connections. To do so, they are often inspired by ancient healing traditions from around the world. According to functional medicine practitioners, the empathy that many traditional healers show their patients is rooted in their own personal experiences of illness, disease, and suffering. Mark explains, "If you look at most traditional medicines, a lot of shamans and healers went through some health crisis, some trauma, some initiatory element to sort of select them to be healers." As demonstrated by the illness narratives of wounded healers, many functional medicine practitioners have experienced similar "initiatory elements." However, the experience of suffering is not generally regarded by conventional medicine as a resource for creating therapeutic connections.

Functional medicine practitioners aim to intentionally break this pattern by publicly recounting their stories of illness and disease, and by empathizing with patients based on the shared experience of suffering. In his conversation with Cynthia, Mark indicates that he suggests to doctors that they share stories of their experience with suffering with their patients: "Don't have this doctor-patient relationship which is . . . very distant and estranged. Be a human! . . . It builds a relationship that helps them know that you have suffered through it."[10] Functional medicine practitioners have learned that the quality and degree of connectedness in the therapeutic relationship matters because it directly influences patient outcomes. To this end, Anup Kanodia—a conventionally trained doctor who now practices functional medicine and is an Institute for Functional Medicine instructor—says, "When you [use] heart to heart connection . . . you have a ten thousand percent chance of them actually doing something, starting a process, completing it, and recover[ing]."[11] From the perspective of functional medicine practitioners, recounting their health struggles and subsequent chronic-disease reversals to their patients deepens the provider-patient relationship, with positive effects for patient outcomes.

The illness narratives of wounded healers furthermore relocate the locus of functional medicine doctors' authority. Instead of providers exclusively forming relationships with patients based on authoritative knowledge (i.e., their medical training), their role as guide and teacher is largely influenced by their embodied knowledge (i.e., their prior struggles with chronic illness and subsequent recovery). Given that patients also possess embodied knowledge based on their experiences of suffering and their agentive quests for recovery, mutuality of embodied knowledge sets the stage for the relationship between them.

DIALECTICAL RELATIONSHIPS BETWEEN PATIENTS AND FUNCTIONAL MEDICINE PROVIDERS

Both functional medicine providers and their patients experience illness and suffering, and both are on a journey toward greater health. Oftentimes, the healing journeys of patients and functional medicine providers intersect. For some providers, treating patients helps them recognize and acknowledge their own diseases. For example, Cynthia describes a consultation she had with the single mother of three children. The patient was working two jobs and was exhausted. As Cynthia went through the checklist for fatigue, she said to the patient, "Oh my God. You are a textbook case for hypothyroidism. I'm going to run these tests." Then it dawned on Cynthia: "Oh my God, her palpitations, her insomnia, her fatigue, her weight loss, her hair loss. . . . Oh my God, I'm a textbook case too." This moment was impactful for Cynthia because she could, almost literally, see herself in her patient's shoes. This example demonstrates how functional medicine providers identify with their patients and, at times, recognize their own disease symptoms through the act of patient care.

At other times, functional medicine practitioners locate answers for patients through attempts to locate them for themselves. For example, Elizabeth says that those who have experienced cancer or other diseases often ask, "Why would this happen to me?" She indicates that in her case, "I really wanted to ask that question . . . because I didn't want it to happen again, and I wanted to recover from it, and I wanted to help my patients get better." Elizabeth stated her simultaneous desires to recover and to help her patients recover together in the same breath. Rangan likewise describes how his exploration into the existing literature augmented his medical practice since it led him to think, "Well, hold on a minute. If this is going to help my son, maybe it can help my patients." Thus, the process of having "found the answers" for themselves or their loved ones on the path to recovery informs the care functional medicine practitioners provide.

Armed with this knowledge gained through experience, functional medicine interlocutors aim to help patients reproduce the positive results they have achieved and avoid frustration and needless suffering. Returning to the primary illness narratives presented at the beginning of this chapter, both Terry and Amy share their personal stories and healing approaches in best-selling books that are accessibly written for a public audience (Wahls 2014; Myers 2015). Terry's recovery inspired her to prove the effectiveness of her dietary protocol through clinical trials. Having received surgery to remove part of her thyroid, it is too late for Amy to live "with [her] body intact," but she has kept other autoimmune issues at bay and has built a functional medicine practice to prevent other patients from facing the same fate she did. She writes, "About ten years ago I developed an autoimmune condition—and conventional medicine failed me. I don't want it to fail you too" (Myers 2015, 3). Echoing Amy, Sarah explains, "I often say that my main motivation for everything I do now is to help people find the answers they need without having to hit the health lows that I did." Jonathan similarly indicates, "I always have this feeling that I want to go out there, teach, and help others, 'Look, it doesn't have to be this way for you. There are options.'" By anchoring their work in their personal experiences as illness sufferers, functional medicine practitioners create the conditions for a renegotiation of patient-practitioner dynamics.

Scholars have previously argued that the distinction between illness and disease and, furthermore, the patient's recounting of their illness narrative in clinical settings, can (re)configure the patient-practitioner relationship. Kleinman ([1988] 2020) distinguishes illness from disease and in so doing is playing a key role in shifting the focus onto patients' experience of suffering. He describes illness as the lived experience of human suffering. Illness encompasses how the sick person, their family members, and their social network perceive, live with, and respond to symptoms. In contrast, disease privileges the practitioner's perspective. Doctors think of disease as altering biological structures or functioning. This distinction between illness and disease has opened the door to viewing the patient's speech acts as a valuable and important part of treatment. Unfortunately, as Elliot G. Mishler (1984, 104) signals, by distinguishing the "voice of medicine" from the "voice of the lifeworld," the clinical encounter is structured in a way that hinders the patient from relating their illness narrative. The doctor often dominates the interaction. To enable the patient to share their lived experience of suffering, the doctor-patient relationship must be realigned in a way that positions the doctor as an active listener and encourages the patient to speak (Clark and Mishler 1992; Mishler et al. 1989).

Wounded healers offer their own illness narratives to emphasize the importance of actively listening to patients and to foster patient-provider relationships based on mutual experiences of suffering. In contrast to the hierarchical nature of conventional medicine, biosociality in functional medicine emphasizes a horizontal dimension since both patients and providers draw authority from their hero's journey and communicate their experiences through the illness narrative. Both roles are anchored in experiences of patienthood—the difference is how, and in what capacity, individuals interact with other patients after recovery.

The Hero's Journey

The illness narratives I heard while conducting ethnographic research on functional medicine fall into a particular category of narrative: the hero's journey.[12] Since recovery from chronic disease may seem more like an ordinary act than a heroic feat, readers may be wondering why functional medicine interlocutors apply the designation "heroic" to their own narratives. Rose Richards (2008) explains that narrative forms in Western culture train readers—and writers—to expect a story to contain an abstract meaning, such as courage under adversity, heroic triumph, or the making of a guru. Wounded healers set out on journeys toward health when faced with chronic and sometimes even debilitating health issues, eventually triumph over their health adversities, and ultimately earn "guru" status in functional medicine. By putting their narratives in the category of "the hero's journey," functional medicine interlocutors critically assert that healing is a "heroic feat" when seen against the backdrop of a health system designed to manage but not reverse chronic disease.

Meanwhile, by decentering biomedical authority and legitimating embodied knowledge, functional medicine positions patients as the heroes of their own health recovery. Providers refer to patients as heroes in email correspondence and on their websites. For example, Shivan Sarna, a former SIBO sufferer turned SIBO expert and Home Shopping Network TV host, addressed an automated email to me, "Hi SIBO Superhero," referring to my small-intestine bacterial overgrowth. Similarly, a banner appears at the top of the gastroenterologist, author, and talk-show host Dr. Partha Nandi's web page for his book *Ask Dr. Nandi: Five Steps to Becoming Your Own #HealthHero for Longevity, Well-Being, and a Joyful Life* that depicts a woman wearing a cape and punching her fist forward, alongside the words "HEALTH HERO: Take Control of Your Health." Next to the image of the book, the web page reads, "YOU CAN BE A #HEALTHHERO." In each instance, the narrative of "SIBO superheroes" or "health heroes" is woven into the provider's or educator's brand.[13] These examples demonstrate how patients are simultaneously interpellated as both heroes and consumers.

Meanwhile, functional medicine advocates interpellate providers as "health care heroes." James Maskell explains that his first book, *The Evolution of Medicine: Join the Movement to Solve Chronic Disease and Fall Back in Love with Medicine*, "sought to inspire doctors and other health professionals to become the hero of their own journey . . . and start their own 'functional micropractice.'" In contrast, his second book, *The Community Cure: Transforming Health Outcomes Together*, broadens the opportunity to be a health care "hero." Maskell writes, "Heroes could be almost anyone deeply concerned by the current state of health care—from hospital administrators to rogue psychologists to community organizers and everything in between." His words point to the valuable roles functional medicine interlocutors play when performing "inclusive" boundary work to expand the role of medicine.

In sum, biosociality within both patient and provider communities is instantiated by a particular discursive form, namely, illness narratives that are structured around the "hero's journey." While wounded healers emphasize their personal health struggles as practitioners and describe how they stepped outside the biomedical paradigm to heal themselves, functional medicine patients are positioned as "the heroes of their own journeys." In the next chapter, I turn to how functional medicine patients are considered the doctors of the future, thus blurring the distinction between the healer and the healed even further. In the final section of this chapter, I explore how illness narratives are relationally constructed through interaction between the narrator and the listener.

ILLNESS NARRATIVES ARE RELATIONAL

Illness and recovery unfold within webs of human connection (see Menéndez [2002] 2010; Molina 2013). The previous health struggles of family members (i.e., one's "family history") partially explain why an individual has fallen ill, while family support (i.e., "community"[14]) contributes to how they get better. Amy links her struggle with Graves' disease to her family's "healthy" diet during her childhood, her mother's pancreatic cancer, and her father's polymyositis. Terry explains how, when she regained physical functions, she, her wife, and her children were filled with relief and overwhelming joy. Andrea relates her Hashimoto's to both her husband's death and her mother's history of Hashimoto's. By the same token, deeper understandings of human biology are enacted relationally—as demonstrated by how Tom encouraged all his siblings and cousins to test their homocysteine levels. Each of these examples indicates that the way we experience, make sense of, and describe our bodies—and our illness experiences—is refracted through our relationships with others.

Situational factors also greatly contribute to the construction of narratives. In particular, narratives are relationally constructed through interaction between narrator and listener. The narrative that is presented at any given moment is just one of many possible narratives that could arise (see Clark and Mishler 1992). The narrator and listener are both active participants in the creation of an "emplotment" (Mattingly 1994) since they are both seeking to connect separate illness events together into a meaningful whole (see Bruner 1986). In the 2020 edition of *The Illness Narratives*, Kleinman explains that patients, families, and practitioners need to interpret illness together to create a dialectic that enhances the treatment and produces an opportunity for the provider's moral education (3–4).

The following ethnographic anecdotes cast a spotlight on how illness narratives unfold relationally among functional medicine providers.

Naturopath Kara Fitzgerald uses multiple platforms to highlight the illness narratives of her colleagues. For example, Kara wrote in her email newsletter FxMed, *"Dear Colleagues: [Marvin Singh's] evolution from a very traditional, academic gastroenterologist, to integrative gastroenterologist, to a cutting-the-edge personalized lifestyle medicine doctor (folded inside his own healing) is a story I think you'll find interesting." While exchanges among conventional medicine colleagues focus on the "professional" and not the "personal," Kara and her colleagues were interested in how Marvin's personal experience of healing led him to transition from conventional gastroenterology to personalized lifestyle medicine.*

On her podcast FxMed, *Kara commented on a new book written by her colleague Vincent Pedre: "It's written obviously from the perspective of being a physician, and you've got lots of really great patient stories in there that I think people will find inspiring and just really illustrative, but you also have your own story. This book is coming from that place as well." Kara then asked Vincent to explain his personal history with gut issues and how that experience informs his current work as an integrative internist specializing in gut health.*

Another time, Kara asked Chris Kresser to share his illness narrative, revealing, "I know you, like many of us, actually myself included, kind of found [functional medicine] in seeking recovery from an illness." Chris responded, "I got really sick in Indonesia and, very long story short, it led to a decade-long recovery process." Chris explained that over the course of his recovery, he learned that conventional medicine is poorly suited to deal with chronic, complex illness. While all the conventional doctors were genuinely trying to help, they did not possess the necessary tools to help him heal. He continued, "If I was going to get better, I would have to take matters into my own hands." In the process, Chris wrote a book titled Unconventional Medicine: Join the Revolution to Reinvent Healthcare, Reverse Chronic Disease, and Create a Practice You Love *about "taking back your own individual health" through changes in diet, lifestyle, and behavior. Kara observed, "It mirrors my own journey. It's a mission, along with our own healing journey, that's so woven in with everything that you're doing."*

Dave Asprey, founder of Upgrade Labs and best-selling science author, told Mark Hyman his personal history of ill health and how he used "biohacking," the practice of improving one's physiology through science and self-experimentation, to achieve "superhuman" health. Mark responded with his own illness narrative, saying, "Personally, for me, I lived in China and got a huge exposure to mercury. I don't have great genes to detox. It destroyed every system in my body." Mark went on to explain how exposure to mercury destroyed his gut, causing diarrhea, bloating, and pain; damaged his mitochondria, leading to chronic fatigue syndrome; harmed his liver and immune system, resulting in rashes and sores all over his body; and impaired his cognition, impeding his ability to think, concentrate, and even remember where he was. Because of his terrible condition, Mark explained, "I literally had to become an expert in mercury, heavy metals, and detoxification." Dave's sharing his story of how he biohacked his way to health elicited Mark's recounting of how he became an expert to heal himself.

Mark listened to Cynthia's illness narrative about her autoimmunity, her fear of being stigmatized as a "difficult patient," and her being sent for a major psychiatric evaluation when her doctors did not understand the full extent of her health issues. He responded, "I was the same story. . . . I knew, going to specialist after specialist after specialist, that this wasn't in my head. I felt depressed, I felt fatigued, I felt unable to cope and manage, but it wasn't in my head. It was affecting my brain, but it wasn't emotional or psychological." The two doctors exchanged fragments of their illness narratives, thus establishing mutual empathy and working to destigmatize chronic disease.

David Sinclair, a Harvard professor who researches aging, explained his research on mitochondrial dysfunction and restoration to Mark. Mark recounted his story again, to David, this time adding details about mitochondrial dysfunction: "I first became interested in mitochondria because mine stopped working. . . . I went from riding my bike one hundred miles a day to not being able to walk up the stairs." Mark explained to David that, as he learned more about functional medicine and mitochondria, he was able to start treating himself by focusing on nutrition, consuming all the co-factors for proper mitochondrial function, removing the mercury in his body, and, ultimately, upregulating his mitochondrial pathways. While Mark had described other features of his illness experience to Dave and Cynthia, he adapted his narrative to focus on David's particular interest in mitochondria.

Finally, Mark indicated to Todd LePine, his close friend and longtime colleague, "We've all personally had challenges with our health and we've used this model to help recover. I remember when I was really sick, you and Dr. [Elizabeth] Boham came to my house and helped me think through what was going on because my brain wasn't working." Functional medicine colleagues become a part of each other's illness narratives. As friends and companions, they guide each other toward recovery.

While the concept of biosociality (Rabinow 1992) has generally been applied to patients, the illness narratives of wounded healers set the stage for novel types of relationships, thus allowing for a medical anthropological analysis of how biosociality unfolds among functional medicine providers and health educators. Kara is a prime example of someone who encourages her colleagues to share their illness narratives. On her platforms she shares how her colleagues' personal experiences have shaped and transformed their practice of medicine, contributing to a sense of familiarity and community among functional medicine providers and educators whose illness narratives unfold together, interspersed in the same discursive realm.

When interviewing Chris, Kara references his finding functional medicine while seeking recovery from chronic disease. She comments that Chris's path is "like [those of] many of us . . . myself included." These simple statements create a sense of unity. Drawing from the philosopher J. L. Austin, I highlight performative utterances like Kara's (Austin 1962); that is, not only do Kara's words describe reality but also her very utterance of these words changes the social circumstances by creating solidarity. Although Kara uses telecommunication technologies to conduct podcast interviews with functional medicine providers across the United States, describing Chris and herself as both belonging to a larger group of "us" is akin to her reaching across the interview table and telling Chris they are one and the same. Illness narratives collectivize the illness experience, thus exploring the social implications of illness.

These unifying speech acts are common among functional medicine providers. For example, chiropractor and two-time international bestselling author Jay Davidson prompts Elena, saying, "You went through—like we all have—you went through your own stories that got us to where we are at." The grammatical errors in Jay's statement point to the thorough intertwinement of "you" and "us." He comments, "You went through your own" before switching mid-thought to "stories that got us to where we are at." In this sentence, Jay switches between referring to Elena's experience and to that of a community of functional medicine providers a total of four times. It seems that for Jay it is nearly impossible to think about "you" independently of "us." Individual wounded healers are embedded in a social community of others who have suffered through similar experiences and have been transformed in the process, so the illness experience is moved from the private sphere into a social context (Hydén 1997).

Furthermore, the illness narratives of individual wounded healers unfold *in relation* to others' narratives. Mark recounts his illness narrative to various other interlocutors. Each time, he emphasizes different aspects of his experience. For example, after listening to Dave's agentive tales of biohacking, Mark describes how he, too, had to biohack his way to health, stating, "I literally had to become an expert in mercury, heavy metals, and detoxification." When he interviews Cynthia, he shares details of his personal experience that validated her fear of being stigmatized by her doctors, indicating that he, too, was shuttled from specialist to specialist, and he says that his case was also not just in his head. Mark and Cynthia connect on the physiological basis of their disease and the experience of having their symptoms dismissed as "supratentorial." During his interview with David, Mark tells his illness narrative vis-à-vis David's research on mitochondria, thus demonstrating his support for David's work by emphasizing how extremely valuable it is for patient care. While Mark delivers multiple iterations of his illness narrative to build connections with the colleagues he interviews, his final telling with Todd indicates how friendships with colleagues are folded into his narrative and, ultimately, his healing journey. These adjustments to his narrative reveal how the stories of wounded healers constitute the basis of biosociality among functional medicine providers and educators; that is, illness narratives are adapted to increase connection between the narrator and the listener. The narrative serves as a strategic device used to achieve certain effects in the social interaction (Hydén 1997).

In essence, my research on wounded healers revealed how illness narratives have emerged as a key discursive form in functional medicine and how the exchange of these narratives undergirds biosociality among functional medicine providers and between these providers and their patients. Bonds among functional medicine practitioners are forged, maintained, and deepened through the relational construction of illness narratives. Furthermore, illness narratives—and specifically, those of the hero's journey—emphasize threads of mutual experience that tether patient-provider relationships along a horizontal plane. In chapter 3, I build upon the themes in this chapter by detailing relational shifts underway in functional medicine—particularly the (re)negotiation of authority in patient-provider relationships.

Interlude

TAKING THE REINS

To provide the reader with access to my lived experience, and with the intent of demonstrating relational shifts in action, I have decided to share my email correspondence with two practitioners on my functional medicine team. Given the digital autoethnographic nature of this book, these emails are a source of raw ethnographic data. My goal is to both *demonstrate* and *describe* the phenomena I have observed as an ethnographer and participated in as a patient. In so doing, I hope to render visible the process of participant observation that informs this book. I then submit these emails to the same critical analysis I apply to all the discourse in this ethnographic study.

Subject: Request and update
Monday, January 6, 2020, 5:00 p.m.

Hi, Janet and Jolene,

I am writing with a request and an update.

Request

I received a message from Genova indicating you have my NutrEval test results. I am unable to access them at this time. Can you send me a copy so I can review the results before our meeting?

Update

I've learned a lot about what is going on in my own body since my last update.

At different points since October, I have taken a few supplements that had negative or mixed effects:
—soy lecithin (highly estrogenic).

—NAD+ (this supplement helped me break my dependency on D-Ribose, and I'm glad I took it—but the specific formula I took is combined with quercetin, which is a COMT inhibitor).
—DIM-Evail and Estrofactors (when taken together, I was surpassing the dose where DIM helps clear estrogen. At higher doses, DIM has estrogenic effects).
—GABA supplement, Mitocore, and Estrofactors (all contain EGCG/green tea extract, which is a COMT inhibitor).

Also, while traveling, the number one methylation adaptogen I had accessible to me was green or black tea. The number one "dessert" that is allowed by MDL was dark chocolate . . . again, COMT inhibitors.

My interpretation of my Comprehensive Hormone Profile is that my "estrogen" levels (E1, E2, E3) are normal. However, they get stuck as Phase 1 metabolites since I have thus far been a poor methylator and have had a limited ability to detox estrogen. Although my body has normal estrogen, an overabundance of Phase 1 metabolites nonetheless leads to a highly estrogenic environment.

I've been focusing on removing the problematic ingredients in my supplements and also avoiding foods that are estrogenic (soy) and high histamine. I have noticed supplements have a much greater effect than diet—therefore, in the long run, I think I can afford a bit of leeway with histamine in my diet after I've sorted out the supplement situation. Nonetheless, I plan to stay aware of histamines in food and choose to limit them, especially around ovulation and pre-menstruation.

Now that I've untangled this problem, I am feeling a lot better and am having a lot fewer allergic symptoms. I will be ready to rechallenge some foods soon, and I expect to get a clearer signal this time.

Hope you had a wonderful Christmas and a Happy New Year!

Looking forward to speaking to you both,

Rosalynn

When reading emails I sent to my providers, you will immediately notice that I address my providers using their first names.[1] I did this with all my providers—physicians and nutritionists alike—regardless of their professional degree or "rank" on the team. The decision to address my providers in this way was intentional. I wanted to be on an even footing with each of my providers, so, from our very first meeting, I chose to address them in a way that would foster horizontal, rather than hierarchical, relationships.

By asking for my NutrEval results (a blood and urine profile that tests for over 125 biomarkers to evaluate a patient's nutritional status) ahead of our meeting, I positioned myself to evaluate the results alongside the practitioners on my team. In essence, I emphasized my vital role on the functional medicine team. In contrast, in the conventional model, patients often walk into the doctor's consultation room empty-handed. It is up to the doctor to explain the results to the patient. This unequal access to the patient's health information sets up a dynamic in which the doctor is the sole authority. It takes away patients' agency and positions them as passive recipients of doctors' expert knowledge.

As a medical anthropologist, I readily acknowledge that medical professionals possess more training in medicine than I do, but I also recognize that I am the greatest expert when it comes to living inside my body, day in and day out. From this standpoint, I gave my providers my interpretation of my comprehensive hormone profile results, and I also explained what I believed to be the underlying etiology of my symptoms. I implemented changes based on my experiences of being in my body, and I indicated the expected outcomes of these changes. Lastly, after describing how I "untangled this problem," I provided a long-term prognosis.

Instead of being put off by my assertive explanations, my providers thanked me for all the valuable information I had provided in the update. They forwarded my NutrEval results for my perusal. After reviewing my NutrEval results, Janet sent me this email:

> Subject: NEW! Test results
> Wednesday, January 8, 2020, 4:26 p.m.
>
> I'm reviewing your NutrEval and have some thoughts for Friday that we'll talk about. I see we have only 30 minutes scheduled so we'll dive right in but definitely won't be able to cover it all. . . . Can you give me your top priorities for our call on Friday? I want to cover those plus my thoughts for next steps.
>
> Thanks for being such an awesome client. You are truly fun to work with!
>
> Janet

With this email, Janet set up a balanced dynamic for our upcoming visit. The thirty-minute visit—considered to be a short follow-up by functional medicine's standards—was to be inclusive of both of our priorities and thoughts. (In actuality, the visit ran over, lasting forty-five minutes). Janet thanked me for being an "awesome client." Here, the word choice of "client" instead of "patient" is indicative. Functional medicine interlocutors suggest that in the conventional medicine model, the role of "patient" is largely inoperative—lacking agency. "Patients" receive "doctor's orders," and if they are not obedient, they are labeled "noncompliant." On the other hand, "clients" are agentive actors. Currently, virtually no functional medicine services are covered by health insurance. They fall into the private sector and are purchased out of pocket by the "client." The "client" pays for the practitioner's services, and the client's role in this economic exchange situates the client in a position of agency.

Janet concluded her email by saying, "You are truly fun to work with!" With this statement she is again establishing a dynamic of equality—especially the preposition "with." If she had said I was fun to "work on" or "work for," these statements would signal disparate dynamics of hierarchical power. By selecting the preposition "with," Janet was again opening up a space for my agentive participation in the relationship.

I needed to decide how to prioritize our time for our upcoming visit, so, to organize my thoughts, I created a three-column table. In the left column was a list of lab markers. In the middle column, I provided information regarding my current approach—the lifestyle changes, supplements, and diet I had already implemented in an effort to produce optimal results for the corresponding lab marker. In the right column, I typed in my plans for adjusting my personal protocol based on the NutrEval results, or, when I was unsure, I posed some potential adjustments and welcomed Janet and Jolene's feedback. To prepare this table, I independently reviewed my lab results, considered individual lab markers in the context of what I was already doing for myself, planned adjustments to my personal protocol, and identified proposed changes that required Janet and Jolene's second and third opinions.

Preparing for our upcoming visit in this way was productive in multiple ways. Between when the NutrEval lab test was conducted and when the results were reported, I decided to introduce a new supplement into my regimen. While I informed my providers of the change, they might not have been as aware as I was regarding how this new supplement overlapped with others I was taking or how it shifted my daily intake of certain nutrients.

After all, as the client, I had physical access to all my supplement bottles and could easily compare labels side by side. In contrast, my providers do not have the same quick access to the ingredient lists and nutritional values for each of my supplements. Thus, as my own functional medicine provider, I self-recommended adjustments to how I was dosing nutrients to bring me squarely within the optimal range. As a patient-self-advocate, I simultaneously indicated my concern when the lab's suggested supplementation placed me at the upper limits of what is considered safe for a particular nutrient. (On a different occasion, my query about a nutrient's upper limit prompted my functional medicine provider to search for published studies on PubMed. He then shared links to these studies with me, thus engaging me as a scientist and positioning himself as a guide.)

I decided that, since I was already obtaining significant amounts of particular nutrients, nutrient deficiencies identified in the lab results were suggestive of poor nutrient absorption. In line with the philosophy of many functional medicine practitioners,[2] if a certain method does not produce the desired result, instead of increasing the dose or using additional force, it is likely more productive to change the format or delivery system. I furthermore identified supplements that could potentially have a two-for-one effect, thus improving biomarkers in multiple areas while also working toward my goal of minimizing the number of supplements in my regimen.

I also offered additional context the lab test did not take into consideration, including details of my health history that potentially counterbalanced the lab's recommendations. In certain cases, I indicated how following the lab's recommendations regarding increased supplementation or further changes to my diet could exacerbate a different health problem. I also cross-referenced the results for specific biomarkers with the results of other recent lab tests, uncovering potential inconsistencies and providing more data when determining the degree of action needed.

Having done all this legwork, I replied to Janet's email regarding my priorities for the visit, copying Jolene:

> Hi, Janet,
>
> Since we will have too much to talk about and not enough time, I want to prioritize my easy questions first (questions where basically I am hoping for a "yea" or "nay" from you). I've highlighted these in green. Other questions involve more discussion (yellow) or require a detailed explanation (red). By prioritizing the green, we can feel very accomplished in a short amount of time, instead of feeling like after

our visit we only got around to the first of several red questions. If we have time, we can move on to yellow. How does that sound?

I am very much looking forward to hearing your thoughts on next steps. I'm sure they will provide me with a clearer direction.

You ladies are the best, and I truly appreciate having you on my team!

Abrazos,
Rosalynn

With my email response, I positioned myself as an active, participatory learner and Janet and Jolene as my health educators. By stating in my email the green items required a simple "yea" or "nay," I indicated I already had in mind a specific plan. By stating the yellow items required more discussion, I indicated there were multiple issues to consider and the topic was up for debate. I would not have sought out their recommendations, and paid out of pocket for their time, if I did not value their training. I was not an expert in their field. At the same time, I was the person with the ultimate decision-making power since I was the one who was responsible for implementing my personalized protocol. From this position, I provided Janet and Jolene with a template for how I wanted to structure our time during the video conference.

In the email, I also highlighted my need for more health education regarding other nutrients and metabolites. By placing certain items in red and indicating these required a more thorough explanation, I readily acknowledged the limits of my knowledge. I asked Janet and Jolene to "please talk me through" several biomarkers on the lab results with which I was unfamiliar. Some of these reflected functional medicine's expertise in metabolomics, which I had never come across when studying medicine or the health sciences. I indicated that listening to their thoughts would provide me with a clearer direction. In so doing, I was still positioning myself as the primary actor but was also acknowledging my need for further guidance.

I concluded the email by expressing my appreciation for having Janet and Jolene "on my team." My choice of the word "team" is operative in the same way as Janet's word choice when she referred to me as her "client." In place of the top-down structure of biomedical authority that has been extensively critiqued by medical anthropologists (see Jordan 1992; Browner and Press 1996; Lock, Kaufert, and Harwood 1998), I was establishing a network of horizontal relationships—a team—within which I was an active participant and leader.

The video conferencing session flew by as we crammed numerous items into a "short" forty-five-minute session—an impossible length of time if we had been subject to the standards of health insurance. After the session was over, Janet sent me an email with notes from our visit, including her recommendations. I responded by providing further context, questions for clarification, and my opinions. For the sake of brevity, I will include only a few here. Janet's recommendations are in boldface and my responses are in regular type.

- **The DIM and Curcumin are dosing/brand recommendations to replace your current one.** I will first finish off what I have on hand.
- **I'd also like to discuss how you feel about some "supplement vacations" every few weeks for a few days/week as well.** I have a few thoughts about this. I would first like to continue dwindling down my supplement list to the ones I truly need. I think, given my relatively lengthy supplement regimen, if I were to have symptoms during a "supplement vacation," I wouldn't know [to which] lack of supplement(s) . . . to attribute them. Also, there are some supplements I feel fine pulsing/pausing (e.g., polypodium extract) and others I feel should be ongoing (the cruciferous blend, for example).

I also included a few points that were not direct responses to the content in her email but were addressing items she included as attachments.

- Other notes: goal #1 seems to have been "achieved" since my last two ANA tests were negative, and my recent EBV PCR was also negative.
- Re: Moving toward Wahls Level 2: I can do anything for 6–8 weeks. However, I would not be willing to do this long-term since it eliminates a lot of my ancestral diets and makes it harder to enjoy the social aspect of eating, like going out to eat and sharing dinner with Rikin.

I responded to Janet's recommendations regarding brand changes for particular supplements by indicating that I accepted her recommendations but I was deferring the changes until after I had finished the remaining supplements I had on hand. During one of our video conferencing sessions, I explained to both Janet and Jolene that, as someone who grew up in an immigrant household, I value non-wastefulness and would rather switch to something different after using up what I have instead of switching immediately and throwing away the "excess." In this way, my personal values were woven into our interactions as legitimate considerations. For her part, Janet gave my personal preferences priority when she wrote, "I'd also like to discuss how you feel about some 'supplement vacations.'"

This focus on what is important to me continued when I signaled that the goals of our therapeutic relationship were changing as I improved and as we "achieved" parts of what we set out to do—at the time, I had recently received my second negative result for antinuclear antibodies (a marker of autoimmunity) and my first negative Epstein-Barr polymerase chain-reaction result (a measure of how many copies of viral DNA are in the blood). During our video conference, I mentioned my goal was now turning to balancing my female and thyroid hormones and preparing for conception.

Finally, Janet had mentioned during the video conference that in the future we might consider transitioning me to a Wahls Level 2 diet. I was already on Level 1 of the Wahls diet—a diet developed by, and named after, Dr. Terry Wahls. The shift to Level 2 meant the additional elimination of grains and legumes. I responded to this suggestion by indicating my willingness to give it a try but also emphasizing what is important to me as a whole person—specifically, social aspects of eating. As a person of mixed Chinese and Mexican heritage, rice, beans, and corn are staples of my cultural cuisines. My husband, Rikin, had recently agreed to eat less processed food as we both prepared for conception, and he was venturing into my diet of mostly plants, some lean protein, and healthy fats. The proposed removal of grains and legumes would make it more difficult for us to share meals, so I raised this issue with Janet.

A few weeks later, I decided to discontinue a number of supplements I considered were interacting poorly with my genome—specifically, the COMT gene. Among these supplements was SAMe—a supplement that donates methyl groups to aid in the degradation of catechols by COMT. Janet and Jolene took turns leading video conferences, and my follow-up to this was led by Jolene. Jolene wondered why I would discontinue a supplement that is geared toward addressing the problem I identified. After another video conferencing session, Jolene sent me follow-up notes and questions, to which I responded the next day in a reply email. I reproduce excerpts from that email exchange here, with Jolene's in italics and the author's comments shown as inline replies.

Subject: Nutrition Session Follow-up
Thursday, February 6, 2020, 7:11 p.m.

Hi Rosalynn,

It was great to connect with you today. Janet and I continue to appreciate being part of your health journey and seeing the amazing work you are doing.

I wanted to follow up with [an additional question] and a recap of our session.

Hi, Jolene,

Thank you so much for your follow-up email!

Can you please clarify your reasoning behind removing the SAMe supplement?

One of Dr. Fitzgerald's episodes of *FxMed* addressed potential problems with supplementing SAMe, especially on an ongoing basis. What I took away from that episode was it may be better to focus on providing the co-factors of methylation through diet than directly providing methyl donors by supplementing with SAMe. This is also emphasized by Ben Lynch in *Dirty Genes*. Overmethylation can also be a problem. (And in other cases, as indicated by Andrew Heyman, focusing solely on methylation won't fix the problem because there are underlying issues with mitochondria.)

In my particular case, I had already been taking SAMe 400 mg for six months at the time the Meridian Labs Comprehensive Hormone Profile (Dried Urine) was done (May-October 2019). That lab result showed very high Phase 1 estrogen metabolites and abysmal methylation. Then, in my December 2019 NutrEval, my methylation was great! I was still taking SAMe at 400 mg, but what changed was my diet. This led me to think that I might be better off continuing to dial in on B vitamins, methionine, magnesium, selenium, etc. to support COMT than simply taking more SAMe.

With all that said, I am not opposed to reintroducing SAMe. I stopped SAMe as an experiment to see how I would feel. In the following weeks after I stopped taking SAMe, I had fewer symptoms, but this could also be due to my stopping a number of COMT inhibitors.

However, I do want to point out I didn't suddenly feel worse without SAMe.

Please weigh in on this. I can easily reintroduce SAMe if that is what you recommend.

You're doing such an amazing job with your nutrition and lifestyle—keep up the great work!

Couldn't do it without you! :)

Thank you and look forward to hearing from you.

Sincerely,
Jolene

Saludos y abrazos,
Rosalynn

This email exchange exhibits continuity in the quality of my interactions with my providers, especially in relation to power and authority. I responded to Jolene's questions as an educated client and provided expert knowledge about the phenomenological experience of being in my body. In her email, Jolene acknowledged that through my "amazing work" instituting changes to my diet and lifestyle, I was primarily responsible for my "health journey" and the chronic-disease reversal I was experiencing. In my email response, I also attributed my steady progress to having Jolene and Janet's support. I continued to seek their opinions and expressed my readiness to accept their future recommendations. The email thread concluded with the same mutual recognition, friendliness, and familiarity. Jolene replied:

Hi Rosalynn,

Thanks for your response. Janet and I have reviewed your email together.

Thanks for the additional explanation with your experience with COMT. We will continue to be mindful with the support you need around this and monitoring symptoms and progress.

Regarding SAMe supplementation, your rationale makes sense. We can test your SAMe level in the future if you'd like.

Sincerely,
Jolene

By valuing my explanations regarding the COMT gene, Jolene and Janet acknowledged my experiential knowledge as valid. They placed themselves in a supportive role and assured me they would be mindful regarding what I had identified as my unique needs. Finally, even though my decision to discontinue supplementation of SAMe was against their initial recommendation and common understandings of how COMT works, they acknowledged that my rationale made sense in my case.

In the next chapter, I turn to functional medicine interlocutors' arguments that patient-led interactions in functional medicine represent a sharp departure from authoritative provider-patient relationships in conventional medicine. These interlocutors suggest that functional medicine reconfigures the roles of patient and provider by casting the patients as the primary protagonists of their own recovery. In this interlude, I have offered raw ethnographic data to demonstrate how relational shifts in functional medicine are redefining the locus of authority, power, and control in the therapeutic relationship. In the next chapter, however, I turn to the larger socioeconomic context within which these shifts unfold and critically examine how functional medicine can sometimes fail to achieve its goals. Who does functional medicine "empower"? Who is excluded, even as functional medicine aims to place the patient in the position of authority?

CHAPTER 3
RELATIONAL SHIFTS

Proponents argue that functional medicine liberates the patient from biomedical authority by valuing the patient's embodied knowledge as authoritative knowledge and positioning the provider as a guide or coach instead of an authority figure. However, my ethnographic research reveals two intersecting problems with this. First, functional medicine encourages patient engagement with wearable technology, suggesting that these devices place valuable insights in the hands of users, who are empowered to turn personalized data into actionable knowledge. But the practice of quantifying the Self renders individuals susceptible to "dataveillance" (Degli-Esposti 2014) and can sometimes reinforce existing power inequalities between patient and provider in unexpected ways. Second, while functional medicine may destabilize existing notions of the patient-provider relationship, it does so through a neoliberal modality of consumption that excludes most and "empowers" privileged "clients." I situate this consumption vis-à-vis the existing literature on the bioeconomy, emphasizing that instead of biomatter, what is for sale in the functional medicine realm is personalized health knowledge. Ultimately, the framing of health as a "choice" and as a "skill set" naturalizes well-being among the wealthy, obscures its socioeconomic underpinnings, and contributes to a recovery meritocracy. In this chapter I interrogate the underlying causes and outcomes of relational shifts that are underway in functional medicine.

POSITIONING PATIENTS AS THE DOCTORS OF THE FUTURE?

Functional medicine proponents suggest that their model displaces the physician as the primary actor in the doctor-patient relationship. For example, Dr. David Brady, a licensed naturopathic doctor and nutritionist with over twenty-five years in health sciences academia, says the key to recovery from chronic disease is not an "omnipotent healer" who provides "some magic pill or some magic fix." Dr. Nalini Chilkov, a doctor of Oriental medicine who specializes in healing cancer, similarly asserts that American patients have been socialized—and misled—into believing that the doctor possesses "a bottle with a solution for us, or a procedure that will fix us." Functional medicine practitioners like physician and sleep specialist Dr. Kirk Robert Parsley contrast conventional medicine, which "consider[s] the gatekeepers of health to be the healthcare providers," with functional medicine, in which, as entrepreneur and functional medicine advocate James Maskell explains, "the patient is participating in their own lifestyle choices and is the most important person in the medical relationship." From a functional medicine perspective, the best kind of provider will foster a true relationship with patients, help patients shift paradigms, and reconfigure their own role as physician to give proactive, health-seeking patients the knowledge and tools they need to take care of their own health.

From a functional medicine perspective, the disruptive potential of functional medicine relies on the agentive participation of individual patients for its fruition since true "preventive medicine" can only be implemented by individuals in their everyday environments, before they ever need intervention from a clinician. Dr. Cynthia Li, a conventionally trained doctor turned functional medicine specialist, indicates, "You don't need a doctor's prescription for health. What you need to do is to make [healthy habits] a part of your life in a natural way." Many functional medicine advocates aim to take health care from hospitals and put it back into people's homes.

Thus, functional medicine providers attempt to cast patients as the heroes of their own healing journeys. Maskell explains, "Helping a patient to feel like the hero of their own journey is actually the best leverage point for creating health." This is accomplished in multiple ways. He elaborates, "[Providers] have to educate patients that there is a different way of doing [medicine] that honors a participatory approach." In this vein, naturopath Dr. Kara Fitzgerald's first general office policy reads, "You are encouraged to ask questions on any health-related topic and to take an active role in your health care." In functional medicine, the patient's outcomes are dependent on their adopting this participatory role since it is up to the patient to implement lifestyle changes that will promote healing.

Functional medicine proponents go as far as to recharacterize patients as their own doctors. In naturopathic physician Dr. Sarah Myhill's words, "People will get better results if they take their health into their own hands because your best doctor is yourself." Sachin Patel, who coaches practitioners on how to create a successful functional medicine practice, similarly sums up the issue, "The patient is the doctor of the future." By positioning the patient as the "doctor," functional medicine proponents propose a thorough reconfiguration of both patient and provider roles in the therapeutic relationship.

This proposal is rooted in functional medicine's critique of how the current conventional medical model conditions patients to relinquish their power and authority. Alex Howard, host of the Fatigue Super Conference, an online conference of experts speaking on causes of and solutions to fatigue, explains, "We have a cultural relationship to the medical establishment. People tend to feel that the power all lies [with the doctor]. It's almost a kind of parent-child relationship." Misty Williams, a patient advocate and health educator, writes to patients from the perspective of a fellow patient in her email newsletter, saying, for example, "We are conditioned in our society to give our power away constantly." Chris Kresser, a health coach and licensed acupuncturist, similarly indicates, "We've been trained to be passive recipients of health care—which in this country is primarily medication, and sometimes surgery." Howard expands by saying that even when the doctor's advice contradicts "everything the patient's instinct is telling them," the patient feels obligated to follow the doctor's orders because, if they do not, it may seem they are not trying to get better. These functional medicine proponents argue that, given decades of inculcation, patients must be retrained. At the same time, one might ask to what degree functional medicine providers are in fact unseating existing power inequalities when they position themselves as the ones to "retrain" patients.

Nonetheless, the arguments presented by functional medicine proponents (unwittingly) reiterate the anthropological concept of "authoritative knowledge." Brigitte Jordan (1992) describes how, given the hierarchical nature of provider-patient interactions in conventional medicine, only the provider has access to authoritative knowledge. Jordan then contrasts authoritative knowledge with "embodied knowledge"—the patient's lived experience. While only the patient has access to the experience of illness, doctors often dismiss this knowledge. From the perspective of both medical anthropology and functional medicine, conventional medical consultations are often characterized by unilateral power and authority instead of bilateral exchange.

In this context, functional medicine interlocutors argue that patients must resist what Dr. Joel Fuhrman, a board-certified family physician and director of research for the Nutritional Research Foundation, calls "bullying" by medical authority figures: "Medical doctors tell them what to do and they think they have to listen to somebody instead of them being their own best advocate and reading, and learning, and making the best choices for their life." Dr. Chilkov similarly opines that a true healing relationship is not characterized by the provider signaling to the patient, "I'm the authority, I tell you, and I have the answers." When patients encounter authoritative providers, Howard notes, "It actually takes a significant amount of courage within patients to self-advocate and stand up for what instinctively they know to be true for them." Williams likewise uses the word "courage" to describe the process of seizing back power through self-advocacy and decision making. In making these arguments, functional medicine proponents characterize themselves as working to destabilize the provider's authoritative knowledge by legitimating embodied knowledge.

This recharacterization of authority, power, and control in the therapeutic relationship returns us to functional medicine's emphasis on the body's capacity to heal. Neonatologist Dr. Mary Newport muses, "I think people give away their power, instead of grasping hold of it and really embracing it. They give away their authority to doctors, instead of relying on the fact that we are all born with the ability to heal." During a conversation with health coach and fatigue specialist Ari Whitten, Maskell notes that patients must undergo a fundamental mindset transformation from thinking a doctor is going to "fix" them to believing they are going to heal themselves with the doctor's guidance. Whitten agrees, emphasizing the critical conceptual shift from locating the power to heal as existing "out there," in the practitioner or in the pharmaceutical, to locating it within the individuals themselves, who all possess the capacity to heal. Taken together, the assertions of these interlocutors emphasize functional medicine's vitalistic approach.

Functional medicine practitioners aim to develop a partnership with their patients and to equip patients to create lasting wellness in their lives. Dr. Brady describes providers as guides to emotional, behavioral, and spiritual change, noting, "We are really on a journey with [our patients]." Dr. Vincent Pedre, a board-certified internist and medical director of Pedre Integrative Health, extends the analogy, saying, "It's like you're taking the patient by the hand and, together, you're walking a journey. You know what the destination needs to be, but you have to help them get there." Functional medicine interlocutors' descriptions of the therapeutic relationship this way emphasize that while patients take on the primary, agentive role in the relationship, providers adopt a valuable supporting role as teacher and guide.

From this perspective, teaching patients in a hands-on way regarding lifestyle changes to improve health will be the most valuable part of physicians' role in the new paradigm. Dr. Brady comments that he likes the model of health coaching "because it really automatically implies that expectation that the patient is going to be actively involved." Internist, endocrinologist, and microbiome expert Dr. Zach Bush's website indicates, "Our phone-based, 45-minute intrinsic Health Coaching sessions are among the most effective parts of Dr. Zach's paradigm-shifting health and wellness protocols." Dr. Mark Hyman concurs when he describes the future of medicine, saying, "I think doctors are going to be more educators. Doctors are going to be less important to the actual delivery of care." This new role ironically goes back to the Latin root of doctor—*docere*—which means "one who teaches" (Prescott and Logan 2017, 33).

This transition away from delivery of care and toward health education is underway and has required some functional medicine practitioners—especially those trained in the conventional medical paradigm—to step outside of their wheelhouse and develop new expertise. Dr. Ayesha Sherzai and Dr. Dean Sherzai—married neuroscientists, best-selling authors, and hosts of the podcast *Brain Health Revolution*—contend that their colleagues must become more comfortable with the role of health educator. Dean Sherzai jokingly used himself and his wife as examples. He laughed, "We have more degrees than a thermostat." Then he admitted that despite all their collective education, they feel uncomfortable going onto a podcast and giving advice about what snacks people should eat—even though this type of practical lifestyle guidance is far more impactful than whatever they do in a clinic.

Many functional medicine practitioners consider self-advocacy to be one of the most practical skills they can teach patients. Thus, these practitioners both advocate for patients and help patients to be more effective when advocating for themselves. Turning to the example of cancer patients, Dr. Chilkov explains that these patients need a functional provider who can help with their decision-making process—a significantly different role than that of the oncologist, who "typically just gives orders." She continues, "I think it's important for the cancer patient, especially at diagnosis and [during the] decision-making process . . . to have someone help you be educated and understand how to make a good decision for yourself." In her view, "An educated patient can lobby for individualized care if they know what to ask for." Within the functional medicine paradigm, educated patients, especially those who have partnered with a physician who lobbies for their interests, are able to obtain a wider array of choices for their care.

In this model, doctors' supporting role involves reassuring patients so they have the confidence to actively engage in their own healing. This, in turn, requires providers to reframe the meanings of chronic disease. Dr. Brady describes what he often tells patients, beginning with, "Listen, you are not alone in this." He then goes on to explain that their chronic-disease diagnosis is very prevalent and is quickly becoming even more prevalent. He furthermore explains that while the patient may have a strong family history of this disease, the patient does not need to succumb to what may seem to be their genetic fate because, unlike their older relatives, they are being equipped with tools that will help them change the outcome. He tells his patients, "We'll work with you. You might have to change a little bit about the way you eat, about the amount of stress you are under, about various things in your life, but these are good things anyway." He emphasizes that by making these changes, the patient will be a healthier person in the long run, with benefits extending far beyond the reversal of their specific chronic disease. That is, the positive outcomes of lifestyle medicine are not restricted to the reversal of chronic disease; rather, chronic-disease reversal is part and parcel of overall health and a long, vibrant life.

According to functional medicine proponents, communicative approaches like Dr. Brady's are integral to achieving positive health outcomes. Physician and BBC star Dr. Rangan Chatterjee explains that to inspire families to change their lifestyle habits, the provider must reframe health using language that is understandable and meaningful to them. Dr. Chatterjee goes on to argue that poor outcomes are generally not due to patients being "noncompliant" but, rather, to the doctor's poor communication. He notes, "So many of my colleagues say, 'Our patients don't listen to us.' I just don't buy it." In his view, the doctor's most valuable skill is being able to communicate with the patient. Similarly, Dr. Brady asserts that what makes a good health care provider is being able to communicate to patients that "you are in their camp. You are their advocate. You are not judging them. You are not there to scold them if they don't do perfectly." From a functional medicine perspective, the provider's ability to communicate and connect with patients is fundamental to helping patients heal. In essence, what both Dr. Brady and Dr. Chatterjee are arguing for is the prioritization of "the art of medicine" over medicine as a "technical endeavor."

Having explored how functional medicine interlocutors characterize relational shifts underway in functional medicine, I now turn to what they identify as powerful tools for empowering proactive, health-seeking patients: wearable devices and personalized health-data apps.

QUANTIFICATION OF THE SELF

Functional medicine is intimately attuned to advances in informatics emerging from the world of technology. The initial conversations that inspired the birth of functional medicine in the early 1990s included about thirty-five thought leaders who acknowledged the role of computational techniques for managing large data sets on individuals' systems biology. Among these individuals was Wayne Matson, a systems biologist and analytical chemist at MIT. According to Dr. Jeffrey Bland, a biochemical and nutrition researcher and a functional medicine innovator, "[Matson] was very good in understanding some of the new statistical modeling that was being done with informatics that was taking us into new things like dendritic analysis, cluster analysis, and complex data set analysis." Commenting on the contemporary moment, Dr. Fitzgerald emphasizes, "We're having the emergence of all these new tools . . . to analyze this massive data." Advances in computational data analysis continue to shape and define functional medicine.

Functional medicine practitioners describe how "disruptive technologies" unfolding outside of the health care system stand to reconfigure how health is sought by individuals and supported by health professionals. For example, Dr. Hyman characterizes online health-coaching platforms as "delivering health care outside of the healthcare system" and indicates that this form of disruption is "happening on a massive scale." From this perspective, if the health care system does not keep up with swift advances in the technological milieu, it will be left in the Dark Ages.

According to functional medicine proponents, self-tracking devices are among the most useful and transformative technological innovations. In basic terms, self-tracking is the monitoring, measuring, and recording of elements of an individual's actions and bodily functions. Some individuals engage in self-tracking for the sake of curiosity, while others aim to use self-tracking to improve their health, physical fitness, emotional well-being, work productivity, or social relationships.

More and more, these wearable devices are ending up in the hands—or on the wrists, fingers, ears, or ankles—of consumers. One example is the Fitbit—a watch-like device that measures data such as heart rate, quality of sleep, number of steps walked or climbed, and other health- and fitness-related data; this product was one of the first personal-data devices on the market and is still being sold. As consumers are increasingly targeted by marketing campaigns for products designed to provide greater insight into their individual biologies, wearable technologies that were nearly unthinkable for the average consumer in the early 2000s have exploded into a booming industry.

At this point self-tracking technologies have extended far beyond wearable devices. The Bloom Health app uses urine sticks and camera phones to gauge fifteen health metrics, including levels of vitamins, minerals, and other essential nutrients. Using this app, bioconsumers can keep track of their health data over time, while making adjustments according to Bloom Health's personalized food and supplement recommendations. Similarly, by combining genetic-profile data with serum laboratory results, Rootine offers "100% Custom Vitamins" for three dollars a day. Another company, Viome, sells kits consumers can use to collect a stool specimen at home and mail it in to the lab to receive microbiome data and suggestions regarding foods to eat, minimize, or avoid either via the company's internet portal or using its smartphone app. Other examples include EverlyWell, which uses Facebook to advertise its at-home lab test that detects sensitivities to ninety-six different foods. The advertisement depicts an image of a young woman smiling down on the test kit in her hands while standing in her kitchen. The caption reads, "No waiting rooms, just answers!" Likewise, fans of the hit ABC show *The Bachelor* are exposed to disruptive technologies: past contestants on the show have accepted sponsorships to promote at-home kits for testing Anti-Mullerian Hormone, a marker of ovarian reserve and a predictor of (in)fertility, and for canine DNA tests to determine a dog's breed and screen for genetic health conditions. This last example demonstrates that consumerism relating to biological technology, services, and information extends to the family pet. Mass marketing of these self-tracking technologies has extended to every corner of the mediascape (Appadurai 1996) and to every aspect of life.

The rise of self-tracking technologies has coincided with the monetization of individualized biological data. However, Dr. Molly Maloof, a health-optimization physician and Stanford University lecturer, foresees that, in the future, value will shift from the data itself to its interpretation. While direct-to-consumer lab tests are readily available to bioconsumers, their price confers access only to the lab report of results; it does not include an interpretation of those results by a health care professional. According to Dr. Maloof, direct-to-consumer lab testing will soon be marketed in a way that monetizes interpretation, not results: "I believe that someone is going to come along and create a lab testing company that is going to be operating at cost, and someone is going to be building apps on top of that data." If her prediction comes true, the interpretation of data will be monetized and sold. Instead of profiting from the test itself, companies will shift to profiting from apps that position the user as a complex data set and a study of $n = 1$ (potentially with the use of artificial intelligence).[1]

The monetization of individualized data is just one of the many implications of digitized self-tracking. The ubiquitous nature of self-tracking has led some social scientists to begin to theorize about the effects of the Quantified Self—how numbers are used to monitor and measure elements of everyday life and, more broadly, practices that have gained momentum in our contemporary era of mobile and wearable digital devices and sensor-saturated physical environments. Minna Ruckenstein and Mika Pantzar (2017) suggest that by defining a new numerical self and promoting a dataist paradigm, popular media representations of the Quantified Self push us to rethink life in a data-driven manner. Ultimately, Ruckenstein and Pantzar detect the merging of epistemological claims, technological devices, and market-making efforts.

Sociologist Deborah Lupton (2014) explores the influences, power relations, and systems of thought that contribute to self-tracking, the ways in which self-tracking is spreading from private to social realms, and the implications of self-tracking for the politics of personal data, or "lively data." Lupton's notion of "lively data" stems from Mike Savage's (2013) use of the term and Dave Beer and Roger Burrows's (2013) work on the circulation and politics of digital data. Lupton contends, "Not only are personal digital data continually generated, as Savage emphasizes, but are fundamentally about the lives of humans" (5). Digital data is "lively" because it provides knowledge and insights into people's bodies and selves; contributes to livelihoods by generating profit for those who use data commercially or facilitate management and governance of people and populations; has its own vitality and social life since it circulates, enacts new forms of knowledge, and is purposed and repurposed in multiple ways (see Beer and Burrows 2013); and produces vital effects by influencing people's behaviors, sense of self, social relationships, life chances, employment, and opportunities.

Functional medicine's intimate embrace of "lively data"—operating with and through self-tracking devices and health apps—appeals to risk-averse and prevention-oriented individuals. The practices, meanings, discourses, and technologies associated with self-tracking are inevitable products of broader social, cultural, and political processes. In essence, the allure of personalized, data-rich medicine unfolds within the context of collective efforts at greater political-economic and material security through technological control, scientific knowledge, and industrial production (see De Courville Nicol 2021). Furthermore, while functional medicine proponents characterize the emergence of self-tracking devices as placing prevention through prediction at the fingertips of users, it can be argued that a neoliberal outlook on health as a personal responsibility—shaped by political and economic stakes in health surveillance and commercialization—undergirds self-regulation.

Surveillance practices lie at the intersection of contemporary projects of security, knowledge, production, and control. Theoretically, self-tracking differs from surveillance since people knowingly and purposefully collect information about themselves for their own review and use. Covert surveillance, on the other hand, produces data sets to which monitored subjects do not have access. People are increasingly surveilled through their transactions online or their movement in spaces that are embedded with sensors and fitted with cameras. They have little knowledge of what data is being collected, where it is stored, and for what purposes it is used.

The line between self-tracking and surveillance is increasingly blurred. Due to the commercial and managerial value of personal data, self-trackers are encouraged, "nudged," or even coerced and enforced to produce data that can also be used by software developers, third parties that purchase this data from developers, data-mining companies and their clients, government agencies, and cybercriminals. When the aforementioned parties harness this data to exercise influence on and control of the behavior of the individuals from whom it was collected, this "dataveillance" (Degli-Esposti 2014) can have disciplining effects.

Over the course of my ethnographic research, I heard functional medicine proponents and providers fail to interrogate the disciplining potential of "dataveillance"; instead, providers describe these emerging bioinformatic devices as practical tools for advancing their craft. In a contribution to Dr. Fitzgerald's email newsletter, Dr. Bland writes, "Smart device informatics . . . capture real time physiological and physical function data, and provide systems-level feedback for personalizing health." Writing for the same newsletter, Dr. LePine concurs, "The rise of $n = 1$ medicine is BIG with apps [and] personal devices. . . . [These] allow people to be engaged in their health and help provide feedback to change behaviors, which is often so difficult to do." Seen from the perspective of functional medicine, self-tracking devices are exemplary tools for gathering the data that enables P4 medicine.

In contrast, we might consider how the impact of self-quantification partially depends on differences among what Jeannette Pols, Dick Willems, and Margunn Aanestad (2019) refer to as "ethico-psychological subjects." Pols, Willems, and Aanestad take an empirical ethics approach when they compare differences in self-quantification in prevention discourse, testimonies from the Quantified Self movement, and empirical work with people with type 1 diabetes. In prevention discourse, self-quantifying ethico-psychological subjects rely on their free will to create self-chosen goals. In this view, nudges from health apps provide support by reminding individuals of what they should want. These apps provide useful data for individuals who are purposefully seeking personalized regimens and eager to follow them. However, Pols, Willems, and Aanestad found that individual will was much more fragile among people with type 1 diabetes, for whom specified aims were translated into so many steps per day and so much weight loss per week. The individuals they observed actively engaged these prescribed goals by either adhering to them or resisting them for other goals, by replacing them with new regimens, or by equivocally accepting or rejecting them (98).

Many of the functional medicine proponents I observed characterized their patients as "prevention discourse" self-quantifying ethico-psychological subjects when they indicated that self-tracking devices and technologies help patients pursue self-chosen goals. Functional medicine proponents support the use of self-tracking technology to upend the relational power structure in which the physician is the possessor of authoritative knowledge and the patient is the unknowing party who must comply with the doctor's orders. Functional medicine practitioners commend emerging bioinformatic devices for delivering data directly to the individual—not the provider—because they give insight into real-time behavior that the individual may be able to control. According to this logic, the quantification of the Self provides these datapreneurial consumers with useful insights for personalized health-optimization protocols.

However, I observed some cases in which goals were prescribed by functional medicine practitioners to patients. In these cases, the data outputs of self-tracking technology were reviewed by health providers to monitor patient behavior, then assessed in conjunction with laboratory test results to determine patient progress. An example is the use of Cronometer—an app that asks users to precisely log their daily consumption of food and subsequently determines the user's percentage of achievement toward micronutrient goals. Some functional medicine patients receive nutrition counseling based on Cronometer data—as often as once a week—to ensure successful outcomes. While there are benefits to technology that produces in-depth data regarding a patient's dietary patterns, I must flag how this technology veers into the territory of surveillance—especially because the data is readily accessible to both patient and provider. As patients complete their daily dietary logs, this information is available in real time to the provider for monitoring. When used in this way, this technology has a disciplining potential that begins to undermine one of the key goals of functional medicine: to place the patient in the primary position of power.

I build on Pols, Willems, and Aanestad (2019) to argue that ethico-psychological subjectivities are relationally constructed and maintained; that is, providers actively contribute to the (re)production of ethico-psychological subjects. Pols, Willems, and Aanestad point to how different relations between facts and desires underlie self-quantification, writing, "Numbers have a strong morality within the socio-material context in which numbers are qualified as adequate, true, boring, evidence of 'bad behavior,' or good or beautiful reporters of the wonders of the body" (2019, 113). While I agree that the subjective interpretation of seemingly objective numbers is an agentive endeavor, I simultaneously point to how the interpretation of numbers is refracted through relational webs of knowledge and authority.

Furthermore, my ethnographic research suggests that while functional medicine proponents emphasize how their work dismantles power imbalances in the patient-provider relationship—especially with regard to authoritative knowledge—functional medicine patients may nonetheless be subjected to other forms of technological control, such as dataveillance. In this vein, Beth Leavenworth DuFault and John W. Schouten (2020) note that datapreneurial consumers may embrace market-provided self-quantification in attempts to agentively liberate themselves from the control of that very quantification. For functional medicine patients, self-tracking technologies may offer the allure of liberation from "hegemonic biomedicine" while simultaneously having disciplining effects.

These disciplining effects may inadvertently unfold through the processes of gamification. Jennifer R. Whitson (2013) applies the lens of governmentality to gamification to show how quantification is leveraged in terms of surveillance. Gamification practices encourage playful subjectivities so that users voluntarily expose personal information, which is then used to drive behavioral change. Gamification inculcates desirable skill sets and behaviors that may be beneficial to the user (e.g., weight loss, educational advancement, etc.) and to others (e.g., workplace productivity and consumer loyalty). Whitson links gamification to the quantification of everyday life, arguing that the production of large quantities of real-time data about users' actions is rooted in surveillance. She suggests that social behavior undergirds self-surveillance to gamify everyday life and participatory surveillance evoked by social-networking services.

In the realm of functional medicine, technology companies argue that consumers are being inundated with external stimuli and, as a result, are less in tune with their bodies than prior generations. These companies are turning to the "gamification" of smart device informatics to apply the structure of a game to the functioning of the human body. In functional medicine, gamification extends to biological patterns such as heart-rate variability scores and sleep quality. As Harpreet Rai, Oura Ring[2] CEO and board member, explains the purpose, "By placing gamification and backing that up with scientific data, people can start to understand their bodies a little bit more and sort of focus back on what's really moving the needle for them or not." Given that the typical cell phone user touches their phone an average of 2,617 times per day (Naftulin 2016), smart-device informatics companies like Oura Ring aim to, rather paradoxically, use "gamification" to help people *reconnect* with their bodies.

Gamification is just one element of a larger trend called biohacking, mentioned in the previous chapter. Dave Asprey—the self-proclaimed "father of biohacking" who has spent over a million dollars biohacking his own body—regularly participates in functional medicine podcasts, docuseries, and summits. Asprey describes how biohacking is used to "upgrade" an individual bioconsumer's biology and make them "age backward." Max Lugavere, a health and science journalist, filmmaker, and author, indicates how biohacking involves taking the reins of one's health and writing one's own destiny. Lugavere characterizes biohacking as "the chance to circumnavigate various flaws that we might have in our genome." Biohacking relies on real-time biological data, and it is thus a major driver behind bioconsumption of disruptive technologies, but it comes at a hefty price.

Functional medicine interlocutors debate the accessibility of modern-day biohacking. Lugavere opines, "Now, thankfully, technology has gotten to a point where it's become cheap enough where each of us can afford to look under the hood of our biology, so to speak." In stark contrast, Maskell indicates, "Look at who can engage with precision things now: the biohackers. Is your average person on the poverty line a biohacker? No! You have to be pretty damn empowered to be a biohacker." This use of the word "empowered" harks back to my argument in chapter 1 regarding the intimate relationship between "empowerment" and socioeconomic privilege. Maskell continues, "You have to be confident enough to order your own labs, and this, and that, and whatever." I agree with Maskell; "confidence" is derived from an advanced level of technological training and health literacy, which, in turn, are markers of economic capital.

Only those who are already socioeconomically and educationally "empowered" are in the position to be informationally "empowered" regarding their own biologies. For example, Mette Dyhrberg, an economist who describes herself as "a little autistic with numbers," illustrates how she used biohacking to empower herself as a patient: "I went home and I turned to the one thing that I've always been able to rely on, which was numbers." Dyhrberg used Excel spreadsheets and built her own algorithm to examine correlations between her behavior and her symptoms. She continues, "I proved in five months that I wasn't a cardiac patient, and then proceeded to think, 'If I can get rid of my first label, I probably can get rid of everything.'" Over the course of sixteen months, Dyhrberg successfully quit her medications, "hypothesis tested her way out of all of her conditions," and normalized her blood work. Inspired by her personal experience of recovery, she transformed her career and is now the CEO of Mymee—a personalized trial and care platform that helps identify patients' specific triggers for autoimmune diseases such as rheumatoid arthritis, psoriatic arthritis, ankylosing spondylitis, lupus, psoriasis, and irritable bowel syndrome, among others—where she continues to work on digital health innovation. Dyhrberg is just one example of how technological training and health literacy (which are indicators of socioeconomic privilege) empower functional medicine participants to agentively take charge of their informational biologies.

SITUATING FUNCTIONAL MEDICINE: PATIENT-CONSUMERS IN THE BIOECONOMY

In mainstream medicine, patients are often limited in their ability to select a physician—their choices are restricted to providers who are "in network" and, in the case of specialists, can be dependent upon receiving referrals from their general practitioners. Patients are not told up front how much the services they receive will cost. Under most insurance plans, the patient receives a bill after medical services have been rendered indicating what portion of the cost has been reimbursed by their insurance and what portion has been deemed the patient's responsibility. Generally, physicians' earnings are not based on the quality of care they provide—that is, physicians are not evaluated based on their percentage of positive outcomes; instead, a fee-for-service structure incentivizes more intervention since this translates to greater income for individual providers.

According to functional medicine interlocutors, the health care system will undergo a much-needed transformation when it repositions passive patients as responsible consumers. Dr. Maloof asserts that the medical system will have to switch from a model in which "broken" patients seek health care as a "fix" to one in which patients claim responsibility for their own health outcomes. Dr. Maloof signals the role of consumption, asserting, "I think the way to make the existing model obsolete is to actually get consumers and patients actually caring about their health." I believe people *already* care about their health; however, they have unequal access to health-sustaining resources through the logic of consumption (see Vega 2018). Furthermore, functional medicine promotes a patient-led dynamic by positioning patients as *clients* within the consumer modality instead of as citizens with a right to health.

Positioning patients as consumers bears some similarities to the Weberian Marxist approach to biocapital.[3] Kaushik Sunder Rajan, an anthropologist, writes, "The life sciences represent a new face, and a new phase, of capitalism and, consequently, that biotechnology is a form of enterprise inextricable from contemporary capitalism" (2006, 3). Rajan simultaneously describes biocapital as one situated perspective of capitalism (among multiple), a symptom of capitalism, and a system of exchange of money and commodities. Stefan Helmreich (2008, 465) critiques Rajan's notion of biocapital, asserting that Rajan's speculative enterprise pays insufficient attention to how the materialities of biologic substances are transubstantiated in the bioeconomy.

Sociologists Kean Birch and David Tyfield (2012, 304) build on Helmreich's perspective when they note that what is often being exchanged in the so-called bioeconomy is health- and "vitality"-promoting *knowledge*, not biomatter. And Rajan (2007) maintains that health itself is the source of value—it does not need to be materialized in labor to become valuable. Birch and Tyfield go as far as to assert that "bio-" be replaced with "knowledge-" since it is "from the application of knowledge to nature, and the subjection of that knowledge to intellectual property rights, and not from the nature itself or from particular biological material" (2012, 315) that value is produced.[4]

Birch and Tyfield furthermore suggest that what have been characterized in Marxist terms as material, commodity-based processes are, in fact, immaterial, asset-based economic processes. To understand this critique, we must turn to Marx. In *Capital*, Karl Marx uses the formula M-C-M', where *M* stands for money, *C* for commodity, and *M'* for the total capital, including the surplus value gained in the profitable exchange of a commodity for money ([1867] 1992, 251). Helmreich applies this formula to biocapital, offering the formula B-C-B', where *B* stands for biomaterial, *C* for the commodity that is fashioned from the biomaterial through laboratory and legal instruments, and *B'* for the biocapital produced at the end of this process, including the value added through the instrumentalization of the original biomaterial (2008, 472). Much of what has been described in the Weberian Marxist approach to biocapital does not fit comfortably in this formula.

I agree with these critiques by Helmreich and Birch and Tyfield regarding inattention to biomatter; nevertheless, some of the existing literature on "biocapital" offers insight into the economic exchanges undergirding functional medicine. For example, Nikolas Rose (2008), as mentioned briefly in chapter 1, observes that the ways in which human beings make sense of their own suffering, attempt to uncover the reasons for it, and aim to be delivered from it, increasingly take a somatic form. That is, human beings identify and interpret their unease in terms of health, vitality, and morbidity. When presenting his concept of the "somatic ethic," Rose suggests that by acting upon their soma, people strive not just to make themselves better physically but also to make themselves better persons (46). Here, "ethic" refers to ways of understanding, adapting, and managing ourselves in our daily lives. Our ethic has become somatic because our soma (our biology, our genome, our neurotransmitters, etc.) possesses heightened salience in the modern bioeconomy. Rose queries the links between biocapital and the ethical work of human beings in the name of health, longevity, and vital existence. While the management of health and vitality once seemed narcissistic, these activities are now regarded as ethically prominent. Finally, Rose suggests that contemporary biopolitics are defined by tension between increasing demand for the products of the bioeconomy (organs, embryos, pharmaceuticals, etc.) in the West and "inequities and injustices of the local and global economic, technological, and biomedical infrastructure required to support such a somatic ethic" (48).[5]

Rajan (2007) sees biocapital as a key index of "capitalism" and, in turn, biosociality as a key index of biocapital. Paul Rabinow's (1996) notion of biosociality centers around adaptable, efficient, self-fashioning, politically agentive, often middle-class subjects who act as consumers of biomedical technology and epistemology, and as consumers on the market. Rajan (2007) contrasts these consumers with subaltern experimental subjects, writing, "It is always harder to form a shared social identification for those *subjected to* capital than for those who are *agents of* it" (172, emphasis in original). Furthermore, Rajan explains that biosociality, and, therefore, neoliberal consumption assemblages, are potentiated by the diagnostic capabilities of biomedicine, which are owed to experimental procedures in the laboratory, on animals, or on humans. He argues that health, articulated through a risk calculus, is the locus of subjectivity for biocapital. Responsible subjects, within this risk logic, become "always already patients-in-waiting" who embrace preventive measures before potential illnesses take place (159).

By turning to the existing literature on biocapital, I am highlighting how the privatization of functional medicine positions patient-clients as *consumers* of biology-enhancing knowledge, substances, and services. These observations are also noted by naturopath and licensed acupuncturist Dr. Michele Nickels, who indicates, "Over the past ten to twelve years, I've seen such a change . . . in the consumers, because this medicine is consumer driven." Dr. Andrew Hill, a cognitive neuroscientist and founder of Peak Brain Institute, recognizes the agentive role of consumers when he says, "It's our responsibility as engaged people that consume healthcare services to actually be part of the treatment team ourselves now." He encourages consumers to ask why they should take recommended medications and to make their own informed decisions regarding treatment plans. He insists that consumers not comply with a particular protocol "simply because the doctor said it was a good idea," elaborating, "Gone is a time when the doctors said, 'This is true,' and we believed them." Instead, consumers must protect their own health by closely managing the recommendations of multiple providers.

Furthermore, in functional medicine, consumers leverage their purchasing power to "choose" the providers with whom they want to work. Functional medicine practitioners provide services that are evaluated by consumers. Whether consumers deem these services to be "quality care" determines the continuity of provider-patient relationships. Stated simply, functional medicine consumers, like consumers in any neoliberal sector, have a choice of where they would like to seek care. They are unlikely to return to the same provider on an ongoing basis if the therapeutic relationship does not produce positive outcomes. Thus, functional medicine "empowers" consumers to sidestep health insurance by purchasing services out of pocket. In so doing, it positions itself as a path to well-being for predominantly privileged individuals.

Furthermore, functional medicine practitioners and supplement companies engage the agentive nature of consumption by creating and distributing in-depth educational resources to "savvy consumers." For example, Ortho Molecular Products pitched their products during the lunch break at the Advances in Mitochondrial Medicine Symposium by describing how they create materials and provide top-notch customer support to "the informed patient." While functional medicine interlocutors describe patient education as a departure from the authoritative provider-patient relationship in conventional medicine, functional medicine inadvertently adopts and expands the neoliberal framework of health care when it markets supplements and lab tests to consumers. Functional psychiatrist Dr. Kelly

Brogan points to how the United States is one of three countries in the entire world (along with New Zealand and Brazil) that permit direct advertising of pharmaceuticals to "consumers, sometimes called patients." In functional medicine, educational resources regarding supplements and lab tests serve a dual purpose since they are effective marketing materials, positioned to capture consumers who are aiming to transform their health through market-based consumption.

While I am wary of how this "new" model reinscribes neoliberal principles, functional medicine interlocutors argue that it unseats long-standing power inequalities in the patient-provider relationship. Misty Williams encourages her readers to make, and budget for, their own health-related decisions instead of relying on the medical system to take care of them when they are sick, on the government to provide dietary recommendations and ensure safety in their food supply, and on health insurance to cover their health expenses. I strongly disagree with her perspective that power can be "taken back" by relying on oneself instead of the medical system, the government, and health insurance. By emphasizing individuals' personal responsibility as consumers, Williams inadvertently deemphasizes the state's obligation to citizens' human right to health and advocates for a model in which individuals will necessarily have unequal access to well-being because of their differing degrees of privilege.[6]

The consumer-driven, neoliberal economic system—in which both conventional and functional medicine are embedded—imbues privileged consumers with power while excluding less privileged individuals who have no other choice but to seek resources through the modality of citizenship. In fact, functional medicine is often even less accessible than conventional medicine since it is not covered by insurance and requires greater out-of-pocket spending. Agentive, careful decision-making is applauded as "mindfulness" by different people within the functional medicine realm; however, consumption is only an option for individuals possessing socioeconomic privilege. In this way, "choice" is hammered together with financial capital.

Functional medicine doctors like Dr. Terry Wahls have been on the receiving end of this type of critique.[7] Recognizing that existing functional medicine delivery models based on one-on-one care, advanced diagnostic testing, and specialized supplements are unaffordable for many patients, Dr. Wahls developed and pioneered a lifestyle-based, group medicine approach.[8] When asked how to make the diet she recommends more affordable, Dr. Wahls explains that, as a physician and assistant chief of staff at the Iowa City VA Medical Center, she worked with patients who were low income and often surviving on food stamps. To help them implement her recommended diet with their income, she would suggest that they go to the farmers market and strike up a deal with the "cleanest" farmer for everything left at their stand at the end of the market. Based on this kind of advice, Dr. Wahls opines that everyone can implement positive, health-promoting change in their lives.

Dr. Wahls and many of her functional medicine colleagues employ the rhetoric of "choice." In a June 2019 email newsletter, Dr. Wahls wrote, "There are so many things you can do, small choices you can make every day." Among the "choices" she listed were cooking with fresh ingredients, eating more nonstarchy vegetables, meditating, gratitude journaling, exercising daily, gardening, foraging for foods, and spending time with supportive people. Dr. Wahls pointed out, "These are all powerful interventions you can implement right now, many for free. . . . The library and the internet also offer plentiful information for free." She encouraged readers to read widely, educate themselves, and find online and in-person communities that can help them "take control" and "take back" their health.

I recognize Dr. Wahls's efforts to alert patients to the lifestyle changes and resources that are likely within their economic reach. Using this approach, she has prompted some patients with less privilege into action, with positive results. At the same time, I want to problematize well-intentioned assertions she made in her email newsletter: "Don't forget that you are in control. . . . You can get started on your healing journey today if you choose." While many patients can afford to implement at least some of her low-cost suggestions, I emphasize that there are other types of functional medicine care many patients simply cannot afford. Dr. Wahls's approach does not make the same care available to everyone, but she has developed a separate model that maximizes cost effectiveness for less privileged patients by focusing on inexpensive lifestyle changes.

Dr. Wahls elaborated on the issue of affordability in her follow-up July 2019 email newsletter, explaining that functional medicine is expensive because it is time intensive. "Just recently, I spent six hours on a patient's first visit—three hours with them and three hours reviewing their labs and writing up the report." During a full evaluation, functional medicine physicians conduct a detailed review of the many environmental, dietary, and lifestyle factors that contribute to health decline.

She also reflected, in the follow-up newsletter, on her past experiences with less privileged patients. "Many people successfully made dramatic improvements to their health without the cost of functional medicine. . . . For the vast majority of people in my clinic at the VA, additional testing was not required." In this newsletter, the distinction between so-called lifestyle changes and functional medicine is clearer. While the lifestyle changes Dr. Wahls suggests are relatively inexpensive, P4 medicine from a functional medicine provider continues to be largely inaccessible to the masses.

The concluding comments of her July email differ from those of the month prior since she indirectly acknowledges that not everyone has the same degree of control: "Do not obsess over whether you can afford functional medicine. Obsess over learning how to cook at home. Obsess over eating what is recommended and eliminating what is harmful. Obsess over what is in your control." By instructing her followers not to "obsess," Dr. Wahls skirts important issues of unequal access.

Almost as if in response to Dr. Wahls, one functional medicine patient expressed on Facebook, "For some, spending the money to work with someone excellent is totally worth it. For others, their financial situation makes that choice a harder one to make. So, instead of spending more money, they spend time trying to learn and find their way." This patient indicated that both approaches are "costly" since neither time nor money is free. This comment elicited a response from another patient, who wrote, "It is just frustrating that so many simply cannot afford it. It is not about not being willing to invest. [There is] a huge difference." These concerns from would-be functional medicine patients highlight troubling issues of (un)affordability.[9]

The rhetoric of "control" and "choice" can inadvertently obscure the socioeconomically stratified nature of access to functional medicine. As one patient put it, "The hardest [thing] is to overcome the panic when you are up against time, without the information, if you have no money." The harsh reality is that patients are left "choosing" the degree of care they can afford to pay for out of pocket (Vega 2018, 10, 15, 63). A political economic approach is indispensable since failing to recognize the financial costs related to health runs the risk of blaming the victim.

HEALTH AS A "SKILL SET": THE UNDERLYING PROBLEM OF BLAMING THE VICTIM

Functional medicine proponents ask consumers—those whom Patel calls "the doctors of the future"—to adopt an expanded role, take greater responsibility for their health, and develop additional skills. In health consultant and entrepreneur Matthew Accurso's opinion, these additional skills include a critical awareness of the pharmaceuticals and surgical interventions that providers recommend to patient-consumers, as well as of the everyday toxins in their environments. From his perspective, consumers should furthermore be able to objectively ask, "What is that going to accomplish for generations to come? Is that going to create stronger genetics? . . . Or is that going to create a weaker vessel that's going to be compromised in the end?" That is, patient-consumers should consider not only the effects of medical, pharmaceutical, and environmental factors on their individual health but also the potential for intergenerational epigenetic effects as well.

This new positioning of patient-as-doctor and doctor-as-educator places a great deal of responsibility on individual consumers' shoulders. Tom Blue, strategic advisor for industry at the Institute for Functional Medicine, asserts that, given our recent understanding of epigenetics,[10] our decisions and actions largely determine our health. He indicates, "If that's the case, the only thing we're left to conclude is that health, more than anything else, is actually a skill set." This is both a valuable and a dangerous assertion.

As someone who has struggled with chronic disease, I identify with Blue's assertion that health is a skill set. I had so much to learn at every juncture of my recovery. When I first became aware of functional medicine, my husband, Rikin, and I dedicated five hours a week to my "Return to Wellness Workshop." We used this time to learn to understand my unique genome, implement changes to my diet, evaluate potential triggers of autoimmunity in my environment, and eliminate harmful toxins in our household. When those five hours per week turned out to be insufficient to meet my health needs, I used ethnographic methods to solve my health issues—thus my personal recovery became the underlying goal of my professional research.

At the same time, as a medical anthropologist, I am very wary of framing health in this way. I am attentive to the potential slippage between "skill" and "merit." I am, by no means, arguing that health is earned. I do not believe those with the greatest skill are the healthiest. In my view, health is not a meritocracy. At the same time, I am vigilant with regard to how the rhetoric of meritocracy can be used to blame the victim and obscure social inequalities (Vega 2018, 187–189).

For example, characterizing health as a "skill set" can be viewed as an indirect assertion that ill health is due to lack of skill. Blue's words can be inverted to suggest disease is due to poor decisions on the part of patients with regard to lifestyle and stress management, and to lack of action with regard to nutrition and exercise. I believe Blue's intention was to empower individuals by arguing health is in their hands; however, statements like his can inadvertently be used to blame people with chronic disease for their suffering.

I, along with other medical anthropologists (Singer 1994; Inhorn and Buss 1995; Carlson 1996), argue that it is an ethical imperative to resist blaming the victim. For those working extended hours and struggling to make a living, a "balanced lifestyle" is out of reach. Families facing food insecurity may prioritize sustenance over nutritional quality as they likely do not even have the option of nutrient-dense food (Hadley and Crooks 2012; Hadley and Patil 2008; Henry 2017). People living in high-crime neighborhoods do not have the luxury of going for a jog in the park and are unlikely to be able to afford gym memberships. In this vein, Dr. Tracy Gaudet, director of the Duke Center for Integrative Medicine at Duke University, asserts, "If you live in a community where you can't get food, or there is trauma on the streets every day, these are the drivers of your health and illness, largely." Thus, the answer for individuals subjected to everyday violence (Bourgois 1998; Scheper-Hughes and Bourgois 2004; Bourgois, Prince, and Moss 2004), social exclusion, stigma, and marginalization is not simply stress management; societal change, rooted in social justice, is required.

In this chapter, I have explored relational shifts underway in functional medicine. Functional medicine's ability to place patients in a position of authority within the therapeutic relationship—to the degree that it accomplishes this goal—is undergirded by how functional medicine first situates patients as "clients" and "consumers." As a result, functional medicine "empowers" privileged patient-consumers while excluding less privileged individuals suffering from chronic illness.

I have furthermore described how functional medicine proponents promote patient engagement with wearable devices. My observations regarding how functional medicine patient-consumers quantify their bodies serve as a preface for my discussion of online patient communities in chapter 4. Rachael Kent (2021) notes the commonalities between self-tracking technologies (e.g., wearable devices and mobile applications) and social media platforms: both are forms of digitally tracking our health and lifestyle, and users increasingly mediate their lives through both simultaneously. While practices such as calorie counting and exercise tracking produce quantitative health data, photographs of the body and of food consumption on social media (fitness "selfies" and tweets with the tag #foodporn) produce qualitative data. In the selfies, healthy identities are carefully represented for the community's gaze (see Kent 2018, 2020). Kent (2021) argues that these mediated, performed, and curated practices engender new ways of understanding our bodies, health, and identity. This process is iterative since body management and the performance of health influence diet and lifestyle.

That is, users' self-tracking and online presence influence health management in their offline everyday lives.

In chapter 4, I turn to how logics of inclusion and exclusion are reproduced or contested within online communities. Digitized social collectives have emerged around specific diagnoses and functional medicine proponents. Patient-organized online social assemblages sometimes enact a "hive mind" to sidestep socioeconomic barriers to functional medicine. In the process, health knowledge—which is often potentiated by economic capital—is reconfigured as a form of social capital. On the other hand, provider-organized and docuseries host–organized online groups can commodify "community," thus reinscribing neoliberal logics of inclusion and exclusion.

Interlude

THE THREE CS

Functional medicine care and the implementation of personalized lifestyle changes are very expensive. As a result, many people are priced out. Over the course of my ethnographic research, I observed how some patients agentively develop strategies to sidestep some or most of the largest expense, one-on-one care with a functional medicine physician. In this interlude, I describe how some of these strategies unfolded in my own healing journey.

James Maskell was a finance banker prior to having a "come to Jesus moment" and asking himself what his true calling in life was. Deciding to dedicate the rest of his career to the betterment of society, he carved out a new path as a functional medicine advocate. Through EvoMed, the company he founded, Maskell is giving conventional practitioners the support they need to take the daring step of opening a functional medicine practice and, further, to make their services accessible to a wide array of people. To this end, Maskell proposes three Cs for cost savings: content, community, and coaching.

Without knowing it, I had cycled through the three Cs Maskell suggests. I did this on my own, out of pure necessity. When I was first learning about functional medicine, I watched online summits, conferences, and docuseries nonstop. These rich sources of information—what Maskell calls "content," his first C—became the backdrop to my everyday life. I listened to them while getting ready for work in the morning, eating lunch, washing dishes—you name it. I gravitated to these sources because they were absolutely free and they provided me with an up-to-the-moment overview of functional medicine knowledge. This "content" allowed me to learn about my own health issues and to identify a few practitioners who had been successful in reversing these diseases when they were personally affected by them.[1] *I learned their techniques and implemented them, acting as my own functional medicine doctor.*

Then my digital autoethnography branched out into the realm of online support groups. This changed everything about how I experienced social media. I joined nine different functional medicine–related Facebook groups and connected with more than 241,100 patients with conditions like mine. I did not know what to expect when I joined these online support groups. I wondered, how do these groups offer "support"? Suddenly, my Facebook feed was overloaded with questions and replies from people I had never met. Initially, the intimate nature of these posts was jarring to me. I scrolled through photos of swollen body parts and rashes and screenshots of individuals' genomic data. Often, I encountered brief descriptions in which patients identified themselves via their web of diagnoses. After adjusting to the new visual and discursive forms that had taken over my feed, I was struck by the immense knowledge possessed by this "community," Maskell's second C. Other patients in the groups were consuming content as feverishly as I was—effectively acting as "patient-anthropologists"—and they really knew what they were talking about. I discovered, more than anything, that these groups operated as a 24/7 question-and-answer board. If anyone in the group had a question related to their health conditions, they would post it, and within minutes a long thread would form with in-depth answers.

I also turned to my close friends and family for support. My good friend David sent me this text message at a critical point in my healing, when I needed the reassurance the most:

> *You're on the right track. Keep looking into your intuition as well as all the info you've collected and sifted through to develop your own personal protocol for healing. I'm impressed with how thorough and dedicated you are in this, as well as your ability to take the risk of forging your own path . . . as you've realized there is no person better to do it than you, especially since you're getting the latest from your conference lectures that put you ahead of the very doctors you would otherwise be consulting with. What a great path you're forging, and look at how brave you are.*

Inspired by his text, I came up with a mantra: "This body was created to heal, and I was meant to heal it." I repeated this mantra to myself every day. David's message reminded me I had a support network—friends and family who loved me and who were rooting for me to get better.

By combining "content" with "community," I was able to adjust my personal protocol to meet my changing needs. I progressed 90 percent of the way to full health without ever paying out of pocket for a functional medicine doctor. Since certain laboratories and supplement companies sell their products and services only through physicians—arguing that this gatekeeping approach strengthens the physician-patient relationship—I used direct-to-consumer laboratories, which tested for the same biomarkers, and I identified supplements that were cheaper than those conventionally recommended but made from similarly high-quality ingredients. To use some functional medicine lingo, I had picked all the "low-hanging fruit" and "pulled all the biggest levers" on my own by the time I had my first functional medicine visit. Thus, the vast majority of my health spending in 2019 was allocated to laboratory testing and herbs and supplements, not provider-based care.

When I began seeking out different practitioners for my functional medicine team, I was no longer in the midst of a health crisis. I was merely hoping to use advanced diagnostics to identify my long-term needs, which would allow me to scale down my health regimen, prevent future health problems, and ensure financial sustainability. When I discovered that the closest functional medicine physician was located five hours away, had a waiting list of over a year, and charged thousands of dollars for just the initial visit, I embraced telemedicine in order to find a comparatively affordable team.

Unaware of Maskell's advice but nonetheless advancing along the path he outlines, my last step was to find "coaching." Maskell refers to auxiliary health personnel as "coaches." While these coaches may include physician assistants and nurses, functional medicine teams most often include functional nutritionists. This makes sense given functional medicine's emphasis on "food as medicine." On the online Fatigue Super Conference, Maskell explains, "Coaching can help you implement all the things that you're learning in the content or through the community." From Maskell's health economics perspective, coaching "creates value" for functional medicine patients because it allows them to have close contact with members of a functional medicine team while paying a fraction of the cost.

At the same time I started receiving coaching, I began working with a functional medicine doctor, so I found functional nutritionists who were able to work with my doctor as a team. Although they were located in different states, my nutrition coaches consulted with my doctor on my case so they could be effective in implementing his care plan. I saw my doctor an average of once every four months at a rate of $400 per hour. The initial visit was ninety minutes, while follow-up visits were thirty to *sixty minutes. I had six total appointments with my functional nutrition team, approximately once every four weeks, at an average rate of $175 per hour. These visits generally lasted thirty to forty-five minutes. Thus, during the height of my direct patient care with functional medicine providers—a period that lasted about eight months—I was spending an average of $210 per month on consultations.*

In this interlude, I have described how I was able to use content, community, and coaching to pay the very minimum in out-of-pocket fees for one-on-one care with a functional medicine physician. While my personal experience demonstrates how the three *C*s can be harnessed to reduce the cost of functional medicine services, these strategies are by no means sufficient for rendering functional medicine accessible to the masses. By pursuing them, I *purchased* my recovery at a fraction of what it would have cost if I had relied primarily on appointments with my functional medicine doctor, but the financial burden on my household for this care and laboratory testing and supplements was still enormous. I am hyperaware that most households cannot afford the nearly $23,000 my family spent, primarily on the lab tests and supplements, to buy back my health. My health is better only because my family could pay the price. Meanwhile, most people cannot explore functional medicine as a potential tool for recovery—not because recovery is biologically impossible in most cases but, rather, because it is financially unattainable. In the next chapter, I turn to how individuals in patient-organized Facebook communities connect one another with content and suggest coaching while critiquing the high costs of functional medicine. These communities engage the "hive mind" to subvert some of the costs of functional medicine and work toward building an alternative media that challenges capitalist structures.

CHAPTER 4
DIGITIZED PATIENT COMMUNITIES

Scholars have published a range of perspectives—from laudatory to overtly critical—regarding the effects of online patient communities on individuals' lives and on society as a whole. My ethnographic research uncovered distinct types of functional medicine online communities, allowing me to consider the complex dialectics between the technical and the social, between digital discourses and health practices, between the political economy of the web and patient self-advocacy, and between self-centered communication processes and network individualism (see Barassi 2015). For each type of functional medicine online community I observed, I explore in this chapter the ways in which these communities either advance communicative socialism and digital communism (Fuchs 2019) or fail to challenge digital capitalism by extracting data and expanding control (Sadowski 2020).

First, I turn to Facebook groups organized by patients. As in the second interlude above, this section of the chapter includes pieces of raw ethnographic data. I weave together extracts from messages posted to social media to *demonstrate* the quality of patient-patient digital interactions and to *describe* how functional medicine patient communities are forged online. I discursively analyze this ethnographic data and identify emerging themes. What motivates individuals to participate in these online communities? What are their hopes and expectations? What types of support do these online communities provide?

Through an iterative process of open coding, I identified how these communities provide mutual encouragement, often through feminized expressions of unity. Group members offer and receive empathy, accompanying one another through seemingly mundane experiences. A hive mind evolves to help solve individual health dilemmas, thus serving as an important source of knowledge outside of clinical settings. These groups also critique the high, sometimes prohibitive, cost of functional medicine and suggest cheaper alternatives to working with an expensive functional medicine practitioner. At the same time, social capital within these groups is indirectly potentiated by economic capital through knowledge of one's own body and medical conditions that can be leveraged to guide others in their healing journeys—what I refer to as (self-)knowledge.

Second, I turn to groups organized by functional medicine providers, health educators, and docuseries hosts. Many functional medicine proponents identify loss of community as a source of individual and societal malaise. In an effort to restore a sense of community, some functional medicine providers and health coaches organize online groups where their patients can receive peer-to-peer support, without active participation from the provider. These providers and health coaches report robust and generative participation among group members and consider these groups to be a key resource for healing. Although these groups are "free," group members often pay significant sums to purchase "salugens" (health-promoting compounds such as herbs and supplements), receive health coaching, partake in healing programs, or obtain personalized care from a provider or health coach. At times, patients are offered access to these online groups after purchasing the provider's protocol.

Functional medicine docuseries hosts also use the rhetoric of community when they use membership in online patient communities to promote docuseries "packages." Over the course of my ethnographic research, I observed how docuseries are often marketed in tiered "packages," with higher tiers offering additional resources and perks. By commodifying membership in online communities, this type of marketing reinscribes neoliberal logics of inclusion and exclusion.

PATIENT-ORGANIZED FACEBOOK GROUPS

In his 1996 book *Essays on the Anthropology of Reason*, Paul Rabinow developed the concept of biosociality, which is the set of unique social interactions that occur between individuals facing similar biological states—for example, among members of a support group who all have the same disease. A focus on a shared biological experience or diagnosis gives rise to unique social forms, bringing individuals together in novel and intimate ways. Interactions occurring in Facebook groups related to functional medicine are all examples of *digitized* biosociality.

At the same time, the digital nature of the support groups in which I participated adds an expanded spatial dimension to the concept of biosociality. Functional medicine patients may not personally know others in their own geographic communities who suffer from the same diagnoses. If they do, those chronic-disease patients with similarly complex diagnoses may not have chosen a functional medicine approach for healing. In either case, functional medicine patients turn to Facebook for an online community that specifically addresses their health concerns. Digitized biosociality allows for connection, rooted in a shared bodily experience, across vast geographic distances and socioeconomic differences.

Although these communities span vast geographic distances, their members share numerous commonalities, allowing for ongoing exchanges of personal stories, comparisons of experiences with alternative therapies, and mutual understandings of disease etiologies. Whereas social media generally allows for a façade of "connectedness," according to functional medicine interlocutors' critique these groups diverge from stereotypical, superficial social media interactions as group members confide intimate health details with one another, mutually encourage one another, and build communal unity.

The following subsections explore four major themes that emerged through an iterative process of open coding of social media data. First, I examine patient-organized Facebook groups as a place for mutual encouragement through feminized expressions of unity. Second, I describe how group members empathized with one another and provided accompaniment through seemingly mundane situations. Third, I note how a hive mind developed in these groups to help solve individuals' health dilemmas. Fourth, I explore group members' critiques of the high costs of functional medicine.[1]

Feminized Expressions of Unity

Hannah offered these words of encouragement for members who were new to the group's nutritional and lifestyle protocol: "The body can heal. It wants to heal and will do so given the right tools!" Likewise, Jennifer reassured new group members, "Don't get overwhelmed by health information—it's a learning curve so just take it bit by bit. You don't have to make changes all at once." As a newer member, Michelle responded to these types of encouraging messages, saying, "I hope to be able to share my success story of overcoming this in the coming months, so stay tuned!" Immediately, a fellow group member replied, "I'm so tuned in to what you say. I recall one of your posts and thinking my story sounds a lot like yours! I can't wait to hear a success story from you. <3"

Paula described her boyfriend's early-stage success. Her boyfriend had had multiple sclerosis for more than ten years and could walk only short distances, and with the help of a walker. He used a wheelchair to go outside of the house. However, in the first two weeks on a new protocol, he told Paula that he had switched off the light. Paula responded, "Well, yes, what's so special about that?" He then showed her that he had walked three to four steps from the sofa to the light switch, without the help of a walker. In the following days, he suddenly began to walk longer distances around the house. Paula wrote, "I was astonished and overwhelmed. . . . I was very surprised when I suddenly saw him in the hallway without a walker." Then, referring to how the group had been a strong source of support before her boyfriend initiated the new protocol, she wrote, "Many thanks again for your support when we were struggling. *Smiley face emoji*"

Jacob, one of the few men who posted during my digital ethnographic research, shared, "Today is the one-year anniversary of me taking back control of my life." In his post, Jacob included a before and after photo collage. Describing a photo of thirty-six bottles, three boxes, and two syringes of medication, he wrote, "[This] picture is what I was prescribed prior to my coma in 2017." He also included a photo of nine supplement bottles, explaining, "The second photo is what I currently take, no prescriptions. I have eliminated all of those drugs since February first." His descriptions were accompanied by emojis of praying hands, a hand making a peace sign, a red heart, and a flexing biceps. At the time I saw the post, it had already garnered 488 "like," "love," and "wow" reactions and had received 116 comments.

Samantha also wrote an enthusiastic post about her recovery. She explained that for years she had suffered from overlapping diseases—some autoimmune in nature.[2] Her diagnoses included hypothyroidism, fibromyalgia, chronic fatigue, irritable bowel syndrome, celiac disease, Barrett's esophagus, osteoporosis, and depression. Samantha wrote, "After much research, I began attempting to repair my gut with a clean, organic food diet, filtered water, cutting out all sugar, dairy and grains." This process allowed her to wean off of prescription drugs and, at the time of her post, she was on the cusp of eliminating prescription drugs entirely. She indicated, "My pain is now minimal. My energy and focus have returned and my IBS is under control. I feel like I'm 30 again!"

Likewise, Victoria shared her story of healing. She exclaimed, "I AM

A MIRACLE!" Her post included a two-page explanation of her painful, decades-long health spiral before detailing her return to health using functional medicine. Victoria was first diagnosed with endometriosis, an autoimmune disease, when she was fifteen years old. She received her second and third autoimmune-disease diagnoses in her twenties: narcolepsy and restless legs syndrome. She was also diagnosed with inflammatory bowel disease, ischemic colitis, gastroparesis, and gastritis in her twenties. Subsequently, she was bitten by a tick and an infectious disease doctor diagnosed her with Lyme disease. In her thirties she was diagnosed with her fourth and fifth autoimmune diseases: thyroiditis and psoriasis. In her late thirties she also developed adult-onset asthma. At age forty, inflammation around Victoria's heart caused her to be hospitalized. She emerged from that experience with her sixth and seventh autoimmune diagnoses: fibromyalgia and systemic lupus erythematosus. By age forty-three, disability forced Victoria to quit her career. However, in August 2014, she embarked on her health journey. Five years into her recovery, Victoria reported to the group, "It has been an outstanding success: I have been free of ALL symptoms of disease for 3.5 years. I am in remission from every condition I listed above." Victoria indicated that her "life was saved" using functional medicine, lifestyle changes, diet changes, faith, stress reduction and meditation, exercise, social support, environmental detoxing, and "biohacking."[3] She continued, "In 2014, I was convinced I would die from Lupus, but now in 2019, I am convinced that I am disease free and will live a long and vibrantly healthy life. . . . I have been able to create the life of my dreams."

When individual members reported positive outcomes to the group, they received cheers of support. Examples include comments such as

GIF of Snoopy dancing
GIF of Charlie Brown placing an arm around Snoopy
"Amazing!!"
"Love this!!!!! <3"
"omg!! This is amazing!"
GIF of an eagle screeching "Go! Go! Go!"
"Fantastic!"
"Oh, I love this!!!! Thank you for sharing!!! <3 <3 <3"
"Look at you glow, girl!"
"Create your own health miracle, sister!"
"You worked hard for this. Take the credit, girl!!!! *Four thumbs up emojis*"

Group members often face disheartening prognoses from conventional doctors and lack examples of healing and recovery in their immediate surroundings. Their diagnoses often include autoimmune disorders that are considered chronic, irreversible, and degenerative. However, as demonstrated throughout this section, group members use their own successful recoveries to inspire others to embrace the healing journey with hope. At times, individuals shared specific lab values to demonstrate the extent of their recovery. For example, Rhonda noted she was able to reduce her autoimmune antibody count by over 94 percent, mostly through implementing dietary changes. Dr. Kara Fitzgerald indicates, "One individual's restoration of health in this paradigm does not stop with that individual. . . . That transformation—just the physical change—it has an impact on people around us." Similarly, Alex Howard comments that "expert-patients" who have gained a strong foothold in their recovery "inevitably feel inspired and want to play a role in helping others." The patterns Dr. Fitzgerald and Howard describe are important since newer group members are inspired by the successes of their fellow group members—the recoveries they witness online give them hope for their own recovery.

Furthermore, Hannah and Jennifer's posts offer welcoming reassurance to newer members. While Hannah encourages newer group mates by sharing a core tenet of functional medicine—that under the right conditions, the body is capable of profound healing—Jennifer emphasizes the importance of patience when learning new health information and implementing changes in one's life. Michelle's post exemplifies how newer members are inspired by encouraging messages to embark on their healing journeys with hope. Through virtually witnessing multiple members of the group recover from chronic disease, these newer members come to believe that their own recovery is not just possible but truly within reach. In this way, online support groups create and sustain hope, even in the face of unknown futures and unanticipated challenges.

The members of these online communities are almost exclusively women. This may be due, in part, to the fact that women are more likely than men to be diagnosed with chronic diseases. While this tendency may reflect biological underpinnings—consider, for example, the relationship between sex hormones and autoimmunity (Borba, Zandman-Goddard, and Shoenfeld 2018; Gaberšček and Zaletel 2011)—it is also likely that men are underdiagnosed for many chronic diseases due to a reluctance among many men to seek out medical care (Galdas, Cheater, and Marshall 2005).[4] But even when the patient is male (for example, Paula's boyfriend), it is often his female family member or romantic partner who actively participates in the online community, a phenomenon that may reflect how women have historically been those primarily responsible for caregiving in the family (Barg et al. 2013).

Given the overwhelming presence of women in these online communities, words of encouragement and cheers of support take on a noticeably feminized form. The use of multiple explanation points and heart emoticons, along with the nouns "girl" and "sister," are discursive characteristics that promote a sense of unity among group members. At every turn, these online "sisters" offer each other empathy and emphasize the importance of hope, often using GIFs to celebrate each other's triumphs. Group members root for each other as women who draw inspiration from other women's progress.

These feminized expressions of unity are undergirded by a special emphasis in functional medicine on women—a focus that is linked to the fact that autoimmunity and chronic disease disproportionately affect women. For example, one email from Dr. Wahls reads, "Super Mom. Super Wife. Super Career Woman or Entrepreneur. Are you exhausted yet?" The email was promoting 50 Ways to Women's Wellness, an online event created for women, by women. According to Dr. Wahls, this "groundbreaking" event was designed to "help YOU cope with the exhausting pressure of being a super woman expected to do everything perfectly, all the time." The seven-day event incorporated fifty-five female speakers and was advertised as teaching the "BEST secrets" for women's health and healing, disease prevention, mental health, weight loss, self-care, relationships, energy, empowerment, and "financial strength." Another example is an email from Misty Williams with the subject "REVEALED: The reason healing is harder for women." This type of functional medicine discourse emphasizes women's experiences, adopts a woman-centric framework, and suggests unity among women based on their shared womanhood.[5]

Empathy: Accompaniment in the Mundane

Adrienne reached out seeking advice on how to explain the extreme exhaustion that many autoimmune patients experience to a loved one who cannot relate. Her post sparked a thread of responses, many of which empathized with her situation. Brooke revealed, "I get so discouraged." The earliest replies to her post included "Me too" and "Me three." When individuals described particularly challenging symptoms and circumstances, these posts received comments such as "I have a lot of the same symptoms" and "I was there."

For members who face setbacks in their healing journeys, Dana posted the image of a handwritten note that read, "Remember when you wanted what you currently have." She captioned this image, "I needed to be reminded of this today, so I thought there might be some here who do too." Dana explained that she had made incredible progress in her health over the past few months, so when she now had occasional "bad days and flares," she had to remind herself that health is a process. When discussing health setbacks, hope was always a part of these Facebook groups' online discourse. For example, Rebecca wrote, "Hope is what will propel you forward. The journey to health is not linear, so do not lose hope at setbacks."

Similarly, Kayla addressed group members who encountered obstacles during the healing process. Her post included the image of a Post-it note on which the following was written: "Read this carefully. You have a good heart. You are a beautiful person. You are doing the best you can. And today, THAT IS ENOUGH." As if responding to Kayla's post, but in a different online group and at a different time, Amanda posted a different quote by Yolo Akili Robinson: "Sometimes I wake up and have to remind myself: THERE IS NOTHING WRONG WITH ME. I have patterns to unlearn, new behaviors to embody and wounds to heal. But there is nothing wrong with the core of me and who I am. I am unlearning generations of harm and remembering love. That takes time."

*Referencing the shared experience of food elimination and reintroduction, Sarah posted, "Can we ever have dairy again? I really miss cheese. *Slanted frown emoji*" She received multiple replies. One group member indicated, "I'm hopeful!" Evincing the global reach of Facebook support groups, a British group member described dairy-free options available in UK supermarkets. Her post was accompanied by a photo. Sarah commented on the photo, typing, "Can you ship me a package to NY? *Laugh/cry emoji*" As if responding to Sarah, Celia posted an image of multiple crisscrossing staircases, asked the group to "focus on the positive," and solicited examples of successful food reintroductions from her fellow group mates. Debbie responded, "Green beans, cocoa, egg yolks, and cumin." Tina posted, "Jasmine rice. Trying peppers at the moment. *Fingers crossed emoji*" Lindsey responded, "Egg yolks, green beans, and peas! . . . I'm pretty psyched that I finally got this far. *Smiley face emoji*"*

Seeking to affordably implement functional medicine recommendations regarding food, Emily asked the group, "What's on your list for Costco?" Her six-word question prompted 104 comments, including in-depth discussions regarding specific ingredients on pantry food labels

> *and numerous photos. Responses came from across the country and around the world—including a group member expressing excitement about Costco opening in her country. One group member responded, "Salmon, avocados, melons, organic blackberries, pink Himalayan sea salt, avocado oil, [and] green beans." Another member shared, "Organic power greens mix, frozen riced cauliflower, frozen organic blueberries, organic frozen cherries, canned coconut milk (when I can't get it at Trader Joe's), mixed nut and seed butter, coconut oil, organic coconut MCT oil, organic onions, organic sweet potatoes, organic spinach, [and] span peas." Emily responded to one of these shopping list replies, "Great list btw lol I'm borrowing it. *Smiley face emoji*"*

Online groups related to functional medicine are filled with expressions of unity, rooted in empathy. Adrienne's and Brooke's posts signal how chronic-disease sufferers turn to Facebook support groups when they need an empathetic community. The sense of belonging these communities create can be especially important for individuals whose family members do not understand the lived experience of a particular chronic disease and cannot relate. In contrast, Facebook support groups are filled with thousands of members who can relate because they have lived through similar experiences themselves. Thus, for many functional medicine patients, Facebook is an ongoing source of empathy—operating at all times of day and night and across great geographic distances.

Group members faced similar obstacles on the road to recovery and offered advice for navigating these obstacles. Group mates inspired each other to focus on the progress they had made while simultaneously acknowledging that progress can be intermittent. In so doing, group members such as Rebecca described hope as the motor that propels individuals through their nonlinear healing journeys. Some of the messages were culled from broad contexts and repositioned within the functional medicine contexts; for example, variations of the image Dana posted of a handwritten note reading "Remember when you wanted what you currently have" have been widely circulated on websites unrelated to functional medicine and chronic disease. The quote, which is occasionally attributed to Nicholes E. Primington, appears on multiple Facebook, Pinterest, Twitter, and Reddit pages and is featured on items for sale at Etsy and Amazon. Nonetheless, the quote resonated with the group's specific experience of recovery from chronic disease. When applied to the context of functional medicine, this quote applied to healing as a *process* and encouraged group members through every stage.

Other posts pointed to the theme of self-acceptance, acknowledging the important role of mental health in the healing process. Variations on Kayla's post of the Post-it note have circulated on multiple Facebook pages (including the page for a clothing line); however, as with Dana's post, its message was particularly pertinent for functional medicine patients struggling with chronic disease. Meanwhile, Amanda's post featured a quote from a writer, poet, counselor, community organizer, and advocate for mental and emotional health among the Black community. In so doing, Amanda extended Yolo Akili's words from their original context in the Black community to an online community of individuals struggling with chronic disease.[6]

Given that food eliminations and reintroductions are a cornerstone of functional medicine, group members often provided one another with support and compared experiences regarding the process. At times, group members sought advice on how to navigate social situations that may become awkward due to food eliminations. One person asked what to do when birthday cake is served at a party. Another person explained that a new beau had invited her over to his house to enjoy a home-cooked dinner. Unfortunately, the dinner he offered to make used ingredients that would cause her to have a flare. These types of conundrums are unique to people with food intolerances but common among the members of the group.

Sarah's post about missing cheese and the responses it elicited exemplify how a shared experience unifies group members, imbuing their interactions with a mixture of empathy and humor. Chronic-disease sufferers use comedy as a way to acknowledge suffering while resisting despair. This complex, paradoxical role of comedy is encapsulated in the laugh/cry emoji. For her part, Celia chose multiple intersecting staircases for the backdrop of her post regarding food reintroductions, emphasizing the progressive and nonlinear nature of recovery. She invited her fellow group members to recognize and share small successes along the way to their eventual goals.

The large volume of group members' replies to Emily's seemingly mundane invitation to compare grocery shopping lists is indicative of their willingness to mutually support one another through the nitty gritty, everyday implementation of diet change. Natasja Kingod et al. (2017) found that online peer-to-peer communities provide the chronically ill with a supportive space for daily self-care. These posts again demonstrate the strong sense of unity and shared experience among group members separated by thousands of miles. This form of accompaniment—the feeling that others are sharing experiences with you, even from afar—creates a digitized space where individual group members who are struggling to resolve a symptom feel comfortable seeking guidance.

Hive Mind

Stacy described her twenty-year history with antidepressants and oral contraceptives. After discovering she is homozygous for MTHFR C677T, she quit taking contraceptives. About six months before she sought the advice of the group, her doctor took her off antidepressants. In the intervening months, Stacy fluctuated between hyper- and hypothyroidism and struggled with feelings of anger and depression. She shared with the group, "I'm depressed, crying over little things. Suicide ideation at times. Wanting to run away from my life. Finding issues with my husband and starting fights. Getting pissed for stupid stuff. I feel better after a blowup or a big cry." After decades of her doctors using antidepressants to manipulate serotonin instead of evaluating all of her neurotransmitters, Stacy decided to take matters into her own hands by purchasing a direct-to-consumer neurotransmitter test. She explained to the group that this would be her first step toward properly diagnosing the issue.

Natalie wrote, "Please help me!! I need help. Desperately. Almost down to a hundred pounds." She indicated to the group that although she had known she has a particular single nucleotide polymorphism (SNP) for years, this genetic variant did not cause any symptoms for most of her life. However, everything changed when she turned thirty-five and common foods started to cause her to break out in blisters. She continued, "I get frustrated because my food is so limited. I don't even want to go shopping for food. So many things I want to eat but can't." In addition to the embodied constraints that determined what she could and could not eat, Natalie faced geographic barriers when trying to obtain the specialty food she needed. Describing how she lived in the "middle of nowhere," with no access to a health-food store, she wrote, "I'm turning anorexic, not by choice, but by frustration." Her local doctors were no help since they did not understand the effects of her SNP. She turned to the group for help because her own understanding was also limited, and the group was one of the very few resources available to her.

Catherine posted a screenshot of her methylation analysis results, which contained multiple SNPs, including the same SNP Natalie has. In so doing, Catherine situated specific SNPs within the context of her genome and her overall health. She explained that despite trying different diets and supplements, she had been feeling terrible for years, with no improvement. Her symptoms included hair loss, rashes, extreme fatigue, blurred vision, gastrointestinal issues, brain fog, insomnia, muscle aches, anxiety, and depression. Catherine wrote, "I have very low quality of life these days. Have to push through everything." Hoping to provide the group with some contextual clues that might help the other members diagnose and provide feedback on her situation, she indicated that she has positive antinuclear antibodies, the Epstein-Barr virus, smooth saline breast implants, normal thyroid levels, and elevated B12.

*Elizabeth posted a photo of a red rash on her forehead, chin, and around her nose to the online support group. She described the rash as bumpy and painful, and implored the group, "I'm so frustrated with my skin! . . . *Frowning face emoji* Any ideas?" Likewise, Madeline posted a photo of cracks and peeling skin on her hand, an issue she described as chronic. She wrote, "Can anyone help me figure out what this is?" Madeline suspected ringworm but was open to other ideas. She continued, "Somebody please help me figure out what this is and how to cure it. . . . Thoughts?"*

Over the course of my ethnographic research, I observed how Facebook groups, comprised of like-minded individuals, are able to build informational resources for chronic-disease reversal through collaborative effort and a hive mind. I use the term "hive mind" to conjure an analogy of how a colony of bees behaves: as if guided by a single intelligence. Other terms for the same phenomenon include collective consciousness, gestalt intelligence, and mind coalescence. When presenting a question to a group filled with thousands of patients who have similar diagnoses or who subscribe to the same approach for healing, the amount of information that can be gleaned from the group is jaw-dropping—what one group member characterized as "INFORMATIONOVERLOAD." The missing space between "information" and "overload" could be a typo—but it is just as likely that the missing space intentionally signals the nonstop flow of information via Facebook groups. The hive is always buzzing.

Individuals use online communities to exchange experiential knowledge that is perceived as extending far beyond what one might learn in the course of conventional medical care (see Kingod et al. 2017). At times, the group responded to intimate, and potentially taboo, questions from members seeking help. Regardless of the question at hand, the Facebook group members took on the functioning of a hive mind in the comments section for each of these posts. Group members responded to each question by seeking a detailed history, suggesting specific lab tests, indicating optimal ranges for biomarkers, making dietary recommendations, and identifying tailored supplements that have worked for them. At times they shared templates and apps used for tracking symptoms and reactions to specific foods.

Questions like Stacy's about her challenges with depression, together with related questions regarding interactions among thyroid medications and antidepressants, were not stigmatized by fellow group members since many of them had faced similar situations. In another instance, a group member posted a 3D image of her armpit, asking if the group had any insight into the underlying cause of what she considered to be a structural anomaly. A different group member asked the group about the underlying causes of a red patch and areas of white coating on her tongue. This post was accompanied by a high-resolution photo and garnered hundreds of responses. Members of the community responded to each of these intimate posts hoping to provide insight and support, not to cast judgment.

Natalie, a "newbie" to the group, received encouragement about her inability to find foods she could eat, as well as functional health education. A member responded to her cry for help, writing, "Thank you for reaching out. . . . That takes bravery." This member went on to explain some foundational functional medicine concepts regarding nutrition absorption, gut health, and the microbiome. She furthermore suggested that Natalie address potential underlying issues such as leaky gut, SIBO (small-intestine bacterial overgrowth), mold toxicity, and autoimmune disorders. In contrast, the hive's response to Catherine's query and her long list of symptoms and lab results was fine-tuned to someone who has a firmer grasp of functional medicine concepts. Thus, comments and suggestions included abbreviations and advanced-level terminology.

In Elizabeth's case, multiple group members agreed, based on location and pattern, that she most likely had a butterfly rash—a lupus symptom—but a diagnosis of lupus would need to be confirmed with a blood test. Multiple group members also agreed that Madeline's skin problem, on her hand, was not ringworm. In all cases, the goal of the group was to provide pieces of information that might help the inquirers to better identify and understand their health issues; to suggest natural, nutrition-based therapies; and to offer encouragement.

During the COVID-19 pandemic, Facebook support groups turned their "hive mind" to so-called long-hauler symptoms of patients who had never been hospitalized for COVID-19 but were nonetheless struggling with long-term symptoms. In an October 7, 2020, news story on *Good Morning America*, ABC News reporter Eva Pilgrim relates, "A lot of the patients that we've spoken to say they've found resources and advice on Facebook support groups, and that is how they've found the clinics and the doctors that they are now going to." Long-hauler symptoms include fatigue, body aches, shortness of breath, difficulty breathing, and inability to be active. Dr. Jennifer Ashton, an expert who was interviewed in the piece, indicates, "We've seen other, similar syndromes after infection, sometimes after viruses [like] Epstein-Barr and chronic Lyme. We've seen it with chronic fatigue syndrome, and we've even seen it after SARS." Many functional medicine patients, myself included, have suffered and recovered from the syndromes Dr. Ashton named, and in the wake of the COVID-19 pandemic, the "hive" continues to buzz to connect chronic-disease patients to the resources they need to recover.

Critiques of the Cost of Functional Medicine

Maxine, a newbie, reached out to the group for advice regarding her daughter's complex web of symptoms. After listing her daughter's many symptoms, she asked the group, "Any advice on where to start to help her?" The very first response was, "I would suggest finding a certified functional medicine practitioner or functional diagnostic nutrition practitioner." In the comments section, the group proceeded to help Maxine identify a practitioner in her area.

Lauren similarly asked the group what type of doctor was most helpful in her group mates' healing journeys. This question elicited a flurry of responses:

> *"[I spent] three years with an [endocrinologist] and nothing happened. In three months I am seeing results [with a functional medicine doctor]."*
> *"Integrative Medicine."*
> *"Functional."*
> *"Functional x 100."*
> *"Myself and doing my own research."*
> *"Functional medicine doctor 100%!"*
> *"Functional med for sure!!"*
> *"Functional."*
> *"I feel like I would have died without seeing my functional medicine doctor."*
> *"My functional MD is the only one I trust."*
> *"My functional doctor gave me my life back."*
> *"I'll never go back to a regular doctor again."*

> *"[My functional doctor] has discovered things I had no idea I had. It's overwhelming, but at least now I have answers."*
> *"[I like functional medicine] 100% more than [conventional endocrinology]!"*
> *"My functional medicine doctor knows more about this disease than my [endocrinologist]."*
> *"I fired SIX conventional doctors before I found [my MD who takes a functional/integrative approach], and I thank God all the time for her!"*
> *"I felt like I was slowly dying going to my regular doctor. If you read all the comments here, no one is saying that a functional medicine doctor was NOT able to help them."*

*While most group members agreed functional medicine produced the best outcomes, many members also expressed frustration with its high cost. Referring to how functional medicine providers often offer packaged recovery protocols that combine health education with lifestyle changes, Susanna inquired whether anyone in the group had been able to make substantial progress without paying for expensive functional medicine "programs." She indicated, "I constantly get the feeling I'm too poor to get healthy. *Laugh/cry emoji*" Responding to the functional medicine recommendation that patients should develop stress-management techniques for the overall betterment of their health, Susanna continued, "Sure, I know that, but can I get there? I don't live on an island with tons of money so I don't have to work or have any problems anymore. So how is that feasible at all? I mean, how do you do it as an average person?"*

Lily agreed with how expense becomes an insurmountable obstacle, mentioning two functional medicine doctors who charge $11,000 to $15,000 for an annual membership that includes one hour per month of online follow-up. Lily explained that the membership price does not include the cost of supplements (the doctor's personal brand), lab work, and other required tests. In a similar vein, Hillary asked her group mates if anyone had sought treatment from a functional medicine doctor that "charges $10,000 to get well?" In response, Ann said she did seek this type of treatment for a few years and saw positive results. However, she was forced to quit her treatment because she simply could not afford the provider's rates or the prescribed supplements. Marissa indicated that she had spent over $18,000 on functional medicine but never got her thyroid problem fully under control. She stopped seeing her functional *medicine specialist because the provider "moved to the ritzy part of town, raised her rates, stopped taking medical insurance, charges for 'reading' your test results, and will no longer work in coordination with my family doctor." Mary noted that she saw a high-cost functional medicine provider for an initial visit that involved blood work. However, the provider wanted $4,000 for a "report of findings and plan of action." She did not go back after the initial visit.*

To be clear, these shocking price tags are not representative of functional medicine costs across the board. In another thread, group members compared prices for the functional medicine services they were actively receiving. While some described being charged $2,000 to $3,000 for a single visit and $4,000 for labs, others indicated that they were paying as little as $75 per visit and $150 for labs. The majority of responses fell between these two extremes.

Group members responded to those facing financial obstacles with cost-saving suggestions, such as working with a functional diagnostic nutrition practitioner instead of a functional medicine doctor. Another suggestion was buying the provider's book, which the member described as "[their] entire life's work in one volume." Individual practitioners' paperback books cost approximately ten to twenty dollars and provide detailed explanations of the protocols they use in clinic, thus allowing self-led patients to implement the protocols for themselves while circumventing the high costs of provider-led care.

As the thread developed, group members who had been following Susanna's post because they shared similar concerns regarding the high costs of functional medicine expressed how helpful their group mates' suggestions were. Susanna responded to these comments by saying, "I . . . think we discussed constructively by finding ways to proceed without having the pleasure of working with one of those experts."

Many members of the online support groups I observed encountered financial obstacles and limitations, leading some to deliver pointed critiques of what they considered exorbitant rates among functional medicine providers.[7] Responding to Ann, Marissa, and Mary, group members called the high prices charged by functional medicine providers "shameful" and a form of "insanity." The frustration that group members expressed regarding the high costs of functional medicine (feeling "too poor to get healthy") points to grave problems of accessibility.

However, not everyone in the group faced the same degree of price-based exclusion. One member responded to the group by saying that she pays $300 per visit and that this amount was not prohibitive for her. Her figure was on a par with what I spent during the latter part of my healing journey, when I transitioned from an entirely self-led protocol to seeking some guidance from a functional medicine nutritionist and a functional medicine doctor. Nonetheless, I argue that for many, the financial barriers are still too high.[8]

Facebook groups harness the "hive mind" to address individual members' concerns, including those about affordability of specific protocols, diets, and lifestyle changes. Without referencing Maskell, these members, myself included, followed his "three *C*s" approach to cost savings. Group members encouraged Susanna to seek out "coaching" from auxiliary functional health professionals who charge much less than their physician counterparts. Furthermore, they suggested that Susanna seek out "content" over care by purchasing the provider's book and implementing the protocol herself, thus offering her "ways to proceed without having the pleasure of working with one of those experts," in her words. The subversive tactics I observed run counter to Kingod et al.'s (2017) assertion that the social ties created in online peer-to-peer support groups supported offline ties and patient-doctor relationships. In the patient-organized online groups I participated in, members recognized the important role of "community" when it comes to accessing health information, and, in so doing, contested the primacy of the patient-provider therapeutic relationship.

Patients like Susanna and me are able to overcome barriers to access and piece together personalized protocols based on coaching, content, and community; however, our ability to do so, in and of itself, signals an intersection of social, cultural, and economic capital (Bourdieu 1984) in the form of online social networks, health literacy, and the purchase of salugens. Without these intersecting forms of capital, many chronically ill individuals are simply priced out of functional medicine care. While digitized biosociality helps certain patients navigate the high costs of functional medicine, it simultaneously creates spaces in which the social determinants of recovery are laid bare.

To clarify this point, I will share my experience attending an in vitro fertilization (IVF) support group and contrast it with the online groups I describe in this chapter. The IVF support group I attended was organized by the clinic where I underwent egg retrieval. Meetings were held in a conference room at the clinic. Everyone in the group lived within the same relative area since they were all patients at the clinic. Furthermore, everyone was middle to upper-middle class—the couples in the group were all working professionals who paid for IVF out of pocket but for whom IVF represented a significant financial burden. Thus, support group members could relate to one another based on their shared experience of IVF, their residency in the same city, and their similar class standing.

The digitized biosociality I observed online was distinct. While members of the Facebook groups were seeking information regarding the functional approach to healing, they did not live in geographic proximity to one another and were often from different socioeconomic classes. I argue that by spanning geographic and class differences, digitized biosociality underscores the lived effects of socioeconomic inequality and, thus, plays a paradoxical role in some group members' lives. On the one hand, group members were offered support and encouragement from like-minded health seekers—people with whom they would have had no contact if it were not for the digital nature of the group. On the other hand, learning about expensive therapies that are out of one's economic reach can cause individuals to feel disheartened, and day-to-day (digital) socialization with people who receive therapies one cannot afford brings issues of inequality into sharp relief. By bringing together individuals with disparate financial means, Facebook groups cause the lesser privileged to be acutely aware of the types of care and (self-)knowledge they cannot afford to purchase. I further develop the concept of (self-)knowledge, and its relationship to different forms of capital, in the next section.

(SELF-)KNOWLEDGE AT THE INTERSECTION OF RELATIONALITY AND CONSUMPTION

When patients take on more agentive roles and make science-informed decisions, they do so as social beings. The knowledge individuals possess and the decisions they make are largely influenced by their community. Turning to food as one example, Dr. Cynthia Li explains that in order for food as medicine to become second nature, individuals must first be exposed to the basic information: "This is something that schoolteachers should be teaching kids, that coaches should be teaching athletes, that doctors should be telling patients, and families should be sharing among themselves." The way people come to know new knowledge is often through interactions with others. In essence, knowledge is relational.

Functional medicine interlocutors value a particular form of knowledge: self-knowledge. By using the term "self-knowledge," I am referring to how functional medicine participants must become experts on their own biologies. The goal of each of the three Cs—content, community, and coaching—is for patients to gather actionable information that can lead to their improved health. Dr. Dan Pardi, a cognitive neuroscientist who has been featured by TED and Stanford Medicine X, explains that individuals are trying to "understand themselves better" and to determine how to "meaningfully augment their day-to-day experience." His words point to the broadly held perspective in functional medicine that one's efficiency in locating and learning copious amounts of health information and subsequently implementing this information as self-knowledge is key in reversing chronic disease.

Given the expectation that individuals will become masters of their own biologies, are patient-organized online groups an example of alternative media? Christian Fuchs and Vincent Mosco indicate that alternative media challenges the commodity character of media since "it aims at a reversal so that use value becomes the dominant feature of media and technology by the sublation of their exchange value" (Fuchs and Mosco 2015, 12). Fuchs and Mosco describe recipients of this media as empowered in questioning the commodified character of the digital world. The way in which members of patient-organized Facebook groups critique the high cost of functional medicine, utilizing a hive mind to subvert existing price structures, suggests that these groups are potentially an empowering form of alternative media.

Scholars have characterized online communities as a good example of how patient empowerment—defined as giving patients the ability to develop mastery over their actions and control over their decisions—occurs independently of and complementarily to the intervention of health care providers and insurers. Victoria Johansson et al. (2021) describe empowerment as both a process and an outcome resulting from participation in online patient communities. Eugenia Lamas et al. (2017, 43) take this argument regarding empowerment a step further when they describe novel forms of "lay crowd-sourced expertise" resulting from the daily exchange among chronic-disease patients and their family members. They assert that this "bottom-up data generation," previously unknown in biomedical sciences, shifts the equilibrium of power away from professionals and toward patients.

Within the functional medicine realm, self-knowledge is portrayed as a form of "empowerment."[9] In an automated email, Shivan Sarna, a SIBO expert, writes, "Hi SIBO Superhero. . . . **You are empowered with the information you need to heal your gut issues once and for all**" (emphasis in original). By addressing email recipients as "SIBO Superhero[es]," Sarna is positioning each recipient as the protagonist of their own healing journey. Her email then directs readers to multiple sources for learning self-knowledge, indicating that she hosts monthly master classes and Q&A sessions with SIBO experts, has "an entire vault of past Masterclasses just waiting for you to dive into," and hosts "Facebook Live" sessions with SIBO experts. Her email implicitly suggests that functional medicine participants are responsible for accruing self-knowledge by explicitly stating, in bold letters, that participants are empowered with the needed information for healing.

While conducting ethnographic research for this book, I felt interpellated as someone "empowered" by self-knowledge. My email inbox was constantly inundated with alerts regarding free master classes. These "master classes" were usually just a "hook"—they merely described the vast amount of powerful, actionable self-knowledge that individuals could accrue by paying for an extended eCourse on the topic at hand. Many functional medicine practitioners' websites include a "Learn" or "Courses" tab. For example, nutritional consultant Donna Gates's website, Body Ecology, has a "Courses" page that reads, "Be educated. Select the course you are most interested in." The page includes a drop-down menu of courses, beginning with "BE101—The Essential Body Ecology Course." This book is, in part, the result of my interpellation—the product of my digital autoethnographic journey.

My observations are supported by the work of Natalie Ann Hendry, a media and communications researcher. Hendry (2022) describes how "wellness emails" circulate content through automated email list subscriptions while potentially escaping social media censorship and public health scrutiny. These emails offer personal and marketized engagement by "promis[ing] an always-ready, abundant space for transforming bodies and optimizing health."

Furthermore, Hendry (2022) describes these "wellness emails" as using time-critical marketing tactics that encourage recipients not to "miss out on opportunities." Similarly, functional medicine online events aggregate interviews from multiple experts, thus delivering hours of video material per day. Interviews "expire" and new interviews are posted each day of the event, thus incentivizing viewers to purchase a "package" so they can view all the material at a less frenetic pace.

In one unique instance, Dr. Jay Davidson, a chiropractor and cofounder of CellCore Biosciences, disregarded this sales strategy when he addressed listeners on the Viral and Retroviral Summit and suggested that those who did not plan to purchase the summit examine the titles and topics and only listen to the interviews that made the most sense for their needs. He said, "It's so easy to be in this state of, 'I need to consume everything!' But what do *you* actually need? What do you need for knowledge?" Dr. Davidson indicated that his goal was to help listeners prevent "paralysis by analysis." This was the only time during my ethnographic research that I observed a functional medicine proponent undermining the self-knowledge-for-sale marketing structure.

In my ethnographic research, I learned that wellness companies and entrepreneurs generally use emails to entice recipients to engage with other forms of self-knowledge media, such as podcast interviews and articles. Viome—a company that uses transcriptomics to evaluate the gut microbiome—sent newsletters that linked to articles, recent scientific studies, and podcasts about topics related to their company. These "informative" resources all pointed to the value of the company's product. Viome's emails are just one example of how wellness companies and entrepreneurs capitalize on individuals' desire for self-knowledge by concealing marketing for products and services in forms of media (e.g., articles and interviews) that are not readily identified as advertisements.

Furthermore, the promise of self-knowledge lures bioconsumers into digital spaces that are designed to create revenue. Before gaining access to the self-knowledge they seek, bioconsumers must navigate around, and through, items and services for sale. One weekly email from Bulletproof, the biohacking company founded by Dave Asprey, provided two links to recent *Bulletproof Radio* podcast episodes. Before clicking on play on either episode, listeners first had to bypass a pop-up advertising Asprey's book, with direct links to every major retail outlet where his book is sold. Next, while scrolling past summaries and links to recent Bulletproof blog posts, email recipients were presented with the summary of an article about "the must-have, go-to, keto and Bulletproof groceries that should be on your list," featuring Bulletproof products. Then, email recipients saw a tantalizing photo with a link to a breakfast recipe. The recipe indicated that "this savory, zingy dish" was created out of a partnership between Bulletproof and a grass-fed, pastured meat delivery service. The self-knowledge "bait"—the podcast episodes—was buried under multiple layers of apparent and inconspicuous marketing.

In addition to emails, I received numerous Facebook messages offering free eBooks that, like Bulletproof's email, interwove potential self-knowledge with advertisements for sponsored products. One such message enticed Facebook users to download a free eBook that was "expiring" the same day. The message boasted over thirty thousand downloads and indicated the eBook contained lessons about "a special oil that inhibits inflammation causing chemicals; soil-derived, natural compound that helps protect your brain; 'golden' spice with an anti-inflammatory effect equivalent to NSAIDs;

freshwater 'superfood' that fights inflammation; and more!" Access to this "free gift" required individuals to provide their names and email addresses. Those who downloaded the free eBook began receiving email advertisements shortly thereafter for a docuseries by Jonathan Otto—a self-described "investigative journalist, filmmaker and humanitarian" who has created multiple docuseries regarding different approaches to chronic disease.[10] Watching the docuseries was also free; however, as I will explore further in the next section, access to the filmmaker's online Facebook community comes at a cost.

In essence, self-knowledge is potentiated by economic capital. Costs that consumers incur on their quests toward self-knowledge include fees for things such as courses, direct-to-consumer laboratory tests, books, salugens, and, at times, in-person conference attendance. For example, in the docuseries *Betrayal: The Autoimmune Disease Solution They're Not Telling You*, Celeste McGovern mentions that she traveled to a congress in Nice, France, when she was "trying to absorb everything she could" regarding celiac disease and autoimmunity. A few weeks before the congress, McGovern, a health and science journalist, saw the speaker lineup on the schedule and thought, "I have got to go there and speak to this [particular doctor] and hear what they are saying." She booked a last-minute flight to Nice. At the congress, she was "gobsmacked" by each consecutive presentation—she could not believe what she was hearing. McGovern's ability to pay for a last-minute flight to France, hotel accommodations, and conference registration is evidence of her "economic capital" (Bourdieu 1984).

Likewise, I was able to attend continuing medical education events, such as the Advances in Mitochondrial Medicine Symposium, because of my socioeconomic privilege. In each case, I tried to save money by using available frequent flyer points from a family member and staying at the most inexpensive hotel within a several-mile radius of the conference site. Nonetheless, these trips cost thousands of dollars. The registration fee alone for the Institute for Functional Medicine's 2020 Annual International Conference was $1,075.[11]

Stated simply, knowledge consumption requires economic capital. In making this argument, I am imbuing the words "knowledge consumption" with a dual meaning—the absorption of information, on the one hand, and the way access to information is often available for purchase, on the other. Over the course of my ethnographic research, I observed how knowledge is doubly consumed in participants' efforts to create their unique protocols.

Since functional medicine participants have overlapping disease etiologies, individual members share their self-knowledge to help other members of the group progress along their health journeys. Thus, I use the partially parenthetical term "(self-)knowledge" to signal how self-knowledge becomes shareable and applicable to others. Members like Natalie are desperately seeking help, hoping someone else in the group will be able to shed light on their personal situations. These members are lacking, and actively seeking, self-knowledge. Meanwhile, members who respond to inquiries like hers are possessors of (self-)knowledge. Their participation in the group provides "newbies" with the valuable information they need to gain a foothold in the functional medicine approach to healing. As (self-)knowledge circulates in online communities, it becomes a form of social capital (Bourdieu 1984; see also R. Putnam 2000).

Furthermore, social capital stands in for economic capital. Those who possess the most (self-)knowledge and, therefore, social capital in online communities are often also those with the greatest socioeconomic resources. They are able to pay for expensive lab testing out of pocket and may work with a functional medicine practitioner on a one-to-one basis.[12] Thus, social capital in online functional medicine communities is often anchored in economic capital. In making this argument, I am building upon and adding nuance to the existing literature on digital capitalism.

Cristina Morini and Andrea Fumagalli argue that our contemporary transition from Fordism to biocapitalism entails a new series of socioeconomic relationships involving the embodiment of relational, emotional, and intellectual capacities and resources; that is, individuals' "ability to activate social links can be translated into exchange value" (2010, 236). For example, Facebook possesses no value without the social relationships and intellectual engagement of its users. Thus, the individual is the coproducer and therefore an unwaged audience-laborer (or "digital housewife" [see Jarrett 2016]) of what she consumes. As Fuchs and Mosco put it, "In recent times, recipients have increasingly become an active audience that produces content and technologies, which does not imply a democratization of the media, but mainly a new form of exploitation of audiences and users" (2015, 11). While commercial mass media is based on low exploitation and high alienation, Facebook, according to Eran Fisher (2015), produces the exacerbation of exploitation and the mitigation of alienation. In this view, the consumption of services, along with the social relationships this entails, becomes an asset for companies. Wittel (2015) suggests that while the means of information production have become more accessible in the digital age, the capitalist class controls the means of information distribution.

While Morini and Fumagalli might consider patients in Facebook groups to be unwaged audience-laborers and Jarrett might position them as specialized digital housewives, I note how possessors of (self-)knowledge are sometimes able to translate socioeconomic privilege into social capital. My ethnographic observations in patient-organized Facebook groups are also suggestive of resistance to exploitation, alongside the mitigation of alienation—and even the appropriation of knowledge "products." The autonomous organization of these online groups safeguards them from companies and entrepreneurs hoping to sell services and capitalize on social relationships. In the next section, however, I explore instances where this is not always the case.

NON-PATIENT-ORGANIZED GROUPS

From a functional medicine perspective, individual patients possess authority over their own healing; however, the outcome of their pursuit of health is largely determined by the degree of care they receive from their community. Maskell shares the following quote by the award-winning writer, researcher, and community organizer Nakita Valerio: "Shouting 'self-care' at people who actually need 'community care' is how we fail people." Maskell points to how Valerio's quote turns the contemporary emphasis on self-care on its head, writing, "The extreme focus on 'self-care' that has permeated the culture in which we live is not necessarily as health promoting as it might seem." Fundamentally, functional medicine argues for a shift in emphasis from self-care as an individual undertaking to community care as a relational endeavor.

Furthermore, functional medicine proponents link society's overemphasis on self-care to a broader context of globalization and the outsourcing of care. Reminiscent of geographer David Harvey's (1990) notion of time-space compression, the expansion of technology has, in some ways, Maskell notes, made our world "smaller." Maskell writes in his email newsletter, "We have become accustomed to sourcing the majority of our products and services from random strangers and corporate behemoths (think Uber, Wal-Mart), rather than sourcing them from people we know in our communities." Individuals feel a need for greater self-care because, unless they can afford paid help, they are now tasked with many of the caring responsibilities (e.g., child rearing and support for elders) that have historically been shared by the community: they are overworking themselves.[13] Functional medicine interlocutors like Maskell argue that what individuals need is not more self-care, but a stronger community.

In this vein, many functional medicine interlocutors contrast the detrimental health effects of loneliness with the longevity-conferring effects of human connection. For example, Vishen Lakhiani—founder and CEO of Mindvalley, a "life transformation platform with a global community"[14]—opines that people in the Western world are lonelier than ever because, despite increased "connectedness" via social media, they lack a sense of community with the people around them. A historical transition toward urbanization has left individuals struggling with the isolating effects of anonymity. In contrast, he cites the lifework of psychological well-being researcher Ed Diener and indicates, "Nothing seems to bring human beings happiness more than the strength of our social connection." He furthermore hypothesizes that the happiness derived from a strong sense of community has life-extending effects.

Within functional medicine discourse, community has furthermore emerged as the antidote to the contemporary ills of urbanization, globalization, loneliness, and anonymity, thus creating new business opportunities for functional medicine practitioners and functional medicine–adjacent entrepreneurs. For example, Lakhiani indicates, "In everything I do at Mindvalley, community is a key part. . . . We bake that into our business model. . . . We're trying to create a product for community." When watching his interview, I was initially confused by the latter part of his statement. I thought he meant that Mindvalley was developing a product that creates community—this interpretation makes sense given Lakhiani's assertion that community is "baked into" Mindvalley's business model. However, as his interview unfolds, Lakhiani indicates that community is the biggest missing piece in people's lives and he critiques how individuals "try to fill this hole by buying craptastic products." It was then that I realized the source of my confusion: at the same time functional medicine–adjacent entrepreneurs critique society's attempts to assuage loneliness through neoliberal consumption, they market and sell access to spaces and events where community *is* the commodity.[15]

In essence, functional medicine interlocutors frame community as a valuable resource for healing and recovery. Maskell describes a presentation Dr. Wahls gave in 2017 regarding her use of groups to scale up the delivery of her protocol. This presentation was deeply moving to Maskell—so much so that it provided the inspiration for his second book, *The Community Cure: Transforming Health Outcomes Together*. Maskell wrote after the presentation, "The group members saw other members of the group who had made progress as even more relatable and inspiring than Dr. Wahls [herself] . . . even though she has fully recovered from the exact issue they were facing and they were following her protocol."[16] From a functional medicine perspective, this finding points to the unique power of peer-to-peer engagement and support. In the following subsection, I explore how functional medicine practitioners attempt to leverage the power of peer-to-peer networks by organizing Facebook groups that bear their names but within which they usually do not actively participate.

Practitioner-Hosted Peer-to-Peer Networks

Recognizing the need for community, some functional medicine practitioners create and host Facebook groups. Patients are invited to join the practitioner's Facebook group after going to the practitioner's personal web page. For example, an automated email from Dr. David Jockers, a doctor of natural medicine and chiropractor who specializes in functional nutrition, concludes with, "P.S. Have you joined our private . . . Facebook group yet? The group was designed to help people (just like you) get answers." Likewise, I received an email from Dr. Amy Myers. The automated email, which contained a photo of Dr. Myers next to her slogan "The Myers Way®," was scripted as a personal invitation to a Facebook group hosted by Dr. Myers's staff. The email read, "Hi Rosalynn, Our community is full of supportive and knowledgeable individuals who have also made the commitment to take their health into their own hands." The email went on to describe this Facebook "community" as a welcoming space to ask questions, read discussions, hear others' success stories, and offer advice. These "personally addressed" mass emails are designed to recruit patient-client-followers to protocol- or diet-specific Facebook groups.[17]

Access to Dr. Myers's group is free; however, the title "The Myers Way Facebook Community Group by Amy Myers MD" serves to market—and create marketing for—Dr. Myers's products and programs. The group feed begins with an invitation from "Amy Myers MD" to share a photo or video of "amazing results" using one of Dr. Myers's products or programs, for a chance to win a $50 to $100 gift card to the Amy Myers Store. The invitation includes a disclaimer that the photos and videos that are selected "may also be shared across our social media channels, emailed to our new customers, and featured on our website!" The rest of the feed is filled with questions and comments from group members about Dr. Myers's books, products, and protocol.

Other functional medicine practitioners and health educators offer access to their Facebook groups after patients have purchased their protocols or participated in their healing programs. For example, Dr. Kelly

Brogan describes how she has created a space for patient-patient support through the Facebook group "Vital Life Project"—an "online membership community for health reclamation." Dr. Brogan argues that the core offering of this program is the community. While membership includes a nutrition and lifestyle protocol, she emphasizes that this is secondary.

As Maskell noted in his comments about the groups of individuals following Dr. Wahls's protocol, Dr. Brogan has also found that providing patients with a peer-to-peer network produces better outcomes than one-on-one care. She believes that witnessing what is possible through the successful health reclamation of others in a collective is the most powerful force for change—so much so that, when comparing the outcomes of her online program to her in-person practice, Dr. Brogan calls her practice "a waste of time." These different outcomes have led Dr. Brogan to appreciate the healing power of community and to embrace Thich Nhat Hanh's quote "Community is the guru of the future."[18] Dr. Brogan's assertions amend the broadly held functional medicine perspective that healing is attained by doing "all the things"—following a protocol, taking supplements, using advanced lab tests, resolving root causes, etc. She is not arguing that "all the things" are unnecessary. However, she has found that out of everything, community is uniquely responsible for helping people get better faster.

Dr. Brogan's online peer-to-peer network unfolds in stark contrast to her private practice since she does not participate in the online group. She describes the online group as "a space, a container, for people to feel held by a collective, for people to be reflected by their highest potential when they're feeling vulnerable." Conversely, the one-to-one care she provides in her practice falls into "the old model"—what she describes as the "master-student, guru-practitioner kind of model"—despite her desire to create a partnership with patients. Comparing the two models, Dr. Brogan indicates, "It's the same exact program, literally. The only difference is the community."

Throughout my ethnographic research, I saw Dr. Brogan's perspective echoed by functional medicine providers and health educators alike. Health coach and fatigue specialist Ari Whitten observed that individuals who had completed his healing program four years earlier continued to be active in his Energy Blueprint members group on an every-other-day basis. Whitten's group is another example of an online community that is available to individuals who have purchased a particular healing program. While functional medicine providers and health educators consider these groups to be a valuable healing resource within their protocol, I signal how they inadvertently commodify "community." In the next section, I turn to how "community" is further commodified by docuseries hosts who include access to online patient groups as part of "packaged deals" for those who purchase their docuseries.

Docuseries-Linked Facebook Communities

Many of the docuseries included in my ethnographic research directly exemplify the commodification of membership in a functional medicine community. In his docuseries *Autoimmune Secrets*, Jonathan Otto describes the "platinum package" as the docuseries' "best value" since it confers access to its private, members-only Facebook group, along with the six-module Autoimmune Recovery Protocol and twenty-five previously recorded Q&A group calls with functional practitioners such as Dr. Jay Davidson, Dr. Elena Villanueva, Dr. Rodger Murphree, Dr. Todd Watts, and Dr. David Jockers. Otto indicates that "survivors" who have reversed their own challenges through engaging with the series are members of the group and that these expert-patients "love answering your questions . . . supporting you and getting to see you get a leg up!" He emphasizes that access to his private Facebook community for one year usually costs $500, but membership is included as a "free gift" in the platinum package—and also saves viewers thousands of dollars on appointments, months on providers' waiting lists, and hours of travel. In response to Otto's final point, I suggest that the *Autoimmune Secrets* Facebook community is an example of how digital communication, characterized by personalization and ubiquitous connection, has resulted in a speeding up of the capital cycle (see Manzerolle and Kjøsen 2015).

Jonathon Otto's tactic was extended by his sister, Sarah Otto, one of the filmmakers of the docuseries *The Gut Solution*, along with her husband, Matt Potts. She indicates in the film that those who "choose to own" the *Gut Solution* platinum package will have access to the *Virtual Health Retreat* as well and that "this is where you find answers, this is where you find a community that supports you."[19] Potts adds that their community allows platinum package "owners" to obtain expert opinions "without having to spend the thousands of dollars that it usually takes to see someone decent." Signaling the couple's social capital, he indicates that one of the doctors whom they know—a popular doctor who appears in the series—has a two-year waiting list. His comment harks back to my observation about how, in the functional medicine realm, docuseries hosts harness the commodification of online groups to accelerate the generation of profit.

Furthermore, Sarah Otto's juxtaposition of the words "choose to" and "own" underscores how functional medicine is embedded in neoliberal ideology. At the same time, online patient groups encourage personal responsibility and evince neoliberal governance. Based on their research on digital self-advocacy in online patient communities, Allegra Clare Schermuly, Alan Petersen, and Alison Anderson (2019) suggest a shift away from "biological citizenship" and toward "bio-digital citizenship." In their view, digital media serves to align contemporary patient communities' interests with those of science and business, resulting in a fundamental reorientation of "activism."[20] In 2021, they noted a shift in patients' conceptions of their agentic selves from "activists" to "advocates" and argued that "digital self-advocacy" limits rather than facilitates health justice (see Schermuly, Petersen, and Anderson 2021). In the realm of functional medicine, "digital self-advocates" sought membership in online groups as part of their drive for personal responsibility in their own recovery instead of engaging in activism around health as a citizenship-based right.

At times, "bio-digital citizenship" was not only encouraged but elicited using manipulative tactics. For example, Sarah Otto's marketing efforts take a disturbing turn in the film when she insists that she and Potts are not "desperate" for viewers to join, saying, "We have so many people that have already purchased . . . that we have to consider closing the doors because it is getting so full. By all means, you are welcome to try and do this on your own." Instead, though, she argues, viewers should want to join because they will not recover their health if they do not join. She goes further, "You can try and find a local doctor. You can try and Google. You can try and ask your spouse, [who] may be thinking that what you are saying isn't even true." With these tactics, she presents viewers with two options: "One, stay as you are, to stay sick, to stay frustrated, and to be without support; or two, you can make the decision to take action and actually see results." Then, in an email to viewers, she emphasizes that viewers have only sixteen hours remaining in which to opt in, writing, "You can either take action today to join a supportive community and gain all of the resources you need . . . or you can continue struggling to find the answers on your own. It's really that simple." Returning to the observation by Hendry (2022) of how time-critical marketing tactics are used in wellness emails, Sarah Otto reiterates in the post-docuseries email, "We encourage you to take advantage of this special offer before it expires. . . . You don't have to. No one is forcing you to. . . . [But] it's going to take you a lot longer to find these answers on your own."

I read these words and felt that Sarah Otto's message was both contrived and threatening. It can be argued that docuseries hosts are motivated by a desire to connect patient-consumers with the providers who helped them and their family members on their paths to recovery, or even that they have a need to recoup some of the cost they incurred to see functional medicine experts.[21] Throughout *The Gut Solution*, both siblings and their spouses share how they have used functional medicine to recover from chronic disease. Furthermore, Potts indicates, "People don't have that time or they don't have that money, and so we wanted to create a community so we can better serve people and actually help them bridge that gap a little bit and connect them with the right people." However, the good intentions he signals are tainted by Sarah's unsettling, manipulative undertone. Whatever their true intentions may be, Jonathan Otto and Sarah Otto have configured belonging in online functional medicine communities as a commodity to be bought and sold.

In this chapter, I have asked whether functional medicine online communities advance capitalist agendas or whether these communities are contributing to an alternative media—that is, alternative ways of organizing and producing media to create critical context that challenges capitalism. Through ethnographic research, I observed how the commodification of community is one way the digitization of biosociality has inadvertently reinforced neoliberal logics of inclusion and exclusion. While the patient-organized communities I describe in this chapter represent a form of resistance to these commodifying tendencies, even these communities can unwittingly reinforce social hierarchies.

The commodification of community described in this chapter prefaces what is to come in the next chapter. Online health forums often double as spaces for the commodification of patient opinion.[22] Deborah Lupton (2014) explores what she calls "the digital patient experience economy"—how patients' opinions and experiences are exploited through prosumption (the combination of production and content consumption), the valorizing of Big Data, and the commercialization of affective labor—to shed light on the growing commercial uses of the data that online health forums generate. That is, companies use social media to obtain data on their market audience and to co-create products with clients (Onomake 2021). In the next chapter, I build on the notion of community as a digital capitalist commodity to examine the multiple tactics functional medicine entrepreneurs employ when interpellating health seekers as consumers.

CHAPTER 5

DOCTOR-INFLUENCERS

In this chapter, I pull back the curtain and expose differences between discourse among functional medicine entrepreneurs and discourse directed at functional medicine consumers. While functional medicine practitioners and health educators interact with one another as entrepreneurs and "visionaries," they interact with consumers as teachers, wounded healers, guides, and "influencers."[1] The distinct positionality of functional medicine doctor-influencers and their patient-consumers results in a "mutual gaze"—with each group hoping to benefit from the interaction (see Baruah 2017).

I furthermore explore the diverse marketing strategies of functional medicine entrepreneurs. In the process, I endeavor to examine functional medicine "influencer pedagogy" (Hendry, Hartung, and Welch 2021)—the mediated processes of education resulting from relatable interactions between influencers and their followers on social media platforms—and how functional medicine entrepreneurship unfolds at the intersection of altruistic motivation and business savvy.

The central argument of this chapter is that the role of doctor-as-influencer is relationally produced and sustained. I therefore explore the three types of relationship that undergird the influencer role.

First, I consider how functional medicine entrepreneurs create an artificial sense of familiarity with consumers by maintaining "constant contact." Consumers receive an enormous number of automated emails that take the form of personal letters, offer "bonus gifts," and use time-critical marketing. Meanwhile, health educators—who also play a role as functional medicine entrepreneurs—use their illness narratives to create an aura of relatability, to leverage their (self-)knowledge as a form of currency via marketing messages, and to serve as what they call "referralists" for functional medicine practitioners.

Second, I analyze relationships among functional medicine entrepreneurs. I argue that the success of individual functional medicine entrepreneurs is dependent on the success of the community as a whole, thus emphasizing the importance of relational ties among these entrepreneurs. Community-based entrepreneurial practices structure relationships among functional medicine doctors and health educators, mutually ensuring their livelihoods. Furthermore, digital platforms recruit functional medicine entrepreneurs, offer overlapping commissions for promoting online events, and facilitate community-based marketing, thus reinforcing relational ties. In essence, relationships among functional medicine entrepreneurs are constituted and consolidated by specific financial structures.

Third, I turn to relationships between individual providers and their corporate sponsors. Corporate sponsors rely on the networking and communication of functional medicine entrepreneurs as a covert marketing tactic. During my ethnographic research, I observed chain-like marketing relationships. Corporate sponsors use familiarity as a strategy for attracting providers to "partnerships," just as providers use this strategy to interpellate health seekers as consumers.

In essence, this chapter details how functional medicine providers are multiply positioned, first as consumers of entrepreneurial know-how, then as entrepreneurs, subsequently as influencers, and finally as brands.

RELATIONSHIPS BETWEEN FUNCTIONAL MEDICINE ENTREPRENEURS AND CONSUMERS

> *I received an email from "Dr. Ryan Wohlfert <doc@upgradedparents.com>." The body of the email newsletter* Upgraded Parents *begins, "I made a mistake last weekend . . . and I'm not repeating it because I want to sleep tonight. *Smiley face emoji* Last weekend, I didn't tell you about Jason Prall's surprise* Human Longevity Project *binge-watch weekend. (And actually, he wasn't gonna do it, but he's having ANOTHER free-replay weekend right now. . . . Geez! It's a replay weekend extravaganza!!)" By admitting his "mistake" to email recipients, Dr. Wohlfert creates a sense of familiarity between himself and the recipient. By placing specifics about Prall's decision-making process in parentheses, Dr. Wohlfert simultaneously alludes to his familiar relationship with Prall—a filmmaker and functional health coach—and casts this behind-the-scenes knowledge as "insider information." The informality of his prose—for example, his use of "gonna" and "Geez!"—further establishes a sense of familiarity with the email recipient. The message reads like an email one might expect to receive from a close friend.*

Dr. Wohlfert continues, "Anyway, back to the main reason for this short email. Another friend and documentary filmmaker, Jonathan Otto (who was a huge part of my Superhuman Brain Masterclass), released a powerful 10-part docu-series called Autoimmune Secrets*.... There.... now I can sleep tonight." Dr. Wohlfert—almost certainly an affiliate of both docuseries—included direct links to* The Human Longevity Project *and* Autoimmune Secrets*. However, by referring to Otto as "a friend," he extends familiarity to a fellow member of the functional medicine community. His email is crafted in a "carefree" manner—the sentence "Anyway, back to the main reason for this short email" is suggestive of a stream-of-consciousness narrative style—thus again signaling familiarity to the email recipient. By writing "I can sleep tonight" and including a smiley face emoji in his email, Dr. Wohlfert frames email recipients as confidants and pals.*

In a different email, Dr. Wohlfert writes, "I ran out of my trail mix, so today I'm making Dr. Nandi's Honey Roasted Almonds. (I hope Dr. Nandi doesn't get mad at me, but I'm giving you the recipe!).... So, absolutely click here to download your free 77 Smoothies & Snacks *eCookbook, and join me for The Slim Gut Summit!" Dr. Wohlfert's inclusion of mundane personal details and use of parentheses again frame this email as private—like a whisper spoken from one friend to another. By simultaneously suggesting a familiar relationship with another functional medicine provider, Dr. Wohlfert once more employs bidirectional familiarity when promoting an online event for which he is likely an affiliate.*

*The tendency to include informal flourishes and emojis is not unique to Dr. Wohlfert. Angel Jockers, Dr. David Jockers's wife and "lead happiness manager" at DrJockers.com, writes in an email, "I wanted to personally introduce myself." Jockers goes on to explain that she has been "assigned to my account" and will be my direct point of contact if I have any questions or need any assistance during the "exclusive showing" of Dr. Jockers's online event. She concludes her email, "I look forward to chatting with you in the future. *Smiley face emoji*" In a subsequent email, she promotes packages for her husband's docuseries and concludes her email with "You're the best!" As Dr. Wohlfert and Angel Jocker's emails illustrate, when casting a net for potential consumers, the net is woven together with fibers of suggested familiarity.*

The amount of effort functional medicine entrepreneurs invest when interpellating health seekers as consumers is impressive. During the two months when I focused my research specifically on this topic, my inbox was constantly inundated with bioentrepreneurial messages. I did not sign up for individual entrepreneurs' listservs. Instead, these entrepreneurs accessed my name and email address after I entered my information while registering for a "free showing" of a docuseries, signing up for a "master class," or unlocking a "free gift." The sheer number of emails I received during these two months was extraordinary—in fact, the daily onslaught overwhelmed my Gmail account and, for the first time ever, I ran out of space. I was forced to manually unsubscribe from each individual listserv and delete large batches of emails to salvage my account.

The experience, however, allowed me to observe how functional medicine entrepreneurs maintain "constant contact" with consumers whose contact information they have gained access to through "gated content" that is unlocked only by entering in one's name, email address, and, sometimes, phone number. Consumers receive invitations to closed Facebook groups and personally addressed emails—some of which include the entrepreneurs' illness narratives, thus establishing a sense of commonality. Consumers often come across video clips and documentaries that further humanize functional medicine entrepreneurs and their work. Consumers may begin to receive text messages from these entrepreneurs and their companies. Simultaneously, consumers begin to see online advertisements for the functional medicine entrepreneurs' products and services. By maintaining "constant contact," these entrepreneurs strategically create an artificial sense of familiarity with consumers. Artificial familiarity is a strategy for attracting consumers—those who ultimately pay for these entrepreneurs' livelihoods.

The Role of Health Educators

Shivan Sarna, a SIBO expert and Home Shopping Network TV host, describes her role as a functional health educator in a welcome email to her listserv, explaining, "I find the innovators—the very best doctors and practitioners from around the world—people like Dr. Allison Siebecker, Dr. Mark Pimentel, and Dr. Steven Sandberg-Lewis (to name just a few) and give YOU access to their research, experience, and insights." Sarna asserts that her training in journalism makes her especially skilled at going to the source and getting the answers and lets email recipients know they can take advantage of her special skill set by participating in the different online events she hosts. She continues, "Every month I host a new Masterclass and Q&As with SIBO experts." Her self-description illustrates how the role of functional health educator is cemented by collaborative relationships with functional medicine practitioners.

In a subsequent email, Sarna uses the Independence Day holiday as a springboard to discuss how outdoor barbecues pose the potential for food poisoning and thus SIBO. After this introduction, she quickly segues into promoting Dr. Siebecker, who was mentioned in her introductory email and with whom she has an ongoing, collaborative, and therapeutic relationship: "I didn't always know these tips and tricks. Many of them I learned from my doctor (turned dear friend) Allison Siebecker, ND." By describing Dr. Siebecker as a "dear friend," Sarna contributes to the positioning of familiarity as an integral feature of functional medicine entrepreneurialism. She then succinctly positions Dr. Siebecker as a wounded healer, writing, "Dr. Siebecker is both a leading SIBO researcher and clinician AND a SIBO patient herself, so she really 'gets' what it is like." With these words, Sarna engages discursive forms that confer legitimacy, authority, and relatability within functional medicine. She explains that over the past couple of years, she and Dr. Siebecker collaborated on multiple classes to "make the powerful information she has taught me (and her other patients) available to YOU." Ultimately, Sarna offers Dr. Siebecker's SIBO educational materials at a "bundled" sale price.

In a different email, Sarna combines a plug for Dr. Jay Davidson's docuseries with elements from her own illness narrative: "For me, Lyme disease AND food poisoning were major triggers for my gut issues. We can't go back and un-infect ourselves. . . . So what do we do about it? Step [one] is to watch The Viral & Retroviral Summit, free and online next week!" Her use of the word "we" establishes a sense of commonality—a shared experience between herself and her email recipients. In yet another email, she promotes the docuseries Betrayal: The Autoimmune Disease Solution They're Not Telling You, *writing, "If you have gut issues like IBS, SIBO, or leaky gut, you should be thinking about autoimmunity, too. That's why I'm so excited to share a chance to watch Dr. Tom O'Bryan's* Betrayal: The Autoimmune Solution *docuseries!" Her "excitement" about potentially facilitating email recipients' ability to prevent autoimmune diseases suggests altruism and concern for their well-being.*

Individuals like Sarna—laypeople who have struggled with chronic illness, have recovered using functional medicine techniques, and have been inspired by the experience to become functional health educators—play a valuable role within functional medicine's entrepreneurial structure by acting as referralists for functional medicine practitioners and their digital content. These health educators do not possess the licensing or credentials to practice medicine themselves; however, by creating online "content" with functional medicine practitioners and offering "bundled savings" on master classes that may potentially illuminate health seekers' paths toward recovery, functional health educators explicitly package self-knowledge as a consumer item (see Birch and Tyfield 2012). Their role as referralists is beneficial for their provider counterparts since "master classes" like the one Sarna describes are an important source of revenue and attract potential clients to the provider's practice.

Marketing tactics employed by functional health educators hint at how their livelihoods are dependent on their ability to effectively refer consumers to functional medicine providers. For example, Misty Williams sent her Healing Rosie email listserv an email with the subject line "Top Secret: I found a functional medicine doctor for you!," writing in the email, "We had an AWESOME Ask-Me-Anything with Dr. Rick Henriksen about gut health, migraines and sleep." She goes on to explain that Dr. Henriksen is one of the MDs at SteadyMD, an online practice where, "for a reasonable monthly fee, you can work with a functional medicine doctor as your primary care doctor." Williams further appeals to her specific audience by indicating that Healing Rosie members can also find a functional medicine doctor who will run labs and help optimize thyroid hormones—a primary concern among group members.[2]

Similarly, Bridgit Danner, host of the DIY Detox Summit, emailed summit attendees to promote the work of Dr. Wahls, one of the featured speakers in her online event, writing, "Hello, Rosalynn! . . . To facilitate an epidemic of health, Dr. Terry Wahls has written several books to help you restore health." After promoting Dr. Wahls's books, Danner shares Dr. Wahls's advice—very nearly a direct match with Dr. Wahls's June and July 2019 email newsletters: "Do what you can. Use the library. . . . Don't obsess over whether you can afford functional medicine. Obsess over learning how to cook at home. Obsess over eating what is recommended and eliminating what is harmful. Obsess over what's in your control."[3] Danner also emphasizes that given the right dietary choices, most people do not need "fancy testing." This example demonstrates how functional health educators can sometimes act as bullhorns for particular providers' messages, thus spreading the word to audiences that the provider might not otherwise reach.

As these examples demonstrate, individual functional health educators enter into collaborative partnerships with multiple physician-entrepreneurs and, additionally, are paid commissions as affiliates for online events. In the process, these health educators become "influencers" who persuade their audience through the conscientious calibration of personae. In making these observations, I am building upon Crystal Abidin's (2016, 387) argument that an influencer's "relatability," or their ability to evoke in their audience the desire to identify with them, is sustained by their accessibility, authenticity, believability, emulatability, and intimacy.

These examples extend my argument from chapter 3 regarding how the functional medicine model represents a shift in hierarchical power by analyzing how self-knowledge as a product is adorned with indications of cultural and social capital and is subsequently bought and sold in the contemporary, neoliberal, online marketplace. In her emails, Sarna switches between sharing details from her own illness narrative and positioning the provider with whom she has a collaborative relationship as a fellow wounded healer. This is an example of how illness narratives of wounded healers are leveraged as a form of currency among functional medicine entrepreneurs.

To make this argument, I turn to Pierre Bourdieu's theory of capital. In his seminal book *Distinction: A Social Critique of the Judgement of Taste* (1984), Bourdieu describes three types of capital. Cultural capital is the things, experiences, and skills that promote social mobility. Social capital is the resources and advantages a person can access based on their social network. Economic capital is simply economic resources, such as cash or property. Using Bourdieu's concepts to build upon his theory, I argue that by sharing details from their own healing journeys, functional health educators demonstrate their embodied cultural capital within the functional medicine community. By describing practitioner counterparts as wounded healers, functional health educators signal their collaborative partners' embodied cultural capital while simultaneously indicating their own social capital. In turn, exerting cultural and social capital produces economic capital.

Furthermore, functional medicine health educators market (self-) knowledge through collaborative relationships with functional medicine practitioners. Alex Howard, host of the Fatigue Super Conference, sent an email to attendees a month after the 2022 conference concluded, indicating, "My close friend, Niki Gratrix, who co-founded The Optimum Health Clinic with me in 2004, and who is an award-winning functional health practitioner, has spent the last 4 years creating something very special." He goes on to describe how, in addition to scouring "literally tens of thousands of studies," Gratrix teamed up with the "brightest minds in the world" regarding overcoming fatigue—"world-renowned psychologists, scientists, physicians, nutrition experts, sleep experts, and neuroscience experts"—to produce the Abundant Energy master class series. He signals that in this series, Gratrix will be sharing powerful strategies for addressing the root causes of fatigue and that participation is "completely FREE." Howard's email describes how functional medicine digital content is both produced and promoted through a social network: he is promoting his friend and colleague's master class series, while she has collaborated with numerous experts to produce the series.

As is usually the case, this free master class was designed as a hook. In the functional medicine realm, master classes are akin to the narrative device that Abidin (2016) refers to as the "advertorial." Their ultimate purpose is to attract consumers to an expensive comprehensive program. Howard's language in a subsequent email is strewn with entrepreneurial jargon. He mentions "investing" in Gratrix's program and talks about her videos in terms of "value" since her insights can help participants "avoid wasting [thousands of dollars] on inappropriate or poorly implemented testing." Master classes are framed as the money-saving option for self-knowledge-seeking consumers, even as they are a money-making strategy for functional medicine entrepreneurs.

RELATIONSHIPS AMONG FUNCTIONAL MEDICINE ENTREPRENEURS

Ocean Robbins is the grandson of Baskin-Robbins cofounder Irvine Robbins. He is also the CEO and cofounder of the Food Revolution Network, Inc. In a June 27, 2019, Food Revolution Network email, Ocean Robbins describes the "fascinating stories of three successful visionary entrepreneurs" and invites email recipients to watch a video compilation in which three of Ryan Eliason's former Visionary Business School students describe their "big visions and big impact." Robbins himself is the first of the three "case studies" in the video. The next day, in an email with the subject line "Make a LIVING and make a DIFFERENCE," Robbins writes, "Hi Rosalynn, My friend and colleague, Ryan Eliason, is a world-leading authority on how to make a good living while making the world a better place." He explains that for the first time, Eliason is opening his "hugely popular leadership program for social entrepreneurs who want to scale up their impact." Robbins describes how Eliason guides students through the process of putting their dreams into action. He personally vouches for how Eliason's training has changed "thousands of lives," writing, "I've seen it help socially conscious businesses—

> *from home-based health coaches to global natural foods enterprises—significantly expand their income and impact." Robbins emphasizes that his June 28th email will be the last time in 2019 that he will be telling email recipients about the business school and warns, "Time is limited. . . . You only have a few hours left to decide." Below these words is the image of multiple countdown timers indicating the amount of time, down to the second, that email recipients have left to respond.*
>
> *The email concludes with two postscripts. In the first, Robbins offers a bonus gift to those who register for Ryan's Visionary Business School by clicking the link in that email. The bonus gift included 120 expert interviews from the 2012–2018 Food Revolution Summits. He indicates, "Normally, you'd have to pay $1,200+ for this collection, but I'll give it to you for no charge if you join Ryan's program using the links I'm providing." The second postscript appeals to email recipients' philanthropic desires. He notes that Eliason will contribute a portion of each enrollee's tuition to support the work of the Food Revolution Network and indicates, "You can be supporting your mission and our work at the same time." These bonus gifts represent a monetary exchange between Robbins and Eliason—Robbins supports his friend Eliason's business school by offering a collection of interview recordings "worth over $1,200," while Eliason supports Robbins's business by contributing an undisclosed portion of students' tuition to the Food Revolution Network.*
>
> *I received so many emails about Eliason's Visionary Business School that I created a separate folder exclusively for promotions related to the school. Within three weeks, the folder was filled with ninety-one items. In one email, Eliason boasts about how his clients, including Robbins, went from zero to seven figures. Other emails invited recipients to view webinars, free videos, and case studies that explain how to "transform your calling to serve into a lucrative business and a lifestyle you love!" The promotional materials indicated that enrollment in the business school was protected by a "60-Day Risk-Free Guarantee."*

Given that functional medicine usually unfolds outside of insurance-based health care, the success of individual functional medicine practitioners and health coaches is dependent on their ability to (re)position themselves as functional medicine entrepreneurs. This introductory anecdote provides numerous clues about the nature of entrepreneurship in functional medicine, including how these entrepreneurs have needed to hone strategies and techniques designed to capture potential consumers. Robbins's including himself as one of the three case studies indicates his personal involvement in the business school. Subsequently, by mentioning extra benefits to anyone who clicks through his email to register, Robbins subtly reveals that his drumming up of enrollment numbers may result in personal gain. The two "bonus gifts" Robbins offers to entice potential enrollees signal that his vociferous support of Eliason unfolds within a context of bilateral exchange. In essence, functional medicine entrepreneurship strategies frame relational ties such as the friendship Robbins describes with Eliason.

This introductory anecdote further demonstrates that individual functional medicine providers and health coaches are interpellated as entrepreneurs using the same strategies that are used to attract consumers. Using automated technology, Robbins's email is composed as a personal letter. By inserting the first names of recipients in the salutations, he created a sense of familiarity in the emails between sender and receiver. Robbins then extended this sense of familiarity to the "product" he was promoting by vouching for Eliason and the business school. He went on to create a sense of urgency by offering a "bonus gift," indicating its enormous value and emphasizing that it was available only for a limited time. He used time-critical marketing again when he stressed the school was enrolling "for the only time this year" and embedded a countdown timer into the body of his email. To remove any lingering doubts, promotional materials for the school indicate enrollment includes a "60-Day Risk-Free Guarantee." In essence, Robbins's recruitment emails position potential business school students as consumers and thus exhibit all the same strategies used to attract (and even lure) consumers to functional medicine online events, services, and products.[4]

Email recipients who enroll in the school will be taught how to use these strategies themselves, thus transitioning them from consumer to entrepreneur. Entrepreneurial models like the one taught by Eliason's Visionary Business School permeate functional medicine and describe the strategies and techniques employed by many "high profile visionary entrepreneurs" in the functional medicine community. Furthermore, entrepreneurialism structures how biosociality (Rabinow 1996) unfolds among functional medicine practitioners and health educators.

How Commissions Structure and Reinforce Relational Ties

I received six emails on the same day from different functional medicine practitioners and educators—including Dr. Ryan Wohlfert, Dr. Sarah

Ballantyne, and Dr. Pedram Shojai (aka the Urban Monk)—alerting me to Dr. O'Bryan's upcoming docuseries, Betrayal.[5] *Thus, I was not the least bit surprised when a subsequent email newsletter from GreenMed-Info—a website for natural health resources—also promoted* Betrayal *by including a hyperlinked logo and photo advertisement for the docuseries.*

In the following days I received more emails touting Betrayal. *Maskell plugged Dr. O'Bryan's docuseries in an email with the subject line "Building community around our future forums," telling recipients, "Speaking of bringing people together, Dr. Tom O'Bryan's autoimmune docuseries* Betrayal *starts Monday, July 29, and it will bring together hundreds of thousands of people to learn about a functional approach to treating autoimmune conditions."*

An email from Dr. Partha Nandi—a practicing gastroenterologist and host of the Emmy Award–winning talk show Ask Dr. Nandi*—also promoted* Betrayal*:*

> *I am sharing this powerful resource that could be one of the most valuable gifts you've ever been given. For a limited time, my colleague and friend, Dr. Tom O'Bryan's powerful (and free!), 9-part documentary series,* Betrayal: The Autoimmune Disease Solution, *will be available online. With over 85 interviews, you're going to hear from experts such as Dr. David Perlmutter, Dr. Joseph Mercola, Dr. Mark Hyman and JJ Virgin, as well as doctors, scientists and survivors from around the globe—United States, England, Portugal, Italy, Germany—to learn of their breakthrough research, life-changing protocols and heart-filling stories. There are scores of breakthrough stories.*

With similar to identical language, a July 6 email from Dr. Wahls reads:

> *Dr. Tom O'Bryan has created a ground-breaking, 9-part docuseries,* Betrayal: The Autoimmune Solution, *that brings together more than 85 autoimmune disease experts. . . . He traveled across the United States, as well as through England, Spain, Portugal and Germany, to consult with the world's leading scientists, doctors and surviving patients of autoimmune diseases. There are scores of breakthrough stories.*

> *When Dr. O'Bryan distributed his own promotional email for* Betrayal, *it hinted at individual functional medicine entrepreneurs' stakes in the docuseries by including PDF "gifts" on killing viruses and fighting cancer from Jonathan Landsman and Sayer Ji—a holistic oral health expert and the founder of GreenMedInfo, respectively—among others.*

How do members of the functional medicine community become involved as speakers in various online events? Furthermore, what motivates individual functional medicine entrepreneurs to promote these events? When I first began receiving overlapping emails from multiple functional medicine entrepreneurs regarding upcoming online events, I was not aware of the commissions individual affiliates receive for advertising events on their listservs. However, I observed obvious social networks among these entrepreneurs and was curious about the underlying financial structure of community-based marketing. Over time, I learned that community-based marketing among functional medicine entrepreneurs—how products and services are marketed by multiple members of the functional medicine community to the mutual benefit of these multiple members—does not occur spontaneously.

When conducting a Google search for the different online events in which a particular functional medicine practitioner has appeared as a speaker, I stumbled upon the website eVirtual Summits. The site includes practitioners' pictures, titles, and biographical profiles. Below this information is the following statement, in bold type: "**If you want to book me as a speaker, fill out the contact form below. If you would like additional information on my upcoming events, please follow me on social media.**" Below that is a fillable form that includes fields for name, email, subject, and message, as well as a captcha. Finally, below the form is a table with all the online events in which the speaker has appeared, their start dates, and their durations. For example, the Healthy Gut Summit started on January 9, 2015, and its duration was 138 weeks. As I continued to explore the site, I realized that most of the individuals I had encountered as speakers in online events during my ethnographic fieldwork, as well as many of the online events themselves, are listed on the site. In this moment, I recognized that the assemblages of functional medicine interlocutors I had been observing had not emerged (exclusively or perhaps even primarily) through organic, person-to-person relationships but, rather, were undergirded by online platforms and financial structures.

Individual functional medicine practitioners and educators promote online events in which they have personally participated. Maskell sent out an email promoting "two upcoming docuseries worth your time," giving his indirect and direct roles in each. He indicates that some of the footage for the docuseries *The Human Longevity Project* was shot at the Journey to 100 event he and his team put on in Guernsey in 2017. He continues, "Tom O'Bryan's autoimmune docuseries *Betrayal* starts Monday, and if you tune in on Monday night you can see my tearful moment caught on camera, where I thank Dr. Tom for his support and belief in me." Maskell's explanations of his own involvement—which are similar to Robbins's indication that he is a successful alumnus of Eliason's business school—point to how self-promotion is collapsed onto event promotion and vice versa.

Online events are further promoted by "affiliates." I received an email from the web platform for functional medicine talks HealthMeans that sought to recruit "health professionals"—defined by HealthMeans as doctors, practitioners, coaches, bloggers, and influencers—to join as affiliates for the upcoming Genius of Your Genes Summit. Explaining how engaging in community-based marketing leads to personal gain, the email reads, "Maybe you're ready to start building online revenue from your practice? Join us as an affiliate to promote The Genius of Your Genes Summit!" Recruitment emails from HealthMeans entice functional medicine entrepreneurs by emphasizing that being an affiliate for multiple events can provide a lucrative income: "This event is taking place on our Health Talks Online/HealthMeans platform, that pays out more than $1 million in commissions each year." They encourage potential affiliates to "start small" and "learn as they go" while promoting the twenty to thirty events HealthMeans holds each year. I also received emails inviting me to be an affiliate for both the docuseries *Betrayal* and the Overcoming Hashimoto's Summit. I did not accept any of these invitations. However, the experience of being recruited for an affiliate role provided me with valuable insight into how digital platforms recruit and pay commissions to individual functional medicine entrepreneurs, thus actively facilitating community-based marketing.[6]

As a consumer who was being marketed to from multiple directions, I was struck by the exact matches in content among emails from various affiliates. HealthMeans's email provided the reason I had noticed these overt alignments, explaining, "There are already several great emails to copy, paste and send (you choose which ones fit your audience best) and plenty of social posts!" To complete their tasks as event affiliates, functional medicine entrepreneurs simply copy and paste from email templates, thus leading to the noticeable overlaps among emails from different individuals.

Marketing emails suggest that community-based marketing unfolds from friendships among colleagues. This is likely true, at least in part; however, it is far from the whole story. The reverse may also be true—friendships among colleagues are constituted and consolidated by underlying financial structures upon which colleagues are interdependent. In either case, due to overlapping commissions, each individual functional medicine entrepreneur is reliant on the community's participation for their success. The community-based logic of functional medicine is fundamentally rooted in entrepreneurialism, while simultaneously reinforcing relational ties.

RELATIONSHIPS BETWEEN CORPORATE SPONSORS AND PROVIDERS

In the lead-up to my attendance at the Advances in Mitochondrial Medicine Symposium in Dallas in 2019, I received an email from an account executive at Ortho Molecular Products. The email began, "Hey, Dr. Vega, I wanted to reach out and introduce myself." The email sender, Robert, goes on to explain that he is the local consultant for Ortho Molecular, a company that partners with providers to sell supplements that are available only through licensed health care professionals, and for the Lifestyle Matrix Resource Center, a membership-based business that provides clinical tools, educational resources, and digital marketing training for clinicians transitioning into functional medicine. Both Ortho Molecular and the Lifestyle Matrix Resource Center frequently sponsor functional medicine providers' blogs, podcasts, and other digital and in-person events. Signaling the partnership between these two entities, Robert writes, "We are so excited to have you at our Mitochondrial Symposium in Dallas. Please stop by the booth so I can introduce myself to you in person." The account executive's word choice—placing "Hey" at the beginning of the email, expressing his "excitement" to have me at the symposium, and indicating his desire to "introduce [himself] in person"—reveals his intention to create a sense of familiarity. This email demonstrates how corporate sponsors also use the discursive strategies analyzed earlier in this chapter to interpellate functional medicine providers as entrepreneurs, who, in turn, use these same strategies to interpellate health seekers as consumers.

When I attended the Advances in Mitochondrial Medicine Symposium, the entryway to the auditorium was crowded with these sponsors' booths. At each booth, medical sales representatives offered pamphlets, free samples, and other promotional materials for their companies. The symposium included multiple meals and snacks per day, and when lining up at the buffet stations, attendees were literally surrounded by sponsors' booths. While presenters were careful not to promote sponsors' products during the portions of the event that were approved for continuing medical education credit, Ortho Molecular Products showed a promotional video to attendees during the lunch break on the first day and a representative from the Lifestyle Matrix Resource Center took the stage during the lunch break on the second day.

My attendance at the symposium provided me with ethnographic insight into how partnerships unfold in a chain-like fashion. Functional health educators promote practitioners, while practitioners promote corporate sponsors. These relationships simultaneously instantiate marketing strategies that move in the opposite direction. Ortho Molecular boasted that its products are available only through a physician; thus, the company's marketing strategy helps to solidify the physician-patient relationship. Corporate sponsors market to functional medicine providers, who, in turn, market to consumers. These economic ties point to how functional medicine providers are positioned as influencers and how corporate sponsors turn to functional medicine influencers as a covert marketing tactic.[7]

Meanwhile, partnerships with corporate sponsors buttress profit streams for functional medicine entrepreneurs. Functional medicine practitioners and health educators use multiple intersecting digitized platforms to directly and indirectly market sponsors' products and services to consumers. Thus, the entrepreneurial framework of functional medicine is not only rooted in community but also buttressed by corporate interests. The power of community-based marketing is harnessed in the production of economic capital.

Reproducing the pattern of overlapping promotional emails I received for *Betrayal* and the Overcoming Hashimoto's Summit, I received another wave of emails from their hosts after registering for these events. An initial email from Dr. O'Bryan credited sponsors—Boomer Natural Wellness, Bio-Botanical Research, and Thrive Market. A subsequent email included a banner for *Betrayal* at the top, but the body of the email was devoted to promoting Thrive Market, a "top event partner." Inna Topiler, the host of the Overcoming Hashimoto's Summit, sent an email with an "exclusive offer" from one of the summit's top event partners—a $100 discount from AquaTru, a company that sells countertop reverse-osmosis water purifiers. In another email, Topiler shared an eBook about "restoring your microbiome" from another top event partner, Microbiome Labs. These examples demonstrate how sponsorships frequently unfold through online events.

At the same time, individual functional medicine practitioners are often supported by multiple overlapping corporate sponsors. Dr. Kara Fitzgerald's email newsletters always end with the logos of her "premier sponsors": Biotics Research Corporation, DUTCH Test, Diagnostic Solutions Laboratory, Dunwoody Labs, Metagenics, Women's International Pharmacy, Genova Diagnostics, Designs for Health, Bio-Botanical Research, T.A. Sciences, and Doctor's Data—each hyperlinked to its respective company's website. And Dr. Fitzgerald's clinic logo is strategically placed on the last row of sponsor logos, along with the text "Interested in sponsorship? Click here!" This logo links to a "sponsor portal" web page on the clinic's site that collects information regarding the potential sponsor and uploads its company logo.

While Dr. Fitzgerald's digital newsletters often include links to emerging research and other items of interest for her email recipients, at times the body of her emails is dedicated to sponsored content. One email featured a graphic titled "Science of Vitamin C" that linked to an extended article promoting CoreMedScience's liposomal vitamin C supplement. Through partnerships with functional medicine practitioners, lab testing and supplement companies promote their products and services to consumers they would not otherwise reach.

As Danner culled from Dr. Wahls's recent content to construct her email regarding Dr. Wahls's work,[8] functional medicine practitioners obtain content from corporate sponsors for their emails to consumers. I received an email from Dr. Wahls explaining the benefits of Biocidin, Bio-Botanical Research's most successful product line. The email included a screenshot of her teleconferencing with a representative from the company, which was hyperlinked to a recording of the conversation. This example demonstrates the chain-like entrepreneurial relationships between functional health educators, functional medicine practitioners, and functional medicine companies.

In a similarly structured email, Dr. Wahls promoted BodyBio by first indicating that she uses BodyBio's PC (phosphatidylcholine) and balance oil. She encourages email recipients to "click the image below to hear my interview with Jessica Kane to learn more about the benefits of PC." Signaling her partnership with BodyBio, Wahls continues, "Wahls Warriors can use the promo code 'Wahls-P' at the checkout at BodyBio.com." In this last sentence, Dr. Wahls instantiates a sense of community by referring to (and branding?) her followers as Wahls Warriors and promotes a company with which she is affiliated. This example demonstrates how influencers develop relationships with companies through sponsorships and in the process they themselves become brands (Onomake 2021).[9] While Dr. Wahls is marketing

BodyBio's PC and balance oil in this email, she is leveraging herself as a brand to brand-loyal "Wahls Warriors," who may purchase the product using the promo code she gives them.

In another email, Dr. Wahls writes about the importance of tea for reducing inflammation and stress as well as supporting cardiovascular, immune system, brain, and gut health. The first 455 words of her email are dedicated to explaining how tea impacts our physiology by supplying prebiotic polyphenols to support the gut microbiome, antioxidants like EGCG to battle free radicals, and L-theanine to boost GABA levels. Her email then takes a precipitous turn as she writes, "My friends at Pique Tea have taken away all the inconveniences and concerns about tea." Dr. Wahls indicates that tea can be a scary carrier of pesticides, heavy metals, and mold—contaminants of which her readers are extremely wary. She continues, "Pique Teas are Triple Toxin Screened for pesticides, heavy metals and toxic mold, so you can rest easy knowing you're getting one of the cleanest, purest teas on the market." Her email includes the hyperlink "Click here to claim up to 28% off + free shipping." As "free" master classes often serve as a hook when enticing consumers to enroll in expensive health education programs, Dr. Wahls's extended description of tea and its physiological effects captured self-knowledge-seeking readers' attention before she turned to promoting her sponsor's product.

Over the course of my ethnographic research, I observed how individual companies sponsor multiple practitioners in order to gain greater visibility and capture the widest consumer base, and, in turn, how multiple functional medicine practitioners and health educators promote the same sponsored products and services to consumers through multiple platforms. For example, Bio-Botanical Research has sponsored Dr. Fitzgerald, Dr. Wahls, and Dr. O'Bryan. Thrive Market sponsored Dr. O'Bryan's docuseries *Betrayal* and is also a sponsor of Dr. Amy Myers. Meanwhile, emails from Maskell, Dr. Fitzgerald, and Dr. Vincent Pedre promoted Fullscript, an online supplement dispensary.[10] These overlapping corporate sponsorships, in part, instantiate the functional medicine community.

At the same time, individual practitioners enjoy the sponsorship of multiple companies. One of Dr. Myers's emails was dedicated to promoting Thrive Market, Kettle & Fire bone broth, and Vital Choice seafood. Dr. Myers's partnerships with these companies point to the role of organic food, food systems, and specialty diets in functional medicine protocols.[11] She characterizes Thrive Market in the email as "Whole Foods meets Costco, meets Amazon!" Dr. Myers tailored this email to the interests and concerns of functional medicine consumers by mentioning how Thrive Market offers "wholesome products," including "healthy foods and toxin-free household products" at "wholesale prices," and she leveraged her brand by embedding "The Myers Way®" into her plug for Thrive Market (see Onomake 2021): "With options for shopping products that are organic, gluten-free, dairy-free, paleo, and more, Thrive Market makes it easier than ever to follow The Myers Way® Candida Control Protocol."[12] As with docuseries promotional emails, Dr. Myers's email offered "free gifts," noting, "Best of all, they're offering everyone participating in the program a FREE jar of coconut oil (just pay for shipping) plus a free one-month membership for all new members, and 15% off your first order!" In this email and others, she contributes to a functional medicine digital marketplace that builds hype around discounts and online sales.

As with docuseries producers, functional medicine entrepreneurs draw from prescripted materials when constructing promotional emails for corporate sponsors. This leads to distinct overlaps in how the sponsors are described. For example, Dr. Fitzgerald promoted her Functional Medicine Clinic Immersion Live Mentorship Program to email newsletter recipients while also including a plug for Fullscript. She explains in the email that Fullscript partnered with her and her Institute for Functional Medicine–trained multidisciplinary team to allow one winner to attend her next Clinic Immersion Program free of charge. She furthermore notes, "Fullscript is doing great work enabling Functional Medicine practices to dispense supplements without inventory." Her mention of Fullscript includes a hyperlink to the company's website. I also received an email from Maskell with three paragraph-length descriptions of "featured resource partners." His description of Fullscript includes some of the same language as that of Dr. Fitzgerald.

My description of functional medicine practitioners' partnerships with corporate sponsors may be read as hypercritical. That is not my intention; in fact, I readily acknowledge that functional medicine practitioners generally partner with companies whose products they genuinely endorse. When Dr. Fitzgerald distributed sponsored content to her email listserv, she expressed her "eternal gratitude" to sponsors who enable her and her team to devote energy and time to writing, research, and education, and she included the following disclaimer: "All the companies who sponsor us are those I trust for myself, my patients, and my fellow practitioners." I take Dr. Fitzgerald's explanation at face value. Having had positive consumer experiences with many of the corporate sponsors mentioned in this section, I do not aim to disparage the products and services these companies offer.

Instead, my intent is to describe the financial structure that supports functional medicine entrepreneurs. Since functional medicine unfolds outside of insurance-based health care, these practitioners must turn to other sources of revenue. Consumers purchase functional medicine products and services in a neoliberal marketplace—one that favors socioeconomically privileged consumers over their less privileged counterparts.[13] I point to the structural context that gives rise to functional medicine entrepreneurial strategies, namely, an insurance-driven health care system that reimburses doctors for the pharmaceutical management of chronic disease while failing to attach financial incentives to lasting recovery. Ultimately, these structural issues create the context in which many functional medicine providers and health coaches are multiply positioned—as consumers, entrepreneurs, health influencers, store owners, and brands.

DOCTOR-INFLUENCERS: WHEN PEOPLE BECOME BRANDS

Maskell, a former finance banker, cofounded the Functional Forum, the world's largest integrative medicine conference.[14] At the September 2017 Functional Forum, Maskell said, "Everyone in this space at this moment is betting on the physician-entrepreneur." Speaking on behalf of Evolution of Medicine, a company he cofounded to equip functional medicine practitioners with practice-building resources, and of the Lifestyle Matrix Resource Center and Ortho Molecular Products, he indicated, "We are in the business of empowering clinician-entrepreneurs to build the medical practices of the future."

In August 2019, Maskell composed an email to his listserv while attending the Mindshare Summit in San Diego. Mine read, "Dear Rosalynn, I've just wrapped up recording episodes for the Big Bold Health podcast with Dr. Jeffrey Bland and female leaders of the next era of health creation. We've recorded some fascinating interviews with people like Dr. Terry Wahls!" The website 10times describes the Mindshare Summit in singular terms as "the conference for health & wellness influencers"—an opportunity for collaboration, innovation, and elevation. The summit's home page on the website Mindshare365 reads, "Meet your tribe. Who are the members of Mindshare? Only the most successful health and wellness entrepreneurs you regularly see in bookstores, on TV, radio, print and online." This quote supports my arguments that community is framed as a commodity in the functional medicine realm,[15] *and health and wellness entrepreneurs aspire to minor celebrity status as influencers.*

Later that month, Maskell emailed members of the functional medicine community to promote enrollment for his Practice Accelerator program, which helps conventional practitioners become functional medicine practitioners, writing, "This only comes around twice a year, in September and February, you can enroll in the program and join the most innovative practitioner community in functional and integrative medicine." He describes Practice Accelerator as Evolution of Medicine's "most prestigious program" and explains that hundreds of doctors have completed the program and "are now running profitable, sustainable low-overhead practices." His email is yet another example of time-critical marketing and the commodification of community.

Then, in March 2020, Maskell piqued email recipients' interest with a provocative subject line: "What if you did a TEDx talk?" In the email, he explains, "Today, I'm joining Taylor Conroy for a webinar about landing a TEDx talk as a functional medicine practitioner." Conroy is a four-time TEDx speaker and founder of the Idea Collective. His organization has helped multiple functional medicine entrepreneurs land their own TEDx talks. Maskell goes on to describe the webinar as a "step-by-step guide to sharing your personal story in a way that naturally leads to more business opportunities, new clients and more."[16] *For many functional medicine practitioners, the "personal story" Maskell mentions is the illness narrative that cements their identity as wounded healers and provides them with a strong sense of purpose as well as helping patients identify with them.*[17] *Maskell further entices his readers with the following hook: "We will even be sharing some TEDx events later in the year, currently looking for speakers." This email points to how the wounded healer illness narrative is intentionally crafted in the functional medicine realm due to its potential for producing economic capital.*

According to Maskell, the Practice Accelerator program is in the business of "empowering" clinician-entrepreneurs; however, I signal throughout this book that "empowerment" is potentiated by economic capital. Practitioners must purchase entry into programs like Maskell's Practice Accelerator or Eliason's Visionary Business School to become functional medicine entrepreneurs themselves. Maskell's emails, like Robbins's earlier in this chapter, simultaneously interpellate functional medicine practitioners as consumers and entrepreneurs. Maskell goes on to plug the Idea Collective, again demonstrating how functional medicine entrepreneurship is a multilevel enterprise. Entrepreneurialism in functional medicine unfolds like a chain reaction: entrepreneurs like Maskell derive income from training practitioners to become functional medicine entrepreneurs themselves.

While Maskell uses "clinician-entrepreneur" and "physician-entrepreneur" interchangeably, I use "functional medicine entrepreneur" to encompass all individuals who derive income from marketing products and services in the functional medicine realm, including physicians, naturopaths, nutritionists, chiropractors, health coaches, health educators, ethnographic filmmakers, science doctorates, CEOs and founders of functional health–related companies, and former patients who have reversed their chronic diseases.

At the same time, I point to the slippage between "functional medicine entrepreneur" and "health influencer." Descriptions of the Mindshare Summit refer to attendees interchangeably as "health and wellness entrepreneurs" and "health and wellness influencers." In our contemporary age, being an "influencer" is often a marker of successful entrepreneurship. Novice functional medicine entrepreneurs seek to become health influencers by participating in summits, online conferences, webinars, docuseries, podcasts, and YouTube interviews, and by securing a coveted TEDx talk. The goal of "influencer" activities is to create a larger "following"—consumers who value their recommendations and are likely to purchase the products and services they offer or recommend.

Functional medicine "influencers" and their audience engage in a "mutual gaze," each expecting returns (see Baruah 2017). Influencers strive for online recognition and engagement, which leads to economic returns through influencer marketing. At the same time, followers anticipate that they can emulate the influencer through the consumption of commodities. This "mutual gaze" is often mediated by what Natalie Ann Hendry, Catherine Hartung, and Rosie Welch (2021) call "influencer pedagogy"—educational and relatable interactions between influencers and their followers on social media platforms.[18]

Functional medicine entrepreneurs engage in "influencer pedagogy" by showcasing their highly cultivated authenticity and expertise on multiple platforms across the digisphere. In this vein, Maskell's email suggests functional medicine practitioners all offer something interesting to TEDx audiences—something that is in the very nature of being a functional medicine practitioner—and that telling their personal stories as practitioners will produce business opportunities. I thus analyze how the illness narratives of wounded healers are recruited as a lucrative resource for entrepreneurialism. By telling their illness narratives, functional medicine entrepreneurs represent themselves as both relatable and knowledgeable, which, in turn, allows them to reach and "influence" their consumer audience.

As entrepreneurs whose goods and services are not covered by insurance, functional medicine practitioners are aware of the importance of "influencer pedagogy" for building a successful practice. Chris Kresser describes how patients follow particular practitioners online, consume their free content, and think, "Oh, I've been reading this blog for the last two years and I've learned a ton and it's helped me tremendously." Eventually, those patients may become "stuck." When they realize they have progressed as far as they can on their own, they make the decision to become the provider's patient. Over the course of two years of training to become an acupuncturist, Kresser used the strategy of delivering "really valuable free content that helped people" in order to help establish his practice. He explains that when he graduated from school and obtained his license, he sent out an email indicating that his practice was open and he was busy seeing nearly the maximum number of patients possible within the next few months. From his perspective, producing free content is an investment that eventually leads to revenue for a clinical practice.

At the same time, health influencers display agility when turning to multiple platforms, producing content in digital and print formats, and taking on different professional roles. As one example, Dr. Pedre is medical director of Pedre Integrative Health, founder of Pedre Wellness, author of *Happy Gut*, and medical advisor to MBODY360 and Fullscript. It is not unusual for functional medicine practitioners to start their own practice, author a trade book, and work as medical advisor to health tech startups.

Health influencers derive further income from being "affiliates," promoting the products and services of companies extending beyond the functional medicine realm to their functional medicine "followers." The products these entrepreneurs market to functional medicine consumers include online grocery subscriptions, supplements, lab tests, water filters, food items, sunscreen, "clean beauty" products, EMF protection, essential oils, home goods, organic mattresses, and baby products, to name a few. As Dr. Wahls embedded a video conversation between supplement company representatives and herself in email promotions to her Wahls Warriors, Dr. O'Bryan promoted Beekeeper's Naturals honey-based products while simultaneously inviting email recipients to a Facebook Live interview with the company's founder. Misty Williams likewise used email to promote toxin-free sunscreen and "organic wine . . . endorsed by health leaders like Dr. Perlmutter, Dr. Hyman, Mark Sisson, Robb Wolf, Dave Asprey, Dominic D'Agostino, Abel James, JJ Virgin, and many more." In so doing, she leveraged social capital to augment the desirability of health and wellness products to functional medicine consumers. Harking back to my observations regarding community-based marketing, her words furthermore hint at an underlying financial structure buttressing overlapping endorsements.

In using the words "affiliate" and "follower," I am applying terms commonly used by other types of influencers to functional medicine influencers. It is important to note that I rarely came across the terms "affiliate" and "follower" while conducting research for this book; however, my ethnographic data suggests that these terms are useful for understanding important sources of income for functional medicine influencers.[19] I observed how these influencers embedded hyperlinks for products they enjoy in their web pages and emails, leading me to suspect these influencers are not immune to the economic incentives that are readily apparent in other realms of influencing.

For example, beauty influencers produce YouTube videos of themselves creating a particular "makeup look" using specific makeup products. Each product is usually listed as a hyperlink in the description box below the video. Whenever followers purchase a product through the influencer's hyperlink, the influencer receives a kickback. Sometimes influencers will also supply an "affiliate code" that confers a discount to the follower in addition to a commission for the influencer. This affiliate structure applies to many different types of influencers. Lifestyle influencers may describe what is on their Christmas wish lists or dedicate videos to what they plan to gift their loved ones for Christmas—and all the while, the products featured were each sent to them for their consideration, with invitations from respective companies to become an affiliate.

When functional medicine entrepreneurs endorse individual products and promote them to functional medicine consumers, these endorsements are often presented alongside their own or a loved one's illness narrative. For example, Ryan and Teddy Sternagel faced every parent's nightmare when their son, Ryder, was diagnosed with pediatric cancer. They detoxified their home and turned to proper nutrition, targeted supplementation, and alternative cancer therapies. Ryder's miraculous recovery inspired the Sternagels to develop the Stern Method—a lifestyle of detoxification. The "What We Use" tab on their website includes hyperlinks to supplements, essential oils, cancer-fighting tools, baby products, nontoxic cleaning products, "anti-cancer" kitchen gear, pantry items, personal care products, water-enhancement products, and other home goods. Ryan Sternagel also uses his email listserv to promote specific products: after the airing of the online event The Anti-Cancer Revolution, Sternagel sent me an email touting a liposomal supplement with "a ton of well-researched solid liver detoxifying ingredients." This email endorsement was interspersed with details from the family's illness narrative; however, there was no disclosure of Ryan Sternagel's relationship with the brand whose supplement he was promoting.

I searched the Stern Method website to see if I could find any such disclosure. At the very bottom of a long list of recommended products, in small type, I finally noticed the following: "Many links on this site, especially those to Amazon, are affiliate links. Should you click on these links and purchase something, the price is no different for you and we earn a small commission. Thank you for your support!" The wording of this disclosure confirms that the affiliate structure that operates in other realms of influencing is also at work in functional medicine influencing.

However, many functional medicine entrepreneurs do not disclose their relationships with brands. Williams promoted EMF-blocking "stickers," writing to her listserv recipients, "Very important! Children's brains are more susceptible to radiation than adults." Since I had attended a lecture on the topic at UC Berkeley while studying for my master's in epidemiology, my interest was piqued. However, as I continued to read her email, I noticed she did not include an affiliate disclosure for the stickers. An email from Katie Kimball at the site Kitchen Stewardship similarly described how small children are more susceptible to radiation from electromagnetic fields (for example, from Wi-Fi, cell phones, bluetooth technology, etc.) and promoted EMF-blocking "stickers." However, in contrast to Williams, Kimball states in the email, "I am an affiliate for this company, which means I'll earn a commission, but it doesn't change your price." While I cannot be certain Williams is an affiliate for the maker of the EMF-blocking stickers, I consider it likely based on the clear overlap in content between her email and Kimball's email.

In society at large, the failure among influencers to disclose their relationships with brands has been sharply criticized by followers. When influencers do not reveal their affiliate relationships with companies whose products they promote, they are essentially advertising to unsuspecting consumers. In 2020, the Federal Trade Commission (FTC) began codifying elements of existing endorsement guidelines into official regulations so that violators could be held liable for civil penalties (Aten 2020). It remains to be seen how FTC crackdowns may impact the functional medicine community, if at all.

As a consumer and participant-observer of functional medicine, I was marketed to by multiple online platforms. I often received emails from unknown addresses. One such email, from "Stephen at MyGreenFills <family@mygreenfills.com>," read, "Hi Rosalynn, Here at MyGreenFills, we LOVE sharing cutting-edge FREE life-changing content about good health." The next line in the email indicated Stephen's affiliate role for a docuseries: "Tonight the *Gut Solution* series begins on Monday, July 1st, at exactly 8 pm Eastern Time and I will be there for sure." Below, the email included a photo of Sarah Otto and Matt Potts laughing—a screenshot from the docuseries. Shortly thereafter, I also started receiving text messages from MyGreenFills on my phone and ads from them on my Facebook feed. Similarly, I noticed sponsorship by Doctor's Data in Dr. Fitzgerald's emails and immediately began spotting their ads in the right column of my Facebook page. These examples demonstrate how, after capturing personal data such as an email address, functional medicine entrepreneurs—and the companies and events with which they are affiliated—simultaneously advertise to potential consumers through email listservs, phone messaging, and Facebook.

Functional medicine entrepreneurs and their corporate sponsors actively create and pay for Facebook advertisements. As I began receiving unsolicited emails from numerous functional medicine entrepreneurs, my everyday engagements with my email inbox shaped the type of advertisements I was exposed to on Facebook. These ads were formatted for Facebook newsfeeds and Facebook stories. They often included video clips to attract the consumer's eye and familiarize the consumer with the entrepreneur's voice and personality, along with a "shop now" button to easily connect the consumer to the entrepreneur's online store. By advertising on Facebook, these functional medicine practitioners infiltrate a key online space where digitized biosociality is occurring, thus interpellating members of online communities (i.e., Facebook support groups) as consumers of their products and services.[20]

Examples of Facebook marketing abound. I saw an advertisement for Quicksilver Scientific that read, "Take control of your health the natural way through effective detoxification protocols and dietary supplements." The ad encouraged potential consumers to "get started on their health journey" by "shopping now." The founder and CEO of Quicksilver Scientific is Dr. Christopher Shade, a functional medicine interlocutor who appeared as an expert interviewee on one of the online summits I attended. In two other ads on Facebook, Dr. Jay Davidson and his colleague Dr. Todd Watts appeared in short video advertisements for their doctor's brand of supplements, Microbe Formulas. One of these ads included a 15 percent discount on a seven-day "challenge" to rid the body of harmful parasites. I scrolled past an ad from Dr. Myers with the text "The Myers Way® Organic Greens taste great, and unlike other brands, they do it 100% organically! You won't find any added sugars, artificial flavors, GMO's, or any other nasty ingredients" alongside a link to order. In each of these examples, functional medicine provider-entrepreneurs turned to Facebook advertising to promote their brands.

Online sales are a major source of revenue for functional medicine entrepreneurs, and they often promote them via email. For example, Dr. Shojai, a doctor of Oriental medicine, licensed acupuncturist, and wellness consultant, emailed *Interconnected* docuseries viewers to promote "molecular hydrogen," an "energy drink" available through his online store. Danner emailed her newsletter recipients regarding the benefits of dry brushing for detoxification. Her email included hyperlinks to her online store, which includes a mix of products and services ranging from dry brushes and supplements to testing and lab-review services for chronic Epstein-Barr virus and thyroid imbalances. Naturopath Carolyn Ledowsky's organization, MTHFR Support Australia, has a similar online store. Under the "shop" tab there, consumers can purchase supplements, MTHFR gene test kits, eBooks, books, eCourses, practitioner webinars, patient webinars, sunscreen, membership, and "products we love." To my reading, "products we love" is influencer code for "companies with which we are affiliated."

Practitioners' stores employ strategies similar to those of other retailers when advertising their products. As a functional medicine consumer, I was constantly being notified of online sales. I received one email from Ledowsky with the subject line "Open for 20% off EVERYTHING in the store!" In the body of the email, Ledowsky used time-critical marketing, indicating that the sale would last for merely one day and advising, "Don't miss it! Be sure to enter coupon code STOCKTAKE on the checkout page to get your discount." On the left-hand side of the email was a graphic of a young girl jumping for joy in front of a pink background, the words "20% OFF; 1 day ONLY" in large type, and a yellow "shop now" button. The number of emails I received regarding online sales exploded around holidays. I received one from Jonathan Landsman that read, "HAPPY 4th of July SPECIAL: SAVE 10% on all NaturalHealth365 Store supplements. Sale ends midnight—July 4." Dr. Krista Burns at the American Posture Institute emailed, "Because you joined us for the Digital Dementia Summit, and in honor of the 4th of July we want to offer you sizzling summer savings of 77% off the enrollment price into the Brain Reboot Program!" These examples demonstrate how functional medicine entrepreneurs' online stores employ the same marketing tactics (e.g., holiday sales and coupon codes) as online stores operating in non-biological realms of consumption. In essence, functional medicine entrepreneurs are not only physicians and educators but also salespeople.

Certain functional medicine entrepreneurs are successfully building their own brands, sometimes succeeding in selling them outside the functional medicine arena. For example, Dr. Josh Axe, a doctor of natural medicine, chiropractor, and clinical nutritionist, has a successful line of supplements, protein, and collagen products that have gone "mainstream." In addition to his online store, Dr. Axe's Ancient Nutrition brand is available in many Whole Foods grocery stores and through Thrive Market online. When advertising her Body Ecology online store's Independence Day Sale, nutritional consultant Donna Gates evinced the central role that branding plays in her marketing strategy. An email from her contained scattered stars and this catchy phrasing: "OH SAY, CAN YOU BE. BE healthy, BE free, and save 20% site-wide with our Independence Day sale! Code: BEFREE20." The capital letters in the word "BE" are the initials of her brand, Body Ecology. In a Google search, her store is listed as "Body Ecology Official Site—Donna Gates," thus hinting at how functional medicine entrepreneurs and their brands are collapsed onto one another.

In Dr. Myers's case, her name is her brand. Her product names appear in bold green type, and each product is also labeled with "AMY MYERS MD®" in sleek, boxy gray type and features the brand's logo—the letters *A*, *M*, and *MD* in a box with two dividers. Her store offers a loyalty program through which consumers can earn points toward future discounts or free gifts through purchases. All store emails—order confirmations, shipping notices, loyalty program updates—are sent from "Amy Myers MD." On Facebook, the banner for the Myers Way Community has a bold green background—the same tone of green as her product labeling, packaging, and her website's menu bar—with a photo of Dr. Myers to the left, wearing a navy blue V-neck top with a gold necklace. The same banner is featured on the home page of her website, and the same photo is superimposed on some of her online programs for sale (e.g., "The Myers Way® Guide to a Toxin-Free Home," "The Myers Way® 30-Day SIBO Breakthrough," and "The Myers Way® 30-Day Candida Breakthrough"). In essence, Dr. Myers is her own brand—her image and her name (and her favorite green color?). When consumers are loyal to "AMY MYERS MD®," their loyalty is to the brand that represents the person.

Like Dr. Myers's, Dr. Wahls's surname is her brand. Emails from Dr. Wahls include a trademark notice that reads, "The terms WAHLS PROTOCOL program, WAHLS diet, WAHLS PALEO diet, and WAHLS PALEO PLUS diet are the trademarks of Dr. Terry Wahls LLC." Also, like Dr. Myers, Dr. Wahls appears in the banner for her Facebook support group, the Wahls Protocol. However, Dr. Wahls uniquely refers to her patients as "Wahls Warriors," thus laying claim to (and potentially branding?) her followers.

Abidin (2016) notes that influencers risk losing their followership if they are perceived as no longer accessible or authentic. This often occurs when followers believe an influencer prioritizes brand alignment over their connection with followers. Since I am not privy to the inboxes of these functional medicine entrepreneurs, I cannot assess how often they are held to task for their entrepreneurial approach to health. However, an email newsletter from Dr. Wahls distributed in June 2019 provides a brief glimpse into how functional medicine entrepreneurs respond to these criticisms. Dr. Wahls writes in the newsletter, "Our society is a capitalist one, in which entrepreneurs create products that the public purchases according to perceived value." She suggests that if consumers do not agree with the capitalist values of their society, they should use their political vote to change society and continues, "The entrepreneurial orientation allows my team to create a lot of content that millions can see for free, more select content that thousands can access with a modest investment, and even more specialized content that hundreds can access for much greater investment." In this way, Dr. Wahls frames her "entrepreneurial orientation" as almost philanthropic—her team helps millions who cannot to afford to pay for content—while also framing exclusive content as an "investment." Dr. Wahls's approach renders information regarding lifestyle changes accessible to many people while simultaneously reinforcing class-based structures and capitalist logic. In response, I underscore the way market ideology and corporate structures have transformed moral values around the right to health (see Abadía-Barrero 2016).[21]

In this chapter, I have highlighted how market-based strategies privilege middle- and upper-class consumers, many of whom are White. In the next chapter, I examine how White functional medicine practitioners frame the traditional healing practices of non-Westerners as a legitimate form of expertise. Meanwhile, functional medicine practitioners of color situate themselves as primarily trained in biomedicine. Furthermore, although salugens are derived from traditional knowledge, racialized Others are not equitably included in profit streams from them. In which ways might functional medicine inadvertently reinscribe "racial" inequality? In what instances might we view salugens the booty of biopiracy?

CHAPTER 6
ANCIENT HEALING TRADITIONS

Functional medicine discourse romanticizes the "ancient healing traditions" of "other cultures" while portraying cultural "Others" (i.e., "non-Westerners")[1] as frozen in an idealized past. While ancient healing traditions are exalted in functional medicine, only individuals who are not from the culture whose tradition is being celebrated can turn to traditional knowledge as a form of legitimate expertise. As a result, functional medicine practitioners of color often situate themselves vis-à-vis this discourse as individuals who are primarily trained in modern biomedicine and do not use or advocate the concepts of ancient healing traditions.

In the process of approvingly citing ancient healing traditions, functional medicine discourse inadvertently glorifies poverty and fails to include racialized Others in profit streams, thus reproducing inequality. I will argue instead for multilateral discourse, which would require functional medicine interlocutors to resist otherization, to view ethnic heritage as a legitimate source of expertise, and to defend the intellectual property rights of the people from whom this knowledge originates. In the absence of these elements, functional medicine entrepreneurship runs the risk of reinscribing "racial" inequality and venturing into the territory of biopiracy. In making these arguments, I draw from Marxist feminist approaches to biocapital.

I begin this chapter by detailing how functional medicine interlocutors idealize the past, and I describe functional medicine as the revival of traditional medicine in a new form. I then explore the relationship between functional medicine's otherization of non-Western cultures and its inadvertent romanticization of poverty. Finally, I turn to what I call the "identity paradox" among functional medicine practitioners and query the politics of inclusion and exclusion in functional medicine.

LONGING FOR AN IDEALIZED PAST

Functional medicine practitioners and health educators celebrate the lifestyles of centenarians living in the "Blue Zones"—regions in the world where, it is claimed, an unusual number of people live longer than average (Dan 2022). According to functional medicine proponents, individuals living in the Blue Zones do not need to "achieve" good health—rather, it unfolds naturally for them. Tom Blue asserts that in the Blue Zones, "it's like health just seems to happen to these folks in a very natural way." According to functional medicine interlocutors like Blue, longevity among individuals living in the Blue Zones can be attributed to their eating traditional foods, living in communities, maintaining supportive relationships, and not "stressing out about small things."

Dr. Rangan Chatterjee supports Blue's assertions when he describes an impactful conversation he had with a centenarian living in Guernsey in which the centenarian described how he maintains his health through simple, unintentional behaviors—as if living in a Blue Zone. Dr. Chatterjee explains, "He grew his own vegetables, and he ate them every day. He would be walking around every day, even on Sundays." While the elderly man enjoyed a glass of wine with his wife every few weeks and indulged in sugary treats at Christmas, neither was a habit. Unlike many of Dr. Chatterjee's young, chronically ill patients for whom achieving health is "very, very complex," this man did not see a doctor until he was in his early nineties. Dr. Chatterjee exclaims, "What's remarkable for me is that he didn't really think about being healthy!" This vociferous admiration of the way of life in the Blue Zones in functional medicine discourse is rooted in a desire for an environment that naturally facilitates health, which, in turn, is imaginatively anchored in the past.

Thus, other functional medicine interlocutors directly collapse "life in the past" onto "nature." For example, Matthew Accurso argues that people can access lifestyles and lessons from the past through experiences in "the wild." For him, the wild is a "place where you can get away from everything, all the distractions of life and really show [your kids], 'This is what it's about. This is where our ancestors are from.'" He suggests that parents transmit "ancestral knowledge" and teach their children about the "ways of life" through activities like hunting, arguing that "if you're a meat eater, showing them that this is where food comes from, it's not a factory line, it's in the woods" is a powerful experience that forges deep relationships based on trust, loyalty, and tranquility among humans. His utopian descriptions hint at the longing among functional medicine interlocutors for an idealized past, one characterized by a natural environment that is in harmony.

Nowhere is this imaginative nostalgia as pronounced as with regard to diet. Dr. Grace Liu, CEO of the Gut Institute, describes the "lifestyles" of hunter-gatherers and the Amish. Her description merges these two distinct groups, thus traversing space and time, on the basis of their shared proximity to "herds, hay, horses, and stalls." Ultimately, she points to how this proximity to animals results in greater exposure to soil and environmental bacteria and asserts that these "probiotics" are associated with microbiome diversity and, therefore, health.

Functional medicine interlocutors contrast idealized microbiomes past with the reality of microbiomes present. Dr. Liu indicates that when laboratory scientists examine stool samples today, instead of finding thousands of bacteria strains, they are lucky to find two to three hundred. She emphasizes, "In the Western world diversity is way, way, way, way down." This may be due to decreasing nutrient density in foods due to soil depletion from monocropping. Certified holistic health coach and environmental toxins expert Lara Adler explains, "If we look at people . . . who are eighty, ninety, and one hundred years old now, the environment that they were raised in is [not comparable] to what we have now." In comparison, Dr. Liu indicates that hunter-gatherers, the Amish, and rural populations benefit from gut diversity that is "really off the chart," leading them to live "cancer free, disease free, autistic free, and free of all of the conditions that would normally affect us chronically at early ages." Seen from this perspective, reconstructing the microbiomes of the past—to the extent this is possible—can produce invaluable protective health effects.

Some functional medicine interlocutors suggest eating unwashed, homegrown produce to increase exposure to a diverse array of microbes. Clinical nutritionist and High Intensity Health podcast host Mike Mutzel explains, "If you look at animals and nonindustrialized humans, they're eating food like this, right? So, you're getting some of those healthy microorganisms." Mutzel argues that while many people think that buying organic, gluten-free, grain-free food at Whole Foods is just as health sustaining, these foods are missing an indispensable microbial component.[2] In his view, reconnecting with nature—including composting and farming with worms, bugs, and bees—is "real feed 2.0." Foreshadowing my arguments to follow, Mutzel reinvents tradition (Hobsbawm and Ranger 1983) when he describes techniques from the past as the way of the future.

When describing ancient wisdom regarding meal taking, functional medicine interlocutors point to historical evidence dating back hundreds or thousands of years. Dr. Jason Fung, a kidney specialist who uses diet and intermittent fasting to manage diabetes, suggests that Jesus Christ, Muhammad, and the Buddha (whom he deems "the three most influential people in the history of the world") agreed on the power of fasting. He then provides examples of religious holidays where believers are instructed to either feast or fast and explains, "These people are not trying to kill off all their parishioners. They're trying to show them [how] to live healthier and better. . . . You've got to have this balance. You have to have feasting and fasting." In recommending this practice from long ago, Dr. Fung indicates that ideas that have stood the test of time—ideas in which different peoples and cultures from around the world have coincided—are wiser than "the latest and greatest idea." His comments again demonstrate how functional medicine discourse destabilizes existing notions of progress from past to present (see Haidt 2007).

Many functional medicine practitioners and interlocutors champion intermittent fasting using evolutionary arguments. Dr. David Jockers indicates, "Our ancestors were dealing with times of food famine where . . . food wasn't prevalent. . . . They had to have incredible drive in order to get it." In the context Dr. Jockers describes, hunger was a mechanism that ensured our species' survival by motivating individuals to hunt and gather. Extending his assertions, an article from Dave Asprey's website, Bulletproof, reads, "In preindustrial times, before we had restaurants and grocery stores, humans were metabolically flexible by necessity." In contrast, humans today have constant access to food in their pantries and refrigerators. According to many functional medicine practitioners, the constant hyper-availability of food has left humans metabolically inflexible, and remedying this situation through intermittent fasting can have incredible health benefits, such as improved energy.

Other functional medicine interlocutors stress that returning to the simplicity of an imagined past involves not only the food we eat and the way we situate ourselves vis-à-vis nature but also the ways we engage our bodies through movement and exercise. Darryl Edwards—who founded Primal Play and formerly worked as a computer programmer for Microsoft, an investment banker, and a financial software writer—argues for the importance of "ancestral evolutionary fitness" for long-term wellness. Ancestral evolutionary fitness encompasses all the movements that humans were "designed" to make in order to hunt, gather, build shelter, and protect themselves and their loved ones. These movements include climbing trees, jumping, carrying heavy items, and walking great distances. Edwards realized that his professional training did not model these movements for him in any way, shape, or form. He thought to himself, "Oh, wow! There's so much that we should be engaging in for movement practice." Pushing back against contemporary sedentary lifestyles, Edwards hopes to integrate ancestral movement patterns into his day-to-day life and, through his Primal Play Method, model them for others. Functional medicine interlocutors agree that, in contrast to lives spent engaging in primal movement patterns, "modern lifestyles" restrict movement.

Functional medicine interlocutors argue that modern-day restrictions on movement affect people of all ages—even small children and babies. Beth Lambert, the executive director of Parents Ending America's Childhood Epidemic (PEACE), bemoans how child-rearing in the developed world limits children's physical exploration of their environment, arguing that this has noxious effects on their mental development. She explains, "We put our kids in these restrictive bouncy seats and we put them in these car seats and we make them lie on their backs to sleep and we do all these things that are artificial." She provides a historical context for her statements on these restrictions on children's movement, asserting that they emerged only after the World War II era. This is one example among many of how functional medicine interlocutors attempt to historicize what they identify as a rupture between an idealized past and a dismal present.

Other functional medicine interlocutors argue that the historical rupture took place during the Industrial Revolution, in part due to the emergence of hourly wage labor. Dr. Kirk Robert Parsley explains, "People were working for six cents an hour, and if they could work in the factory for two more hours, they made twelve more cents. And that was a difference between feeding their kids tomorrow and not." Dr. Parsley suggests that the Industrial Revolution marks a shift to a modern world system that equates time with money (see Polanyi 2001). He continues, "People realized that they could survive on less and less sleep. And regardless of how badly they felt, they could push through it." As a result of this shift, individuals withstood hunger, lack of exercise, stress, and self-doubt to be more productive workers—with obvious consequences for human health and well-being.

Functional medicine providers furthermore decry the environmental dangers of living in the modern era, likening a recent boom in toxic exposures to what individuals were subjected to during the rise of industrialization. Dr. Christopher Shade points to negative effects from contemporary physiological stressors such as toxins in the food supply, radiation from electromagnetic fields, and blue light exposure. In his view, we are surrounded by a sea of chemicals, which accumulate within us and cause damage. Emphasizing a dystopian shift in our environment, Adler maintains that in comparison to individuals born in 1900, "We're not even on the same playing field anymore with regard to . . . the chemicals that we are exposed to." In her view, reducing chronic disease to the level experienced by individuals born at the beginning of the twentieth century will take significant effort in our current context since "they never had to fight against radioactive nucleotides in their drinking water because of hydrofracking. . . . They didn't have to deal with polychlorinated chemicals and bisphenol A in their plastics." Echoing some of these points, Dr. Deanna Minich, a clinical nutritionist who holds a PhD in nutrition, opines, "Now we really amped up and we've got different toxins to be thinking about—like electromagnetic field toxins and other things that we've created over time." From a functional medicine perspective, we are now living in an era of unprecedented toxicity.

These historicized approaches by functional medicine interlocutors frame bleak descriptions of contemporary life. Summing up "the modern lifestyle," Chris Kresser concludes that we live in a way that is fast paced, distracted by technology, undernourished, stressed, and lacking in social connection. Cognitive neuroscientist Dr. Dan Pardi remarks, "The world in modern life is different than it's ever been in all of human history. . . . We're born into a world that is really different than what our biology expects." His assertions point to a core tenet of functional medicine: chronic disease in the present day is due to a fundamental mismatch between the environment and human biology.

These practitioners additionally caution against contemporary forms of stress. Dr. Minich describes how pervasive, subtle, and underlying stress in our contemporary society "wears on our reserves, it wears on who we are as people." In essence, she describes how we have become acclimated to experiencing life as "on this fast track" and "kind of a rat race." Dr. Pardi further points out that "modern forces" exert pressure on individuals, thus shaping their aspirations. Dr. Shade extends these comments, saying, "All we have is this constant competition going on and this constant politics of scarcity, where we have to achieve, we have to make money, we have to secure our space here." In his view, individuals' perception of their positionality in society and surrounding environment, combined with a lack of social support, leads to neurological stress. From a functional medicine perspective, these multiple aspects of society have shifted individuals into chronic sympathetic overdrive, thus diminishing their ability to detoxify.

Functional medicine proponents' critiques regarding the negative consequences of industrialization on individuals' psyches dovetail with their criticisms regarding the overuse of technology in the present day. These interlocutors attribute the omnipresence of technology in our everyday lives to capitalist interests. Dr. Pardi critically observes, "There are many organizations, companies, and [venture capitalists] investing in technologies." Turning specifically to wearable technologies, Dr. Parsley contends that it is these companies' goal "to entirely take control of how the person is living. 'We're going to tell you what to eat [and] when to go to sleep.'" He deems this a "misappropriation of potentially useful technology." While many of the functional medicine proponents I observed critiqued the omnipresence of technology, few applied this critique to wearable devices. Dr. Parsley's assertion harks back to my argument in chapter 3 that self-tracking devices are paradoxically marketed as helping consumers to become more in touch with their bodies while disassociating well-being from individuals' internal cues.

Nonetheless, functional medicine proponents' critiques of technology extend to the use of technology in the practice of medicine. Blue comments, "It's to me striking how the presence of high-tech medicine doesn't seem in any way to correlate to longevity." In his perspective, higher-tech medical interventions often lead to more complications and side effects. Returning to functional medicine's admiration of people's way of life in the Blue Zones, Blue points out, "These folks have managed to avoid [disease] and, in doing so, have created astounding longevity—even without access to high-tech, acute care." Kresser builds on Blue's assertions by indicating, "We have a lot to learn from traditional people." In his view, it is functional medicine providers' job to understand how elements of "the modern lifestyle" are antithetical to health and to mitigate their negative effects, as well as to reframe elements of traditional medicine as "the future" of medicine.

FUNCTIONAL MEDICINE: THE REMAKING ANEW OF TRADITIONAL MEDICINE

When critiquing contemporary life and expressing reverence for traditional wisdom, some functional medicine practitioners argue that science is simply confirming what others have known all along. According to Dr. Andrew Heyman, an MD who is highly regarded for his research in the area of integrative and functional medicine, traditional healers have observed over the course of millennia the subtle features of how humans experience illness; however, medical researchers are only recently able to interpret these observations using scientific tools. He explains, "What was thought to be unscientific from a certain perspective, is now being revitalized." In practice, this means "the observational component to managing the disease process, which was more empirical in nature in the past, is now being given a biological reality—an objective explanatory model." As a transcriptomics researcher, he is acutely aware of how the "-omics" field marries pattern shifts, observed in clinic, to a "biological reality" that can be measured in very discrete ways, according to contemporary science. Functional medicine practitioners like Dr. Heyman support functional medicine's role in using emerging scientific tools to validate what ancient healing traditions have known for thousands of years.

Functional medicine practitioners further link ancient healing approaches to functional medicine when they describe pattern analysis as a primary skill that functional medicine doctors use to deliver clinical care. Dr. Heyman has explained in multiple venues that traditional medicines—ranging from ancient healing traditions such as Traditional Chinese Medicine and Ayurveda to comparatively "newer" traditional medicines such as homeopathy—use pattern analysis to make diagnoses in clinic. As he describes it, "In all of these older healing approaches, what they attempted to do was, through the power of observation, understand the stages that a person goes through . . . from health to illness." He elaborates, "What they were talking about were these patterns that you can observe, define, treat, and try to get the patient back to homeostasis." Providing specific examples, Dr. Heyman notes that practitioners from different ancient healing traditions might analyze the patient's pulse, tongue, and reported symptoms in an effort to capture all the subtle findings that define an illness complex.[3] While functional medicine providers locate data for pattern analysis in the patient's inclusive history (i.e., using the functional medicine matrix to evaluate antecedents, triggering events, and mediators of an illness) and in advanced diagnostic laboratory results, they similarly seek to observe, define, and treat a pattern to restore the patient to health.

Pattern analysis, an important skill from a systems biology perspective, is thus described by functional medicine interlocutors as a diagnostic method that was established by the ancient healing traditions and yet is a cutting-edge method. Functional medicine proponents consider ancient healing traditions like Traditional Chinese Medicine and Ayurveda to be the primordial systems biology approaches, and functional medicine doctors demonstrate their reverence for these approaches when they search for patterns among multiple symptoms to identify and treat underlying, systemic causes. While functional medicine in general is known for immediately incorporating emerging scientific discoveries into patient care, it is simultaneously characterized as a return to the enduring wisdom of ancient healing traditions. According to Dr. Heyman and Dr. Robert Naviaux, a mitochondrial medicine expert, functional medicine is always culling from the past while also setting the stage for the future of medicine. The mutual inflection of past and present in functional medicine is a sort of "remaking anew of traditional medicine" (Vega 2018)—a concept I introduced to disrupt Euro-American notions of chronological progress in science and medicine. In this vein, Dr. Naviaux notes, "Part of medicine [in the future] will involve pattern recognition." Dr. Heyman throws the supposedly linear nature of medical progress into question and describes "the convergence of the old and the new." The way in which functional medicine practitioners characterize ancient wisdom and practice as "version 2.0"—the next big thing—defies existing notions of science as progressing linearly toward greater "truth."[4] In this view, instead of moving toward a truer reality in the future, the truest wisdom can be accessed only by returning to some of what has been established in the past.

In the process, some functional medicine interlocutors are reframing what counts as evidence.[5] Razi Berry—publisher of the *International Journal of Naturopathic Medicine* and *Naturopathic Doctor News & Review* and founder of NaturalPath, "a community online for people to find their health naturally through the principles of naturopathic medicine"—points to the hubris of science (see also Hård and Jamison 2005) when she explains, "Anything in science when we try to create or prove something in a lab is really a way that we're trying to . . . harness nature or capture nature or trump her in some way." Building upon Dr. Heyman's point regarding how emerging scientific methods are validating the knowledge of ancient healing traditions, Berry continues, "Most of everything we do is just really going back to the empirical evidence that many of the people you've spoken to all around the world from many cultures, the plant medicines that they've used." Providing one example, Berry argues that scientific research on curcumin, a biochemical substance present in turmeric, has simply proved what people have known for generations: turmeric has powerful healing effects. From a functional medicine perspective, the use of salugens is rooted in valid evidence, even when scientific findings lag behind established empirical knowledge.

At the same time, functional medicine's validation of prior knowledge also extends to past scientific discoveries. Dr. Benjamin Chan, an associate research scientist in the laboratory of Yale School of Medicine biologist Dr. Paul Turner, describes how the inception of their current research on bacteriophages (viruses that infect bacteria) was akin to picking up a leaf from the past. Phages were discovered around 1915 by Franco-Canadian microbiologist Félix d'Hérelle at the Pasteur Institute in Paris and bacteriologist Frederick Twort at the University of London (see d'Hérelle 1917; Twort

1915). *FxMed* podcast host Dr. Fitzgerald comments on this, "One of the things that I looked at when I was reviewing [d'Hérelle's] book, again, is that they used phages for cholera and for typhus. . . . I mean, pretty extraordinary infections, with good outcome." Dr. Chan points out that despite these successful attempts approximately a hundred years ago, the approach fell out of favor until he and Dr. Turner began focusing their attention on using bacteriophages as a potential strategy for managing bacterial infections. Dr. Chan and Dr. Turner characterize their research as learning from the past to produce better treatments in the future.

Finally, functional medicine proponents cite epigenetic science to argue that the past is embodied in our present medical practice. GreenMedInfo founder Sayer Ji asserts that, based on "racial" or cultural heritage, individuals have epigenetically coevolved with specific dietary patterns. He furthermore suggests that individuals should eat according to their heritage.[6] While I am aware of the science upon which Ji's assertions are based, I am leery of how this ethnocentric approach may contribute to the exoticization of non-Western "Others."

THE OTHERIZATION OF NON-WESTERN CULTURES AND THE ROMANTICIZATION OF POVERTY

Functional medicine interlocutors sometimes simultaneously and inadvertently exoticize cultural "Others." Kresser indicates that his institute trains health care practitioners in functional medicine, ancestral diet, lifestyle education, and health coaching. When explaining what he means by "ancestral diet" and "lifestyle," Kresser praises the positive health outcomes among the Tsimané of Bolivia—a subsistence-farming group that follows a traditional diet, walks approximately eight miles a day, lives in close contact with nature, and maintains close-knit social groups. In contrast, he describes "getting heart disease, diabetes, and obesity" as "conditions that characterize *our* old age" (emphasis added). When functional medicine interlocutors like Kresser contrast "traditional cultures" with "us," they unwittingly otherize (see Brons 2015) "nonmodern" societies.

Some functional medicine interlocutors extend the idea that cultural differences are responsible for health outcomes to disparate cancer rates around the world. Cancer survivor and health coach Chris Wark describes a study that suggests that 70 percent of cancers in the United States are due to lifestyle choices such as smoking, "the Western diet," and environmental pollution. He points to a second study suggesting that up to 95 percent of cancers are preventable and are "caused by our diet and lifestyle in the Western world." Comparing cancer rates in the United States to those in less developed countries, Wark asserts, "If you move to Mexico and live, and fully embrace yourself in Mexican culture, you're going to drop your cancer rate in half." He emphasizes that cancer rates are even lower in other parts of the world, such as rural Africa, where "the rate of colon cancer is fifty times lower." Dr. Servan-Schreiber also concludes that cancer rates are worse in the West, pointing out, "The cancers that afflict the West—for example, breast, colon, and prostate cancer—are seven to sixty times more frequent here than in Asia" (2009, 8). He is quick to signal that these disparities are likely not due to differences in the prevalence of precancerous microtumors.[7] Instead, he argues, "Something in *their* way of life prevents these microtumors from developing" (8, emphasis in original). Then, turning to how the cancer rate among Japanese people who have migrated to the West increases to that of other Westerners within one or two generations,[8] Dr. Servan-Schreiber writes, "Something about our way of life weakens our defenses against disease" (8). He characterizes the "Traditional Western Diet" as aggravating inflammation and labels the Mediterranean diet, Indian cuisine, and Asian cuisine as "reducers" of inflammation (48). These examples demonstrate how functional medicine interlocutors homogenize all "traditional" cultures, uniformly deeming them cancer-protecting and contrasting them with "our" harmful diet and "way of life." In addition, functional medicine interlocutors portray differences between "us" and "them" as unfolding through a series of binaries: developed versus underdeveloped, urban versus rural, and Western versus non-Western.[9]

Functional medicine interlocutors turn to cutting-edge science to bolster their argument that divergent health outcomes are attributed to cultural differences, not genetic inheritance. Kresser explains, "We share the same genes as these traditional cultures that don't develop Alzheimer's for the most part. They're not developing [Alzheimer's], we are. What's the difference between *them* and *us*?" (emphasis added). As if responding to Kresser, Wark states, "[Other cultures] don't have a genetic advantage, but their diets and lifestyles are different." From a functional medicine perspective, diet and lifestyle predominantly determine health and disease, and while "they" have a health-promoting lifestyle, "we" are experiencing an epidemic of chronic disease.

Functional medicine proponents also emphasize differences in movement between "us" and "them." Wark comments that "a lot of them get more exercise naturally" due to walking instead of using motor vehicle transportation and climbing stairs instead of taking elevators. Jason Prall similarly distinguishes "Indigenous cultures" for having active lifestyles and contrasts this with our culture, which relies on the gym for artificial forms of physical activity. According to Lambert, Americans could learn a lot from observing how children in developing countries are able to interact with nature. She opines, "I would love for Americans to go spend some time in developing countries where children are allowed to grow and develop the way that they've been growing and developing for thousands of years." Lambert's description of how these children crawl and explore their environment imposes the ancient past onto present-day life in less developed countries. Taken together, functional medicine descriptions of how "Others" move their bodies conflate all peoples living outside of the United States with indigeneity and the past.

Functional medicine interlocutors similarly glorify non-American diets. Dr. Fung contrasts Okinawans with "us"—the majority of North Americans for whom highly processed food is a consistent part of everyday fare. He intervenes on the so-called macro-nutrient wars by arguing carbohydrates and saturated fats are not the problem. To substantiate his argument, he turns to "traditional diets" that are high in carbohydrates, indicating that Okinawans ate a lot of sweet potatoes and the Chinese ate a lot of rice into the 1980s, and both populations enjoyed good health and longevity. Like many functional medicine practitioners, Dr. Fung argues that the problem is actually highly processed "fake food." Pointing to how "fake foods" increased the consumption of trans fats, Dr. Fung contends that whenever food is manipulated away from its natural state, it produces the potential for health problems since the human body is adapted to eat real food. Many functional medicine practitioners agree with Dr. Fung and argue that while "traditional diets" have been followed for millennia in many places around the world, Americans are essentially the "inventors" of processed food—products that "we" then marketed to the rest of the world (see Otero 2018; Gálvez 2018). The binary distinctions functional medicine interlocutors make between "our" and "their" diets belie the reality of transnational marketing and the global food system.

Otherization of non-American cultures in functional medicine extends beyond exercise and diet to how relationships are constructed and maintained.[10] Contrasting true person-to-person connections with social media "connections," Wark indicates, "A lot of cultures with long lifespans have very close social networks. Not Facebook—I mean they really are very social, and spend a lot of time with family and friends." Sachin Patel extends Wark's comments when he contrasts individualism in the United States with Italy, Greece, and Japan, where people are motivated by a common goal and seek to create healthy, happy relationships among "the entire village." Patel opines, "I think the level of difference [between these countries and the United States] really comes from this idea of working together for a common good versus competing with each other." Patel attributes the "competition mindset" in the United States to capitalism, saying, "We seem to have this weird ideology that we should do things on our own or that it's better if we do it on our own." While Patel named capitalism, he and other functional medicine interlocutors are actually diagnosing a lack of deep social connections as a pathology of neoliberalism.[11] They align neoliberalism with the United States, but I argue that neoliberalism is a world system (Polanyi 2001).

While functional medicine proponents portray non-Western cultures as investing time and energy into creating harmonious relationships with others, they describe people in the United States as inordinately focused on "the superficial," with detrimental effects to their health. Adler discusses how Western society's "superficial" culture contributes to individuals' overall toxic burden. Referring to the numerous toxins in many personal-hygiene and beauty products, Adler notes, "We have this onslaught of exposures that are happening due to [these] really superficial, societal dictates about beauty norms . . . and our bodies are struggling." From her perspective, women in other cultures do not face cultural pressure regarding their appearance and, therefore, are less exposed to chemicals and experience less anxiety and stress. As she speaks, she shifts her body to the right to emphasize a contrast between "our culture" and "other cultures," indicating, "And then you look over here and you see these populations of people who are like, 'Yeah, I don't really care about that stuff. You know, family is really important to me. Connection and community is really important to me, and whatever about the rest.'" Her comments pose authentic connections with family and community versus inordinate focus on superficial beauty standards as an additional layer in the many binary distinctions functional medicine interlocutors make between "us" and "them."

Overt admiration in functional medicine for diverse cultural heritages may inadvertently lead to the romanticization of socioeconomic inequality. Specifically, by celebrating the diets, movement patterns, "lifestyles," and values of "non-Westerners," functional medicine interlocutors unwittingly glorify global poverty and food insecurity. When describing the diets of "other cultures," Wark indicates, "A lot of them eat plant-based diets. . . . They're not pure vegan, but they eat mostly plants because they're in a much lower socioeconomic bracket. They're poor, and plants are cheap." Although he briefly acknowledges poverty, Wark goes on to say in his next breath that "we" should start modeling "them." Similarly, Adler opines that individuals who live in "cultures" that have to travel large distances to get water develop "an incredible respect and reverence for [nature] because [the experience] allows you to see in a really clear way [your] very intimate connection with the environment." She argues that living in these "cultures" imbues individuals with a sense of gratitude for natural resources, thus leading them not to waste or take natural resources for granted. In contrast, she points out, "We take everything for granted." I argue that Wark and Adler mistake scarcity for "culture." People living in poverty cannot afford to waste resources because they face food insecurity and lack reliable access to clean water. Given global issues of food insecurity and lack of access to clean water, gratitude for meeting one's basic human needs for survival in impoverished settings is not something that should be romanticized.

Nonetheless, poverty is romanticized by functional medicine interlocutors in indirect, and sometimes direct, ways. Molecular biologist Dr. Sherry Zhang—a woman whose overarching goal is to "reverse the obesity epidemic by using nutrigenomics to change how people access food and nutrition"—shares the following story in her email newsletter *GenoPalate*:

> There was a boy, whose family was very wealthy . . .
>
> One day his father took him on a trip to the country, to show his son how poor people live. So they arrived at a farm of a very poor family, as he considered. They spent several days there. On their return, the father asked his son if he liked the trip.
>
> "Oh, it was great, Dad," the boy replied.
>
> "Did you notice how poor people live?"
>
> "Yeah, I did," said the boy. The father asked his son to tell in more detail about his impressions from their trip.
>
> "Well, we have only one dog, and they have four of them. In our garden there is a pool, while they have a river that has no end. We've got expensive lanterns, but they have stars above their heads at night. We have the patio, and they have the whole horizon. We have only a small piece of land, while they have endless fields. We buy food, but they grow it. We have a high fence for protection of our property, and they don't need it, as their friends protect them."
>
> The father was stunned speechless.
>
> Then the boy added, "Thank you, Dad, for letting me see how poor we are."

This anecdote romanticizes economic poverty and allows social inequality to be mistaken as benefiting the "have nots." It exemplifies how functional medicine discourse often mistakes structural factors (e.g., socioeconomic differences, political context, environmental issues, etc.) for "culture." Functional medicine interlocutors attribute disparate health outcomes to "culture" when, in fact, poor outcomes are due to the social determinants of health. In the next section, I turn to how functional medicine may inadvertently exacerbate existing inequalities by excluding the very people whose cultures it idealizes.

INADVERTENT EXCLUSIONS AND POTENTIAL BIOPIRACY

Dr. Christiane Northrup's website celebrates her as a New Thought Walden Awards honoree and identifies her as a "visionary pioneer and a leading authority in the field of women's health and wellness." The website includes a picture of Oprah Winfrey wrapping her arms around Dr. Northrup, alongside the tag "Oprah Winfrey Network 'Super Soul 100 Soul Igniter.'"[12] Dr. Northrup, an ob-gyn, author, and public speaker, earned this distinction for using her voice and talent to "awaken humanity." In 2013, *Reader's Digest* named her one of the "100 Most Trusted People in America," her website notes.

When describing her interest in using herbal medicine for gynecological health, Dr. Northrup indicates that while the Thai people have been using one powerful herb for seven hundred years for this purpose, this herb was "discovered" by the Germans in the 1970s. She comments sarcastically, "Don't you love it? Someone always discovers what the hill tribes of Northern Thailand had only been doing for seven hundred years—and now it's a big 'discovery'! Not for them!" With these words, Dr. Northrup asserts how unjust it is for Western "discoverers" to lay claim to non-Western traditional ethnomedical knowledge.

At the same time, her referring to the "discoverer" as "someone" and "the hill tribes" as "them" contributes to processes of otherization and reinscribes existing binaries. Functional medicine interlocutors describe "them" as living in either tribes or villages. I am wary of the slippage between "tribe" and "savages" and between "ancient" and "uncivilized." Dr. Northrup's description coincides with understandings of non-Western peoples as nonmodern. It inadvertently essentializes others, suggesting that non-Westerners are frozen in the past. This portrayal is inaccurate. Over the course of my experience as an anthropological fieldworker, I have observed how traditional healers have increasingly incorporated markers of "modernity" into their lives and their ethnomedical practices (e.g., technologies such as cell phones, digital cameras, and Facebook and behaviors associated with biomedicine such as the use of IVs and sterilization practices). Practitioners of traditional ethnomedicine are not exempt from the transformative processes of living in a globalized and digitized world.

When Dr. Northrup goes on to describe her company, her explanation is ironic, given her pointed critique of Western "discoverers." She says, "I, myself, started a company called A Model Life when I heard about this herb from Thailand." She explains that this herb provides a phytohormone that "works so well for menopause that I started a company to bring this into the public consciousness." According to her other comments, the "hill tribes of Northern Thailand" had already been using the herb for seven hundred years; however, she does not include these "hill tribes" in what she deems "public consciousness." Thus, Dr. Northrup fails to extend her own critique of how Westerners "discover" what has already been known to native peoples to how her company brings traditional knowledge into the "public consciousness."

My point is not to personally attack Dr. Northrup. I am not privy to the inner workings of Dr. Northrup's company, but I am concerned that the "hill tribes" may not be equitably included in profit streams. It may be that Thai people significantly contribute to the company's vision and daily operation while also equitably reaping profit. However, without further information, I am left to reflect on how Dr. Northrup's entrepreneurship profits from traditional ethnomedical knowledge while potentially excluding the very people whose intellectual property she celebrates (and has usurped? [see Vega 2018]). Moreover, how might the production, marketing, and sale of salugens in functional medicine be indicative of biopiracy?

In asking this question, I turn to Marxist feminist approaches to biocapital. Most desirable biological resources (e.g., "tropilogicals"—organs for transplant and wombs for rent) originate in the economically deprived Global South, leading to an exacerbation of age-old inequalities in the new "bio-informational economy." Medical anthropologists, including Margaret Lock (2001, 2002) and Charis Thompson (2005), drawing on Marilyn Strathern (1992a, 1992b), Donna Haraway (1997, 2007), and Paul Rabinow (1992, 1996), have similarly studied how "biologicals" are stabilized, dominated, stored, accumulated, distributed, and converted into novel forms of property, thus teasing at the contested relationship between biological collection and its commodification. Examples of biocapital include patentable biodiversity (Hayden 2003) and biobanking of human DNA, human tissue, human embryos, and human stem cells (Parry 2004). Kalindi Vora (2015) asserts that contemporary commodification of life and vitality[13]—the substance of the activity that produces life—is framed by earlier, colonial modes of exploitation, including the racialization of labor.[14]

In functional medicine, salugens are created from biological compounds that have been isolated from herbs and foods traditionally consumed by people around the world for their health-promoting benefits. Examples include curcumin from turmeric, ECGC from green tea, and resveratrol from red grapes. These "biologically desirable resources"—examples of "substances that produce life" and their commodification—originated outside of the United States. The ways in which they are portrayed and sold by functional medicine entrepreneurs resembles earlier, colonial modes of exploitation.

When individuals accept recognition for knowledge that originates in a different culture, without including the "ethnic others" who gained the knowledge originally, they inadvertently marginalize the originators of that knowledge, thus reifying economic and political inequalities. "Thought leaders" like Dr. Northrup are recognized for the work they do to "empower" others. According to the New Thought Walden Awards web page, these awards "honor those who use empowering spiritual ideas and philosophies to change lives and make our planet a better place."[15] The questions become: Who is in the position to do the "empowering"? Who are the "empowered"? And who is excluded from the equation entirely—rendered invisible? My concern is that the original possessors of "spiritual ideas" (and ethnomedical knowledge) may be excluded, not only from profit streams but also from recognition on a global stage.

While bioentrepreneurs use community-based marketing within the functional medicine realm,[16] their community is constituted by and for people of socioeconomic and often "racial" privilege. Functional medicine community-based marketing is not the community-based entrepreneurship "centered on ethnomedicine, enhancement of local livelihoods, gender empowerment, and conservation and enhancement of traditional knowledge through community capacity building" that sociologist Maria Costanza Torri describes (2010, 40; see also Dana and Riseth 2011). Functional medicine's entrepreneurial community unfolds at a social, political, and economic distance from the communities where "traditional" knowledge, lifestyles, and ethnomedicines are woven into the fabric of everyday life.

THE IDENTITY PARADOX

While in chapter 2 I argued that functional medicine decenters biomedical authoritative knowledge and instead privileges the patient's embodied knowledge, in this chapter I describe how some functional medicine practitioners and health educators position themselves as experts regarding traditional ethnomedicines. More specifically, non-Western cultures, and with them their "ancient healing traditions," are romanticized by individuals who are either from a different culture or have been trained in the biomedical paradigm. I do not argue that individuals should practice traditional medicines according to only their "racial" and ethnic heritage. I do ask, however, who is able to build a functional medicine career based on expertise in traditional medicine? How does this intersect with individual practitioners' ethnic and "racial" upbringing?

In search of a more holistic approach to health, certain functional medicine practitioners have either considered or received training in Traditional Chinese Medicine (TCM). As someone who learned through personal experience that "conventional medicine [is] poorly suited to deal with chronic, complex illness," Kresser, a White man, indicates that he "decided to go back and study Chinese medicine because that was the closest thing that I had encountered in my journey back to health [that had] a more holistic framework in it." Kresser was not aware of functional medicine at the time, although it already existed. At present, Kresser's training in TCM informs his perspective as a licensed acupuncturist, functional medicine practitioner, health coach, author, and ancestral nutritionist. Dr. Heyman, also a White man, was likewise trained in TCM. His background in TCM shapes both his mitochondrial research and his functional medical practice.

In contrast, Dr. Cynthia Li,[17] a Chinese American, practiced conventional medicine until she faced health challenges that it could not heal. After a two-year hiatus from work and slowly recovering her health, she sought advice from colleagues on how to return to practicing medicine. She describes how she told one colleague, "I really love the Traditional Chinese Medicine way of thinking. It makes so much sense to me—the systems thinking . . . being the foundation of healing and how ancestral health figures into it." While Dr. Cynthia Li was interested in seeking further medical education in TCM, her colleague's response diverted her attention elsewhere: "It sounds like you are interested in functional medicine." This response shocked Dr. Cynthia Li, who until then had never heard of functional medicine. Her colleague recommended that she take a course with the Institute for Functional Medicine; she took her colleague's advice and never looked back.

How might Dr. Cynthia Li's conversation with her colleague have unfolded differently if her interest in TCM had been rooted in her own Chinese identity? What would have happened if she had emphasized, "I would like to combine my training in conventional medicine with wisdom from the medical system that my Chinese ancestors have been using for millennia"? As a person of mixed Chinese heritage[18] who was raised with TCM and as a young adult considered pursuing a doctorate in Oriental medicine, I listened to Dr. Cynthia Li's story with deep interest. Who is encouraged to turn to TCM as a source of legitimate expertise?

This curiosity continued when I listened to a conversation between Dr. William Li and Dr. Hyman. Dr. William Li begins to quote a Confucian teaching from Japan that instructs people to eat until they are 80 percent full when Dr. Hyman interjects, supplying the saying: "Hara hachi bu."[19] Dr. William Li nods in agreement and indicates that avoiding metabolic stress by exercising moderation at the dinner table is a common denominator for cultures that exhibit high longevity. He furthermore suggests that people are more likely to eat at a slower pace when they socialize while eating, thus recognizing their satiety cues before gorging themselves, and notes that people in Mediterranean countries and the Blue Zones eat with others.

During the interview, Dr. Hyman, a White man, engages his interviewee as a person of Chinese descent. He says, "You are Chinese, and in Chinese, the word for 'take your medicine' is *chur yao*, which means, 'to eat your medicine.'" Dr. Hyman's ability to speak Mandarin reflects his time living in China. He continues, "[This] is a very interesting way of framing it. They don't take your medicine as a pill, they eat their medicine." Turning specifically to TCM, Dr. Hyman explains, "Traditional Chinese Medicine is actually a system of thinking in the body, as a system. And that is what functional medicine is. It is a systems-thinking approach." Dr. William Li concurs, "In Traditional Chinese Medicine, you view food and medicine and herbs all in continuity. . . . All the things that we are now rediscovering using science." By using the word "we" to describe those engaged in scientific discovery, Dr. William Li resists Dr. Hyman's identification (and potential otherization) of him as a representative of China and instead (re)aligns himself with Western approaches to knowledge.

Dr. William Li further frames himself as a scientific researcher and a biomedically trained physician when he mentions, "I'm a researcher, so I'm always looking at the latest new thing." He agrees with Dr. Hyman's view, saying, "I think there is great value in looking back at the ancient cultures and the ancient recipes. We've probably forgotten more than we have [learned]." However, he again uses "we" to indicate that he is among the learners who have forgotten the wisdom of ancient cultures. Throughout the conversation, Dr. William Li comments from the position of a biomedically trained physician who has researched the benefits of TCM, not as a Chinese man who was raised with TCM.

In the same vein as my queries about the identity politics surrounding Dr. Cynthia Li, I wonder if Dr. William Li would be as celebrated if his primary training were in TCM. Would he still be a world-renowned author and TED speaker? Would his work have garnered the interest of *Good Morning America*, CNN, MSNBC, NPR, Voice of America, the *Atlantic*, *Time*, and the *New York Times*? Perhaps even more provocative is the following question: would he be as successful and well regarded in functional medicine as Kresser and Dr. Heyman, White functional medicine practitioners whose training is in TCM? I have noted that, within functional medicine discourse, traditional ethnomedicines are rarely represented by the people who come from the cultures from which the ethnomedicines originate.

During the course of my ethnographic research, I observed how functional medicine practitioners of color avoided recommending ethnomedical remedies related to their personal heritage in order to ensure their legitimacy as practitioners. At the Advances in Mitochondrial Medicine Symposium, Dr. Shilpa Saxena, a board-certified family physician and functional medicine expert, described how she incorporates functional foods in the form of meal-replacement shakes into her practice in Lutz, Florida. She indicated she would love to be able to recommend ashwagandha, a traditional Ayurvedic herb, but exclaimed, "I can't do that!" Then, emphasizing her Indian heritage by slowly enunciating every syllable of her name, she said, "I am Shil-pa Sax-en-ah." Dr. Saxena went on to explain that, given her Indian heritage, recommending Ayurvedic herbs would be considered too "woo woo" by her clientele. Dr. Saxena's livelihood is dependent on her maintaining a safe distance from Indian ethnomedicine. For her, being of Indian descent is not a source of authority but a potential threat to her legitimacy.

In contrast, I frequently observed phenotypically White individuals being positioned as experts in traditional, ethnomedical knowledge.[20] Brian Vaszily, host of the Your Best Years Start Now online event, describes Nick Polizzi as "today's leading ancient and Indigenous medicine expert" and explains that Polizzi "is going to share his [three] secrets you need to know to look and feel your best, and live long doing it, from his unique set of expertise." Polizzi is the founder of the Sacred Science, a "website and blog dedicated to explorations of alternative healing modalities and Indigenous healing traditions," and the executive producer of the docuseries *Remedy: Ancient Medicine for Modern Illness*. Similarly, a description of Prall's interview for the Fatigue Super Conference indicates that Prall shares "powerful lessons from Indigenous cultures" and teaches viewers how to "integrate these lessons into their own lives." Both Polizzi and Prall are phenotypically White. Polizzi's surname suggests Italian heritage, while Prall identifies himself as a "Northern European white guy." While neither claims to be Indigenous or a traditional healer himself, they are both portrayed in promotional content for online summits and conferences as Indigenous medicine experts. Furthermore, the very terminology of "Indigenous medicine" and "Indigenous healing traditions" is problematic since the knowledge it references is not specific to a place or people but can be multiply located around the world.

Other times, phenotypically White individuals lay claim to racialized identities.[21] For example, the docuseries *Remedy* features Karta Purkh Singh Khalsa. According to Khalsa's website, he is "nationally credentialed to teach herbalism, yoga and bodywork, including Ayurvedic massage and spa techniques."[22] He appears in *Remedy* wearing white robes and a turban. Despite his name and ethnic clothing, he is phenotypically White. While I cannot speak to Khalsa's ethnic heritage, his self-identification as an expert in Ayurveda left me wondering who is allowed to speak as a representative of ethnomedical knowledge (see Spivak 1988).

During her appearance in *Remedy*, Dr. Tieraona Low Dog is similarly portrayed as an expert in Indigenous medicine. In addition, Dr. Low Dog, who has partial Native American heritage, has sometimes been referred to as a "medicine woman" in the media.[23] When asked by an interviewer for *Alternative Therapies* if her interest in botanicals comes from her Native American heritage, she resists how she has been identified by this term, saying, "I am not a 'medicine woman'" (Gazella 2005). Dr. Low Dog is phenotypically White, and, according to her website, "she studied midwifery, herbal medicine, massage therapy, and martial arts before earning her medical degree from the University of New Mexico School of Medicine."[24] The way in which Dr. Low Dog contests being labeled as a "medicine woman" signals the importance of i(nter)dentification (Vega 2017b). Identities are relationally constructed, not only through how individuals identify themselves but also through how they are identified by others.

This pattern of functional medicine practitioners of color avoiding claims to ethnomedical knowledge and phenotypically White functional medicine interlocutors positioning themselves as experts on indigeneity and ancient medicine persisted throughout my ethnographic research. However, as the COVID-19 pandemic sparked critical analysis of "racial" disparities in health outcomes, I noticed two indications that a reexamination of identity politics may also be underway in functional medicine. First, in June 2020, Dr. Low Dog responded to a reference to her "lineage" by Maskell by indicating that she is not the representative of any nation or people and can speak only from her own experience. Listening to Dr. Low Dog's disclaimer regarding her "lineage" was like a breath of fresh air. She went on to indicate, "Here in New Mexico, our Navajo and Pueblo peoples" are disproportionately affected by the pandemic. Her response then shifted into police brutality against Black individuals and how intergenerational trauma is passed down in certain groups of people.

The second example indicating a reexamination of identity politics in functional medicine occurred in April 2020, when Dr. Fitzgerald explained in her newsletter that TCM was being used in China across "all settings" (spanning biomedical and traditional) for COVID-19, with strong preliminary data to support its use.[25] Dr. Fitzgerald noted how TCM had previously been used to prevent and treat SARS-CoV-1, with very, very strong outcomes. She sat down with Dr. John Chen on her podcast *FxMed* to explore the topic of TCM further. Dr. Chen holds doctoral degrees in pharmacy and Oriental medicine and is a licensed acupuncturist. In his biographies for both Evergreen Herbs, an online company that sells herbal products for which Dr. Chen serves as a medical consultant, and a webinar for Lhasa OMS,[26] Dr. Chen links his authority in Chinese herbal medicine to his "family tradition." While he lives and works in the United States, his hybrid professional identity renders him the perfect person for, in Dr. Fitzgerald's words, "actively following TCM in China and shar[ing] his experience, insight, and observations with all of us." Dr. Fitzgerald emphasizes that Dr. Chen effectively "fram[es] TCM in language clear for the Western-trained clinician" and that his role is that of a bridge between "us" and "them."

How did the COVID-19 pandemic facilitate this unique exception in which an individual positioned himself as a representative of the traditional medicine associated with his own "racial" heritage? To answer this question, I point to the arc of racializing narratives regarding Chinese individuals throughout the COVID-19 pandemic. From the very outset of the pandemic, Chinese people were discriminated against as vectors of disease and were targeted for hate crimes.[27] As reported on ABC News, a March 2020 FBI Intelligence Report indicated, "Hate crime incidents against Asian Americans likely will surge across the United States, due to the spread of coronavirus disease . . . endangering Asian American communities" (Margolin 2020). Asian Americans reported being coughed at, spit on, told to leave stores, refused by Uber and Lyft drivers, and verbally and physically assaulted (Kandil 2020). Racialized rhetoric surrounding the coronavirus—most notably, President Donald Trump referring to the infection as "the Chinese virus" and the "kung flu"—fueled and legitimated acts of "racial" violence and discrimination.

When Andrew Yang, a 2020 Democratic presidential candidate, became the target of racism, he took to the *Washington Post* to publish an op-ed titled "We Asian Americans Are Not the Virus, but We Can Be Part of the Cure."[28] In his "call to action," Yang describes how Asian Americans should respond to "racial" hate, arguing, "We Asian Americans need to embrace and show our American-ness in ways we never have before." He furthermore urges Asian Americans to "demonstrate that we are part of the solution" by helping neighbors, donating gear, funding aid organizations, voting, volunteering, and "wearing red, white, and blue." His article received significant backlash from readers who argued Yang placed the burden on Asian Americans to prove their deservingness as Americans.

As an Asian-Mexican-Native American, I have observed how many Asian Americans have climbed professional ladders, thus securing positions in the middle and upper classes. While debates on racism and discrimination tend to focus on African Americans and Latinos—Black and Brown people, including myself, who have been targeted by atrocious forms of "racial" hate—it is as if the Chinese Exclusion Act and the Japanese internments are long-forgotten notes in history. However, while some Asian Americans have secured a degree of economic power, they are far from equally represented in seats of political power. A few days of global pandemic is all it took to reveal the ugly truth: Asians living in the United States are still racialized beings.

After China swiftly controlled the spread of COVID-19 among its citizens and the United States became the nation with the greatest number of confirmed COVID-19 cases, a counternarrative emerged. While China was accused of concealing the extent of the pandemic, it was simultaneously reframed as an example to the world of how to rapidly and effectively control the spread of infectious disease. The Chinese government's approach to the coronavirus pandemic saved the lives of millions of Chinese and potentially tens or hundreds of millions of people around the world. In addition to the Chinese government's actions, China's success was attributed to the Chinese culture and, as evinced by Dr. Fitzgerald's newsletter, Traditional Chinese Medicine.

I must signal that Dr. Chen's anomalous inclusion in functional medicine discourse as a representative of the traditional medicine with which he was raised was *rendered possible only* by his training in Western pharmacy. His hybrid professional identity and his ability to explain TCM concepts to "the Western-trained clinician" earned him a seat at the functional medicine table. However, this "entering and exiting" of hybrid individuals (see García Canclini [1990] 2009) has not been repeated with other traditional ethnomedicines, including Ayurvedic medicine.

A few short weeks before Dr. Fitzgerald's newsletter, Maskell sent an email from India to his listserv recipients. In this email he describes his visit with "the founder of one of the biggest companies in India," explaining that reading Maskell's book was the first time his unnamed host saw how Ayurveda and pharmaceutical Western medicine could complement each other through the bridge of functional medicine. While functional medicine practitioners who are not of Indian descent often applaud the healing powers of Ayurvedic herbs, Ayurvedic practitioners in and from India have not been included in functional medicine discourse.[29] Maskell elaborates, "Currently, the country spends less than 4% of the GDP on health care, and without the barriers of pharma influence and, dare I say, materialism, there's a huge opportunity for India to create the perfect healthcare system, much like the opportunity America had in the 1950s." His words are uplifting, and, at the same time, they run the risk of romanticizing India's health care system as belonging to an idealized past.

In this chapter, I described how functional medicine practitioners and health educators tend to romanticize non-Western or non-US cultures with which they do not personally identify. On the one hand, "we" are described as Western or US societies that are modern, unhealthy, high tech, stressed, lacking social connection, and distracted by a fast-paced lifestyle. In contrast, "they" are nonmodern, traditional, healthy, low tech, calm, slow-living people who benefit from close-knit relationships and an ancestral diet. This binary approach homogenizes all "non-Western" and "non-US" cultures from a "Western" and "United States" perspective. Idealistic descriptions of "them" are permeated with inadvertent otherization. Functional medicine unfolds at a political and socioeconomic distance from the ethnomedicine it celebrates, and as a result functional medicine entrepreneurship verges on biopiracy while potentially reinscribing "racial" inequality.

Instead, I argue functional medicine must embrace multilateral discourse, engage people from around the world as equals instead of racialized "Others," celebrate ethnic heritage as a source of legitimacy and expertise, and ensure intellectual property rights of the people from whom knowledge originates. In the next chapter, I focus this social justice lens on a macro scale and explore the systemic shifts that must occur in the pharmaceutical and health insurance industries to ensure equitable access to the resources that reverse chronic disease.

CHAPTER 7
BIG PHARMA AND HEALTH INSURANCE

Now I turn to the voices of the functional medicine practitioners who speak from a place of experience as former conventional medical doctors when they critique existing funding structures of pharmaceutical research and financial incentives in hospital systems. I also draw from the perspectives of interlocutors who leverage their training in economics to advocate for health justice. Finally, I consider direct critiques of the health insurance system by providers who derive their income from medical insurance billing, who are rare. By weaving these critiques together with perspectives from medical anthropology, I outline systemic shifts that are required to ensure equitable access to strategies and techniques that create health and reverse chronic disease.

Functional medicine providers point to the health care system's inherent conflict of interest: by operating through a fee-for-service model, providers are incentivized to manage, but not heal, disease. Specifically, functional medicine practitioners and proponents highlight how, by focusing on ameliorating symptoms while failing to address the root cause of disease, the pharmaceuticalization of medicine has effectively turned physicians into drug dealers. Patients are caught in a vicious cycle of symptoms and side effects, creating greater dependence on an increasing number of medications and greater profits for pharmaceutical companies. At the same time, functional medicine proponents assert that health insurance does not facilitate access to health. Instead, it is merely a method of paying for conventional medical interventions, meaning that for most people health insurance acts as a "prepaid drug plan."

Functional medicine discourse emphasizes the importance of switching to value-based care—that is, paying doctors based on positive patient outcomes instead of the number of services they provide. I engage functional medicine proponents' arguments for value-based care by identifying both challenges and opportunities for the change they propose. To achieve meaningful change in the health care system, the funding structures for academic research and, indeed, our very understanding of what constitutes legitimate science must also undergo change. The current funding structure, which is party to the interests of the pharmaceutical and health care industries, determines which are "fundable" research questions, thus constraining what scientists can study and therefore what they can discover. To remedy this problem, I suggest that the state prohibit pharmaceutical companies from funding medical research, both directly and indirectly. Instead, I argue for state-sponsored research (see Moynihan et al. 2019) that focuses primarily on the creation of health instead of merely finding new ways to treat disease. At the same time, I document significant inroads with respect to the insertion of functional medicine into state-funded health care.

FUNCTIONAL MEDICINE'S CRITIQUE OF THE PHARMACEUTICAL INDUSTRY

As a whole, those in the functional medicine community are very critical of what they view as the overuse and misuse of pharmaceuticals in conventional medicine. According to functional medicine proponents, the hegemony of the pharmaceutical approach obscures consideration of dietary changes that would address root causes without the dangerous side effects of medication. Diabetes specialist Dr. Jason Fung asserts, "The wrong answer, if you have too much insulin, is, 'Let's give more insulin.'" He compares the conventional approach to treating type 2 diabetes to treating an alcoholic with alcohol, explaining, "The short-term symptoms are going to be better, because if you're an alcoholic and you're starting to shake, that alcohol is going to make you stop shaking. But it's not going to make the alcoholism get better." Returning to type 2 diabetes, he advocates for lowering insulin levels through lifestyle and diet. Functional medicine practitioners like Dr. Fung argue that while dietary approaches can produce lasting results, they are often ignored because they are not profitable to the pharmaceutical industry, and that industry exercises enormous influence over how medicine is practiced.

Others have critiqued the pharmaceutical industry through the lens of the opioid epidemic. For example, Dr. Anna Lembke asserts in a TEDx talk that the opioid epidemic is first and foremost an epidemic of overprescribing. Dr. Lembke is associate professor and medical director of addiction medicine at the Stanford University School of Medicine and chief of the

Stanford Addiction Medicine Dual Diagnosis Clinic. She describes a historic transition from the 1950s to the 1990s wherein doctors went from being reticent, in the earlier years, to prescribe pain medication to anyone because they were afraid of addiction to, "by the end of the 1990s, . . . dispensing opioids like vending machines to anyone that came in and said, 'I have pain.'" She provocatively queries the TEDx talk audience, "How did healers become dealers?" From Dr. Lembke's perspective, this transition was buttressed by a cultural shift in medicine that views pain as dangerous.

Dr. Lembke goes on to describe the role overprescribing has played in this "public health crisis." She notes, "The United States consumes over 80 percent of the world's supply of opioid pain pills despite constituting only 5 percent of the world's population." She argues that while a "small subset of pill mill doctors" contribute to the opioid crisis—doctors who willfully and nefariously exchange prescriptions for cash—the majority of the crisis can be attributed to "compassionate doctors meaning to do well, caught in a system gone awry, harming patients who are showing up who really want help." Her comment about a "system gone awry" evokes a recent study in the *British Medical Journal* that identifies "medical error"—which the article classifies as "death from medical care itself"—as the third leading cause of death in the United States, outpaced only by heart disease and cancer (Makary and Daniel 2016, 353). Foreshadowing some of the comments in the section of this chapter on conflicts of interest, Dr. Lembke opines that the problem is not individual doctors' moral failings but, rather, this health care system that has gone wrong.[1]

Functional medicine doctors describe how their perspective on prescribing pharmaceuticals changed when they distanced themselves from conventional medicine. Dr. Steven Masley, a conventionally trained MD and fellow of the American Heart Association who is also a clinical nutritionist and certified densitometrist, states simply in the docuseries *Betrayal*, "When I have to put someone on a medication, I feel like I've failed them." He explains, "It's not that I'm anti-med. But it means that I didn't find the underlying cause and there probably was one that probably would have actually been their true solution, and probably would have done it without medication." Functional medicine doctors like Dr. Masley recall their education in conventional medicine and how they were trained to use the prescription pad as their primary "tool" in clinical practice. When considering the prescribing patterns of their conventional medicine counterparts, this shared experience allows them to empathize with their counterparts' hope to alleviate the patient's pain and symptoms with medication. Thus, when arguing that functional medicine is better equipped to reverse chronic disease than conventional medicine, functional medicine practitioners do not doubt the good intentions of the individuals who practice conventional medicine. Ari Whitten asserts, "The entire medical system—every layer of it—from the actual care that you are receiving; to the insurance; to the actual research; is being conducted by very well-intended, altruistic, great, very smart people who are . . . trying to help people."

In essence, functional medicine proponents diagnose the *systemic* pharmaceuticalization of medicine, resulting in a patient population that is increasingly dependent on multiple drugs because their conventionally trained doctors are trying to help them as they were trained to do. Tom Blue describes how this process occurs in an archetypal patient. An otherwise healthy patient goes to the doctor and discovers they have high cholesterol. The doctor tells them not to worry and prescribes them Lipitor. That patient takes Lipitor and is compliant with their cholesterol-management plan. Their cholesterol numbers come down. The next time they come to the doctor, they are congratulated for restoring their good health! However, the next year, when they return for a checkup, their blood pressure is high. The doctor puts them on a blood pressure medication. They are compliant with the management of their blood pressure, and their blood pressure numbers come down. Again, they are congratulated for restoring their good health! Blue concludes, "And then, it's your blood sugar and then it's stomach acid. And then, these things begin to conspire with one another to create some new symptoms that we can then suppress with new technologies and new innovations." Blue's description points to drug interactions and side effects as well as the progression of chronic disease in the absence of "root cause" treatment.

Blue goes on to link expanding health costs to a definition of health as the mere absence of symptoms. In Blue's opinion, this definition of health will inevitably produce more cost, unsustainability, and dependency on the health care system since it places no restrictions or conditions on how an absence of symptoms is achieved—a situation that is exemplified by his archetypal patient. Reducing health costs will require major structural changes to the health care system.[2]

According to functional medicine proponents like Blue, the pharmaceuticalization of medicine blocks conventional doctors from getting to the root causes of disease. In the next section, I interweave medical anthropology analyses and functional medicine practitioners' critiques of health insurance in the United States.

HEALTH INSURANCE IS NOT HEALTH CARE

In the United States, health care coverage is provided through a combination of private health insurance and public health coverage (primarily Medicare and Medicaid) since the US government does not provide universal health care to citizens. Health care in the United States is very expensive—for example, the average three-day hospital stay costs approximately $30,000.[3] In 2020, the US national per capita health care expenditure exceeded $12,500.[4] Most hospitals are privately owned and are reimbursed for the services they provide by insurance companies.

Health insurance serves as a lens for understanding how people seek security against life's calamities, how risk is distributed, and how the US health care system is structured (see Ericson, Barry, and Doyle 2000; Lehtonen and Hoyweghen 2014). Most Americans have health insurance to mitigate the risk of significant debt if they fall ill or become injured. People under the age of sixty-five obtain insurance via their employer or a family member, by purchasing health insurance on their own, or through government assistance based on income (Medicaid). Individuals over sixty-five are eligible for Medicare.

In general, insured individuals make monthly payments, called premiums, to private health insurance companies for a health insurance plan that will pay some or all of the cost associated with specific interventions, provided that the insured seeks care from a provider that is in network with the health insurance company. In this fee-for-service model, the insured may pay a deductible (a minimum out-of-pocket amount before their insurance benefits take effect) or a fixed percentage of the service fee, according to their plan details. Insured individuals often must pay a co-pay (a fixed fee) at the time of service. Co-pays are generally lower when seeing a primary care physician and higher when seeing a specialist. Insurance plans offer differing amounts of prescription coverage—some prescription medications may be covered fully, some may not be covered at all, and others may need to be paid partially out of pocket by the insured. Insurance plans usually have spending caps, meaning that once a patient's annual spending reaches a certain limit, the responsibility for the cost reverts to the patient. Most plans also have exclusions—services that are not covered by the plan and must be paid out of pocket by the insured.

In 2010, the Affordable Care Act (ACA, commonly known as Obamacare) prompted major changes in health insurance. The ACA promised to broaden access to quality care by offering coverage options to the uninsured and underinsured.[5] However, ethnographic observations suggest the law has failed to meet its goals. The ACA endorses high-deductible insurance plans, signaling the considerable financial responsibility individuals must assume for their own care. Rebecca Adkins Fletcher's (2014) observations of unionized workers in an urban central Appalachian community illustrate how increased cost sharing, high deductibles, and unstable employment can leave even insured individuals in a state of precarity. She describes growing disparities among differently insured working families. At issue is limited access to *appropriate* health care and growing medical financial burdens for many families. In a context of shifting eligibility and coverage, Christina M. Getrich et al. (2018, 248) describe immigrant-serving providers in New Mexico as "safety-net providers" who play "critical buffering roles" in a fragmented health care system. Safety-net providers are often responsible for negotiating emerging bureaucratic barriers for insured patients. These examples show how differing levels of deductibles, co-pays, prescription coverage, spending caps, exclusions, and premium rates lead to disparities among the insured (see Adkins Fletcher 2014). By broadening access to insurance while increasing disparities among the insured, the ACA both lessens and exacerbates social inequality.[6]

Both medical anthropologists and functional medicine interlocutors argue that the ACA has led to fewer health care dollars being spent on actual health care provisioning. Its plans are financed by government subsidies and individual premiums but operated by private insurers in competitive markets. Maskell describes how the ACA has inadvertently incentivized increasing health care prices since insurance companies can only earn a capped percentage of the price of services: "What you find out is that they are negotiating everything upwards—not downwards! Because everyone is in on the scam." Jessica Mulligan, a medical anthropologist, explains, "Financial techniques obfuscate how much health care costs [and] foster widespread gaming of reimbursement systems that drives up prices." Money is funneled away from actual care provisioning and toward administrative costs and investor profits using creative "representational techniques" (Mulligan 2016, 37). As if responding to Mulligan, Maskell deems increasing financialization of the $3.8 trillion health care industry—that is, the process by which the health care market and its financial institutions have increased in size and influence—"the most powerful scam in human history." Referring specifically to pharmaceutical partnerships, referral quotas, and reimbursement-led decisions, Maskell asserts, "It's not fair that your health is secondary to a system's financial bottom line." Both Mulligan's and Maskell's arguments build upon the work of medical anthropologists who explored the relationship between managed care, market-based medicine, and inequality in the early 2000s and noted the depoliticization of ill health and poverty through bureaucratic and technocratic means (Nelson 2005; see also Rylko-Bauer and Farmer 2002). Given my ethnographic observations, and responding to Amy Dao and Jessica Mulligan (2016), I might suggest that contemporary insurance techniques in the United States promote individual responsibility at the expense of social solidarity and, far from facilitating the right to health, merely facilitate the right to purchase health.[7]

Functional medicine practitioners and proponents distinguish having health insurance from having appropriate health care. They emphasize that health insurance is simply a method for paying for health care. Their explanations destabilize the assumption that health insurance is the only possible method of paying for health care while simultaneously pointing to the economic interests that led to the reification of this assumption over time. Functional medicine proponents furthermore argue that the pharmaceuticalization of medicine has taken an "insurance product" and reconfigured it in a way that betrays the very meaning of "insurance." Maskell explains, "If you have a car or home insurance, you know that in the statistically insignificant chance that you have some sort of disaster, this third party company that you contract with [will] give you money back for the premiums that you have paid to insure your risk." In contrast, functional medicine interlocutors describe health insurance as a prepaid drug plan. Building on Blue's critique, Maskell indicates, "The standard of care [is] to give everyone a ton of drugs that is all covered by insurance." These financial structures reinforce conventional medicine's drug-based approach to chronic disease. Thus, functional medicine proponents' critique of the health insurance structure dovetails with their critique of the pharmaceuticalization of medicine.

As a result of these processes, functional medicine interlocutors argue, health insurance does not confer access to the kind of care that can reverse chronic illness. Maskell explains, "If you have insurance, and your only way of interacting with health care is to use the people that are insurance-billable, you have no access to a kind of care that can reverse your chronic illness."[8] Not only do functional medicine interlocutors decouple health insurance from health care, they furthermore divorce health care from health. In this vein, functional medicine proponents argue that once patients experience the holistic interventions that functional medicine offers, they will no longer consider disease management with pharmaceuticals to be adequate care.

I identify with this perspective. As someone who has reversed multiple overlapping chronic diseases, I know healing is possible for many people like me. Speaking to my sentiments, Blue notes, "The tragedy of [ongoing pharmaceutical management of chronic disease] is . . . disease reversal really is very possible." He continues, "We have legions of people that have basically been sentenced to a life sentence on a disease management protocol when they very easily could be accessing disease regression and even disease reversal programs." I disagree with Blue's word choice in this latter statement; I argue that while disease regression and reversal are "very possible," they are *not* easily accessible to most people. That is the crux of the matter.

The issue of unequal access to healing therapies looms large in my mind and haunts my conscience. The fact that six in ten adults in the United States have one chronic disease and four in ten have two or more feels terrible, wrong, and almost criminal. As a medical anthropologist who practices hyper-self-reflexivity (see Kapoor 2004), I am achingly aware of how my healing was potentiated by my socioeconomic privilege. I purchased chronic-disease reversal, and I would not be better today if I had not had the financial capability to do so.

Many functional medicine interlocutors argue that while functional medicine could help many millions of American adults suffering from chronic disease, at present their care is largely inaccessible due to limited pathways for its insertion into existing health care structures. Dr. Anand Parekh, the Bipartisan Policy Center's chief medical advisor and former deputy assistant secretary for health (2008 to 2015) at the US Department of Health and Human Services, explains, "If you are a drug or a device, there is a pathway in this country for that intervention to be scaled. But if you are an evidence-based program—either prevention or treatment—lifestyle-focused . . . there is no pathway in this country like there is if you are a drug or a device." Dr. Mark Hyman adds that while there are billions of dollars spent on research and development of pharmaceuticals in the United States, there are no funds to support research into nutrition and lifestyle interventions. In a similar vein, Paulette Jordan—a former Democratic member of the Idaho House of Representatives (December 2014 to February 2018) and a 2020 Democratic candidate for the US Senate—notes, "We're not collecting any data [on reversing chronic disease]. . . . We're not really operating off of a model or a method that is going to move our country forward to address the root problem that we're facing." Functional medicine interlocutors agree that evidence-based nutrition and lifestyle interventions should be encouraged to reverse the steady progression of chronic disease in America.

It may be that functional medicine has not gained purchase in the existing health care system because the inclusion of functional medicine in primary care would actually *lower* health care spending and *improve* outcomes overall. While this argument may seem counterintuitive, especially given the ways in which I have represented functional medicine as unaffordable except for privileged consumers, I assert that the money spent on reversing chronic disease pales in comparison to the health care costs associated with a lifetime of chronic-disease management.

Unfortunately, the current health care system shifts the responsibility for cost and labor of care onto "de facto disentitled" patients (López 2005; Willging 2005), and care is rationalized through "medical necessity" (Wagner 2005). Under "Necessity for Treatment" in the *Medicare Carriers Manual* (part 3—Claims Process, section 2251.3), the policy indicates that "services that seek to prevent disease, promote health and prolong and enhance the quality of life, or maintain or prevent deterioration of a chronic condition" are *not payable* under the Medicare program since they are *not medically necessary*. Functional medicine proponents are extremely critical of disease-focused policies like *MCM* 2251.3, arguing that they lead to a health care system that fails to support health.

CONFLICTS OF INTEREST: COST VERSUS OUTCOME

Functional medicine practitioners often critique the American health care system for trailing behind those of less developed countries. On his podcast *The Doctor's Farmacy*, Dr. Hyman indicates the reasons Americans should expect to have the best health care: "We have the best hospitals, we have the best technology, we have cutting-edge treatments and drugs for a whole multitude of problems. . . . We spend more than twice any other nation on health care." However, turning to outcomes, he ultimately paints a dismal picture: "We have pretty crappy life expectancy. . . . We have health disparities. And we're lagging behind almost every other country in health metrics, including infant mortality, life expectancy." According to Dr. Hyman, American citizens' poor health is linked to uneven quality of care and unequal access.

This mismatch between expectations and reality inspired Dr. Hyman to assess value in American medicine by looking at outcomes and cost. He recounts how, after being named the director of the Cleveland Clinic Center for Functional Medicine in September 2014, he attempted to obtain data from payers regarding the total cost of care. His attempts were quickly thwarted as he encountered an utter lack of transparency—an experience he describes as being in a "no man's land." He emphasizes, "We don't have evidence-based medicine, we have reimbursement-based medicine. I think that is a reality we have to face." The experience made Dr. Hyman realize it is impossible to effectively measure outcomes for value in the conventional medical system.

According to many functional medicine interlocutors, the "no man's land" Dr. Hyman describes has been created by design. Referring to a Goldman Sachs report that points to curing patients as an unsustainable business model (see Kim 2018; Martyn 2018), Maskell elucidates, "On the one hand, you have customers for life, and on the other hand you have people independent of the medical system." Dr. Parekh extends this when he explains, "You can't make as much money on prevention as you can on treatment." Maskell's and Dr. Parekh's comments indicate that, as openly stated in *MCM* 2251.3, the health care system is engineered to provide ongoing disease management, not disease prevention or reversal.

When making this critique, functional medicine interlocutors point to the important role of economic incentives. Maskell notes it is "no wonder" natural health has not been incorporated into the health system, and clarifies, "No one is incentivized to get people off medication and keep people healthy. . . . And, ultimately, incentives matter." John Robbins, cofounder and president of the Food Revolution Network, coincides with Maskell when he indicates, "Medicine is a business and there are powerful commercial forces involved. There is a lot of money at stake, and the incentives haven't always been aligned with patient well-being" (Robbins and Robbins 2013, 10). In essence, our neoliberal health care system capitalizes on patients' suffering.

Hospitals and insurance companies are primarily concerned with increasing profits. Acknowledging this fact, functional medicine proponents argue that chronically ill patients are highly profitable for the health care industry. As Blue puts it, "Dead's not profitable. Healthy is minimally profitable. Chronically ill is a very profitable state to keep a population in." Referring to Sachin Patel, Maskell elaborates, "People say health care is broken, but it's not. It's fixed. . . . What that reframes in your mind is that [the health care system] is a profit maximization machine that has been oiled for years and is working perfectly." The result, according to Dr. Dean Ornish, a physician, researcher, and clinical professor of medicine who founded the Preventive Medicine Research Institute and has been identified by Forbes as "one of the seven most powerful teachers in the world," is that "we pay for things that are dangerous, invasive, expensive, and largely ineffective" (Robbins and Robbins 2013, 10). The profit-oriented health care system leads to exorbitant expenses while undermining patient well-being.

This is especially a problem in the United States. In a TEDMED talk, "Why Your Health Care Costs So Much," health economist Irene Papanicolas indicates the United States has some of the highest prices in the world for medical goods, services, labor, and drugs. Papanicolas explains that Crestor, a cholesterol-lowering drug, costs double in the United States what it costs in other, similar countries. She notes that American primary care physicians are paid just over $200,000 per annum—about double what physicians are paid in other high-income countries. Likewise, procedures including CT scans, MRIs, and colonoscopies cost more than double in the United States. Explaining that higher prices do not coincide with higher quality, and signaling, "MRI machines in Geneva are every bit as good as those in Boston, but the US price is three times as high," Papanicolas asserts that the US health care system has a "price problem." Harking back to Dr. Hyman's experience of trying to evaluate cost based on value, she notes, "Finding price data in health care is difficult, and that points to another reason why health care costs are high." When buyers are unable to find out what prices are, sellers are more likely to charge higher prices.

Worse yet, from a functional medicine perspective, higher costs do not result in better quality. Maskell observes, "It was super confusing to me that health costs were rising and yet the return on that healthcare investment was incredibly, painfully low." As if responding to Maskell, Blue elaborates, "Technologies have evolved to really magnify and multiply the effective investment. Except, in the totality of health care." Stated differently, other industries rely on technology to increase quality while reducing cost. But in health care, costs are intentionally kept high. Furthermore, this situation unfolds with total impunity. Clinical nutritionist Dr. Peter Osborne indicates, "From a business perspective, medicine is the only business that continues to grow at an exponential rate despite failing miserably its customers. What other business can you think of . . . that has that track record?" His comment builds on Papanicolas's argument that "customers" (i.e., patients) should understand health care costs by furthermore suggesting that they demand value-based care.

At present, few health care institutions focus on delivering value—meanwhile, the Cleveland Clinic Center for Functional Medicine delivers value at a loss. Describing a program at the center called Functioning for Life, Dr. Hyman explains, "We take people living with chronic disease, we change their lifestyle, we change their diet, we actually—through social support—help them change their behavior." The program has produced extraordinary results including weight loss and the reversal of diabetes and heart failure.[9] Despite these positive outcomes, Dr. Hyman reveals, "We are saving [insurers] so much money and we're not getting paid for what we do.

We get paid thirty cents on the dollar, and we're lucky if we make a hundred bucks on a patient." Although the Center for Functional Medicine is providing enormous value to the health care system—to the benefit of Medicare, Medicaid, and private insurers through reduced reimbursements—their work is so poorly reimbursed that it does not cover the cost of running the center. As Dr. Hyman concludes, "The whole system is kind of rigged and not incentivized to do the right thing." His words hint at medical anthropologists Amy Dao and Mark Nichter's (2016) explanation of how "moral hazard" unfolds among providers and administrators—due to erroneous incentives, some providers and administrators game the system to maximize reimbursements; meanwhile, preventive health care services are not reimbursed.

Functional medicine interlocutors also identify significant issues with how health problems are named, arguing that medical nomenclature conceals the true nature of health care costs. Turning to a specific example, Blue explains that the sickest 1 percent of working-age adults (defined as adults under sixty-five) account for about 25 percent of total health care spending and the sickest 5 percent account for a little over half of total spending. This data led Blue to ask himself, "What is it about that 5 percent [that is] driving more than 50 percent of the costs of the whole working-age population?" He clarifies that these sick individuals are not expensive because of infrequent catastrophic events—"They're expensive every year. And getting more so every year." Blue says he found the answer to his question when he discovered that this population is characterized by a high prevalence of autoimmune disorders. He goes on to note that in 2016, four of the five top-selling drugs by dollars were immunosuppressive biologic drugs. From his perspective, autoimmunity is a "quiet epidemic" that has been concealed by a naming convention that makes different autoimmune conditions seem like discrete entities.

While there are currently more than one hundred distinct autoimmune diseases,[10] people do not tend to think of them as belonging to one, unifying category. For this reason, the cost burden of autoimmunity is concealed. Blue explains, "It's not like cancer, where you can really easily roll up the total cost burden of cancer because things are conveniently tagged with the word 'cancer.'" He asserts that the growing autoimmune epidemic is the most addressable high-cost chronic condition in American society. Speaking to the treatment protocols employed by functional medicine practitioners, he emphasizes that autoimmunity is addressable and "doesn't involve shutting down your immune system and exposing you to risks of dying of pneumonia at the age of sixty-five." According to functional medicine proponents like Blue, the "autoimmunity epidemic" is a huge cost driver that can be easily defined, targeted, and addressed.

While Blue points to more effective, lower-cost treatment methods for an expensive—and often concealed—category of disease, Papanicolas argues for systemic shifts in health care as a whole. She attributes the problem of high costs to three main things: "First, lack of data on prices and lack of cost transparency. Second, decreasing competition with little price regulation. Third, a system that is fragmented and administratively complex." Her observations echo those of Mulligan (2016). Papanicolas then turns to "fundamental prescriptions" for the problems of price, decreasing competitiveness, and administrative inefficiency, indicating, "The first prescription is about encouraging real price transparency in health care for patients and providers." Papanicolas explains that when patients seek care, they have no idea how much the services they receive will cost until they receive the bill. She argues that consumers in any other industry would not tolerate blank price tags, so health care consumers should not tolerate lack of price transparency either. She continues, "The second prescription goes out to US government agencies like the FTC and the Department of Justice, and it's about enforcing antitrust laws in health care." Specifically, Papanicolas points to hospital mergers being on the rise and how less competition allows for price gouging. Finally, she says, "The third prescription is about improving administrative efficiency." While in her view there is "a lot of low-hanging fruit," I agree with Mulligan (2016) that administrative inefficiency is by design.

However, some functional medicine interlocutors believe change is on the horizon—not due to a sudden surge of altruism in health care financing but, rather, due to the utter unsustainability of growing health costs. Papanicolas affirms, "When you compare the US to other countries, one fact comes into sharp relief. The US healthcare system today is on an unsustainable trajectory." Responding to these calls for change, I note the obvious: reducing the rate of chronic disease not only would lower costs, it also would improve the quality of life of millions of patients, ease the burden of their caretakers, and increase the disability-adjusted life years (DALYs) of the population at large.

LOWERING COSTS WITH FUNCTIONAL MEDICINE?

Functional medicine proponents view health care costs through the lens of "the therapeutic order"—a concept originating in naturopathy. Maskell explains, "We should use the least costly, least invasive approaches first, and then work our way up." According to this logic, surgery and ongoing management with pharmaceutical drugs are the most expensive forms of intervention and should therefore be used as last resorts. In comparison, the advanced diagnostic testing and lifestyle-based treatment protocols offered by functional medicine are intermediate costs, and prevention strategies are the most cost effective.

Thus, according to "the therapeutic order," lower-cost interventions should be "upstream," while higher-cost interventions should be "downstream." Maskell notes that the majority of costs in the health care system—$4.3 trillion per year—are incurred after the primary care doctor refers the patient to a specialist. Therefore, the majority of health care costs could be avoided if health problems were resolved at the level of primary care. He explains, "The cost of . . . diabetic neuropathy is way different and way bigger than dealing with the upstream factor of creating stability in your blood sugar." In essence, the earlier disease is prevented, the less costly it ultimately is. Unfortunately, developing health issues are usually not addressed until disease etiology has progressed past the point of prevention.

In a 2019 study in the *Journal of the American Medical Association* (*JAMA*), "Association of the Functional Medicine Model of Care with Patient-Reported Health-Related Quality-of-Life Outcomes," Michelle Beidelschies et al. conducted a retrospective cohort comparison of functional medicine patients with propensity score–matched conventional medicine patients. Their findings support many of the arguments presented by different interlocutors in this chapter. Like Blue, Beidelschies et al. (2019) point to the simultaneous increase in incidence of chronic disease and health care–related costs, writing, "Chronic disease is challenging health in the United States with nearly 100 million people having 1 or more chronic conditions in 2014. These individuals contribute to 90% of the nation's annual healthcare expenditure."[11] They assert, "Without new approaches that focus on reversing chronic disease, our current healthcare model will become economically unsustainable."[12] The study, which included 7,252 patients from the Cleveland Clinic,[13] found that after both six and twelve months of care, functional medicine patients demonstrated improvements in their PROMIS Global Physical Health score that were significantly greater than those of conventional medicine patients. PROMIS is a psychometrically validated system that is funded by the National Institutes of Health Roadmap Initiative and measures self-reported health across multiple areas. These results led Beidelschies et al. to conclude that the functional medicine model of care represents a viable delivery system for reversing illness, promoting health, and optimizing function.

Immediately after its publication, the Beidelschies et al. study took on a social life of its own. In an article titled "Cleveland Clinic's Functional Medicine Outcomes in *JAMA*: Six Perspectives," integrative practitioner and editor in chief of the *Journal of Alternative and Complementary Medicine* John Weeks called the Cleveland Clinic Center for Functional Medicine "a pilot based on a largely untested belief that functional medicine could outperform regular medicine, and at lower cost" (Weeks 2019). Dr. Weeks is both the article's author and the interviewer of the six contributors featured in it. As a contributor, Dr. Melinda Ring—a clinician and researcher who serves as director of the Northwestern Osher Center for Integrative Medicine and a core faculty member at the Duke Leadership Program in Integrative Medicine—critiqued Beidelschies et al. for not including the financial aspects of functional versus conventional medicine. Dr. Ring asked, "What does it cost the system when these functional medicine doctors spend more time with patients? They don't generate as much revenues as regular primary care doctors in short visits." Dr. Weeks indicates that during his interview of Dr. Ring, he noted that while her concern is valid in the current volume-based industry, there is no clinical data to support the assumption that shorter visits have more valuable impact on patient care and better long-term cost savings when compared to longer visits.

In response to critiques like Dr. Ring's, functional medicine proponents argue that increased investments early on produce long-term cost savings. In this vein, Dr. Ornish points out, "The opportunities are really ripe now for industries to realize that a new paradigm of medical care can be much more sustainable, and even profitable" (Robbins and Robbins 2013, 17). Returning to his critique of pharmaceuticalized health care, Blue asserts, "Symptom suppression medicine is essentially the greatest cost driver in health care." However, despite functional medicine proponents' assertions that addressing the root cause of disease is cheaper in the long run, functional medicine has made limited inroads into the health care system. At present, there are only a few examples of integrative medicine operating in large health systems. Maskell indicates that "most of those examples are failures" and explains, "You can't make as much money getting people well through nutrition as you can doing heart stents." Since integrative centers do not produce as much money per square foot as acute care centers, the latter are prioritized to maximize profit.

In conventional medicine's current fee-for-service model, profits are based on the volume of services offered (tests, procedures, and labs) irrespective of the outcome or quality. Maskell explains in the docuseries *The Human Longevity Project*, "There are lots of people who want to increase those costs. Health insurance, pharmaceuticals, hospitals, they actually have no incentives to reduce costs at all in the American system." Integrative family medicine doctor Jeffrey Geller, founding member and past president of Integrative Medicine for the Underserved (IM4US), explains the doctor's perspective: "If I have a patient who is sick and they come eight times, I earn eight times more than [for] a patient who is well." Dr. Geller's words were not meant to incriminate doctors but, rather, to signal how doctors are cogs in a system that prioritizes volume.

Emphasizing the systemic nature of the problem, Dr. Lembke similarly describes how physicians practice "assembly-line medicine" in "healthcare factories"—what she calls "the Toyotaization of health care." She succinctly notes, "The throughput of bodies is more important than whole person health. The health care system's emphasis on volume puts tremendous pressure on doctors to palliate pain and perform procedures because that is what pays." To fix this situation, Dr. Lembke, a sharp critic of the opioid epidemic, wants to reprioritize the patient-provider relationship over time so that medications do not come to stand in for that relationship.[14]

Functional medicine interlocutors seek more radical change than this, arguing a systemic problem requires a system-wide transformation. Dr. Parekh indicates he would like to see a "value-based insurance system" that promotes "high-value preventative services." This transition would involve shifting from paying doctors for the services they provide to paying them for the value they deliver. Maskell and Dr. Geller similarly suggest that a capitated, value-based health care system would reduce illness by incentivizing doctors to produce good health outcomes among their patients—a stark change from the current system in which providers profit from patients' ill health. Dr. Geller pleads, "Let us, physicians, have some money for keeping people well." Together, functional medicine proponents are pushing for a switch from volume to value in health care.

Functional medicine proponents are optimistic that change is within reach. Maskell writes, "One of the most significant changes in the way healthcare is being paid for is the shift from fee-for-service to fee-for-value. This shift, especially in America, has been very slow to materialize until now" (2020, 62). Maskell further expresses his excitement regarding what he sees as a transition in medicine toward rewarding practitioners for delivering value in health care. At the same time, functional medicine practitioners are cognizant that change will take time. Dr. Hyman notes, "We need to do [value-based care] across a whole spectrum of Medicare and Medicaid. . . . I think that we are not there yet." Dr. Parekh likewise acknowledges, "Value-based healthcare transformation with the focus on payment based on outcomes, as opposed to volume . . . is going to be in the long haul." However, Dr. Parekh cites the Center for Medicare and Medicaid Innovation's recent confirmation of the diabetes prevention program's cost-effectiveness as one significant success. Functional medicine interlocutors like Dr. Parekh call for bipartisan support and "targeted investments" for evidence-based prevention in public health.

While Dr. Hyman notes, as discussed above, that functional medicine services at the Cleveland Clinic are not sufficiently reimbursed by insurance, he is nonetheless hopeful for the future. Dr. Hyman points out that functional medicine unfolds in the uncharted territory between existing reimbursement structures and reimbursement based on value. As if responding directly to Dr. Ring's inquiry about the financial impact of functional providers spending more time with patients, Dr. Hyman continued, "I don't think we are going to do ten [randomized controlled trials] and convince the world about functional medicine. . . . I think that the way it is going to change is by showing value." In his view, demonstrating that functional medicine delivers better outcomes at lower cost to a wide population will prompt a change in reimbursement structures, which, in turn, will shift the focus of the entire health care system. Functional medicine interlocutors like Dr. Hyman argue that functional medicine is uniquely positioned to solve the problem of value.

While it is up to functional medicine providers to demonstrate the superior value of functional medicine, health care "buyers" must also opt for the value-based alternative. Blue indicates that self-insured employers might play a key role in the transition toward value-based care since their economic interests cut against those of the current health care system: "Self-insured employers are the ones most likely to . . . lead the charge in putting an end to this nonsense. . . . Every dollar they're spending on health care that they don't need to, is a dollar taken out of profits." Self-insured employers are motivated to make sure their employees are productive and loyal to the company.

Ultimately, functional medicine interlocutors argue that change will activate from the bottom up. Blue contends that the pendulum of cost will be pushed in the direction of value by employers and the legions of consumers who are becoming educated about functional medicine. Maskell says a lot of patients and providers have identified the "scam" of increasing health care costs, and this, in turn, will drive a transition toward value-based care. In the next section, I elaborate on the specific challenges and opportunities framing this transition.

TROUBLING THE WATERS: "FUNDABLE" RESEARCH QUESTIONS AND "REIMBURSABLE" INTERVENTIONS

Harking back to the pharmaceutical industry's undue influence over health care, I argue that the potential of value-based care has thus far been obscured by a lack of research funding to prove its benefits. My argument is informed by functional medicine practitioners' and health educators' critiques of how industry sponsorship leads to conflicts of interest in medical research. As Dr. Christopher Gardner, a nutrition scientist and the Rehnborg Farquhar Professor of Medicine at Stanford University, explains, fundable questions tend to be reductionist—for example, studying one molecule for its effect. While Dr. Gardner notes that this tendency pits rigor against generalizability, I add that it disfavors a holistic health care approach.[15]

In essence, research on creating health, as opposed to that on managing disease, is not occurring because there is no funding to support it. Dr. Zach Bush, a conventionally trained internist and endocrinologist with expertise in the human microbiome, explains that virtually all health research funding in the United States "goes into chronic disease management and chronic disease treatments rather than [asking,] 'What is the fabric of health? What is a healthy human body?'" Dr. Emeran Mayer—director of the G. Oppenheimer Center for Neurobiology of Stress and Resilience; codirector of the Digestive Diseases Research Center; and professor of medicine, physiology, and psychiatry at UCLA—similarly writes, "Federally funded biomedical research is almost exclusively focused on unraveling disease mechanisms and not on identifying the biological and environmental factors that contribute to a state of optimal health" (2018, 266). These two doctors' comments hint at the interrelationship between federal research funding and the pharmaceutical industry.

Describing the specific pathways that consolidate these connections, Dr. Bush explains, "Public money is through the National Institutes of Health in the United States, which is all disease-based. . . . The NIH is broken up into different sectors . . . but they are all disease-based."[16] According to a

2018 study by Ekaterina Galkina Cleary et al., "NIH funding contributed to published research associated with every one of the 210 new drugs approved by the Food and Drug Administration from 2010 to 2016" (2329). During this time, the NIH provided more than 200,000 years of grant funding, totaling more than $100 billion. Of this funding, more than 90 percent was for "basic research related to the biological targets for drug action" (Cleary et al. 2018, 2329). The later stages of pharmaceutical research and development—widely referred to as "applied research"—are predominantly funded by industry. Commenting on these relationships, Dr. Bush laments, "If you can't tie yourself to the profit margins, you can't get the money, and you can't do the research."

Since the financial interests of the pharmaceutical and hospital industries shape how medical research is conducted, they also shape public perception of truth. Turning to an increase in chemical exposures in our environment, Dr. Bush addresses how a lot of people think "science must be kind of bunk science or it must be conspiracy theory, because if all of it was that toxic, then certainly the universities would have figured that out by now." Responding to this widespread assumption, Dr. Bush says, "No, they won't. They can't figure it out because they aren't getting paid to figure it out!" With this example, he explains how what the public thinks of as "legitimate science" is, unbeknownst to the public, determined by funding structures.

This begs the question, what is the solution for the wellness research funding crisis? According to Dr. Bush, wellness research should be funded with private money by inventors like himself. His assertion is informed by his own experience. He notes, "I didn't have that luxury in seventeen years of academia. I could never ask any question I wanted. I had to ask questions that were compelling in an area that could get funded." For him, "fascinating" research questions leading to "some of the most compelling stuff I've ever done" became "askable" only once he created enough "profit centers" to fund his company's research lab. As the result of his successful entrepreneurship, Dr. Bush now has a lab that is internally funded that allows him and his team to ask "all kinds of interesting questions."

Novel questions produce novel results. Dr. Ornish elaborates on Dr. Bush's points by describing the impact of his own research. "We use these very high tech, expensive, state-of-the-art measures working with first-rate scientists to show how powerful these very simple, low tech, and low cost interventions can be" (Robbins and Robbins 2013, 10). Every one of his research groups' studies have demonstrated that lifestyle and diet changes facilitate enormous improvement in health outcomes.

While I respect the work of researchers like Dr. Bush and Dr. Ornish, I point to the shortcomings of pharmaceutical industry–funded research to argue that private funding, tied to private interests, is not the answer. Private interests, whether they belong to pharmaceutical companies or entrepreneurs, are prone to shaping research questions and determining research outcomes based on potential profit. However, as an academic and a health scientist, I agree with Dr. Bush that something must be done to remove the constraints on health research. Instead of sidestepping the system for public research funding, an appeal must be made to decision makers for public research funding to study wellness. While privately funded research may initially serve as evidence to support this appeal, directing public funding to basic science studies on creating health is important because doing so places responsibility for ensuring the health of citizens in the hands of the state, instead of in the hands of individual citizens themselves.[17]

Individuals related and unrelated to functional medicine are already engaged in a struggle to recast existing funding structures. Liam Mannix, a science writer, introduced these issues into the public sphere when he pointed to a "global campaign" to separate medicine from Big Pharma. Referring to an earlier publication by Ray Moynihan et al. in the *British Medical Journal*, Mannix (2019) points to how "doctors are being unduly influenced by industry-sponsored education events and industry-funded trials for major drugs." In their article, Moynihan et al. assert, "Endemic financial entanglement with industry is distorting the production and use of healthcare evidence, causing harm to individuals and waste for health systems" (2019, 1). Their assertions are supported by a systematic review of seventy-five papers published in the Cochrane Database of Systematic Reviews, which reads, "Industry sponsored drug and device studies more often had efficacy results that were favorable to the sponsors' products . . . compared with non-industry sponsored drug and device studies" (Lundh et al. 2017). Ultimately, Moynihan et al. argue that trials for drugs and medical devices should be funded by the government, not by industry. I will add that public funding should prioritize research on creating and sustaining health.

The conversation between functional medicine proponents and political actors regarding the state's role in providing the necessary resources for creating health is already underway. During a 2020 interview on his podcast *The Doctor's Farmacy* of surgeon and former Republican senator Dr. Bill Frist, Dr. Hyman, a Democrat, turns to the Democratic push for Medicare for all, indicating, "Everybody should have a human right to health care, but it's a disaster if we load up the system with a chronically ill population instead of fixing the reason why people are in there in the first place." Then he asks Senator Frist what can be done "beyond better coordination, our health IT, improving efficiencies, [and] improving payment systems [to] deal with the real issue." As many other functional medicine interlocutors do, Dr. Hyman argues that becoming more efficient at treating disease will always be a losing battle unless the health care system learns to take prevention and health creation seriously.

Senator Frist engages in this conversation with Dr. Hyman with zeal. In addition to being the former US Senate majority leader, Senator Frist is a heart and lung transplant surgeon and the author of over one hundred peer-reviewed medical articles. His medical training provided him with a unique perspective among US senators. When he was elected as a senator from Tennessee in 1994, he became the first physician in the US Senate since 1928. Thus, while Senator Frist and Dr. Hyman belong to different political parties, their commitment to medical science unites them, and, in this podcast interview, they are able to agree on the state's role in creating wellness.

Responding to Dr. Hyman's questions, Senator Frist indicates that bipartisan consensus regarding the importance of investing in wellness can be achieved by framing chronic disease as an economic problem. The right language will discuss chronic disease in terms of productivity costs and loss of the American Dream. In contrast, he asserts, "If we show that their improved health leads to more productivity [and] less absenteeism, and you take that data and you give it to the appropriate people in Congress, they will act." As a Republican, Senator Frist notes that creating health must be presented as important for economic growth.

Senator Frist then turns to Medicare Advantage—a program that currently covers half of the forty million people on Medicare. He comments, "We've seen a certain receptiveness of Congress to things like Medicare Advantage . . . a program that I helped start back in 2005." Through Medicare Advantage plans, private health care providers are under contract with Medicare and receive bundled payments for their work. These providers receive the same amount whether their patients are sick or healthy, thus dismantling the noxious incentive structure of the fee-for-service system. Senator Frist indicates, "Medicare Advantage has begun to open up to nutrition, to transportation, to some of these nonmedical determinants for reimbursement in the future." In response, Dr. Hyman expresses his appreciation for how legislation is catalyzing a shift among providers' behavior, leading them to address social determinants, nutrition, and lifestyle.

Senator Frist opines that Medicare Advantage plans are popular with insurance companies because they give them the flexibility to issue reimbursements based on data and outcomes. He provides the example of medically tailored meals for people with diabetes, hypertension, and other chronic diseases. In response to a meal preparation company's request for reimbursement through Medicare Advantage for their services, Senator Frist relates, he asked the company to first collect data proving the effectiveness of their meals. He explains to *Doctor's Farmacy* listeners that after two years of data collection, "they found that medical admissions fell by 30 percent if you were on these meals for, like, three to four months. . . . Chronic conditions fell by about 50 percent." Using this data, the company was able to demonstrate that providing healthful foods tailored to patients' chronic conditions could reduce patients' overall medical cost by 37 percent over a period of six months. The meal preparation company presented their data to Congress, and, beginning in 2019, their services were approved for reimbursement.

Although Senator First signaled potential benefits of Medicare Advantage, it is important to note that Medicare Advantage has also recently come under fire for the restrictions these plans place on patients, while increasing public health care spending. Medicare Advantage plans often have limited networks of doctors, hospitals, and other essential facilities, typically covering only the patient's home area. In contrast, nearly all doctors and hospitals are available to patients without a referral through Medicare. Furthermore, while Medicare enrollees can purchase supplemental coverage to help cover out-of-pocket expenses, Medicare Advantage enrollees are often barred from purchasing supplemental coverage. Medicare Advantage insurers—including UnitedHealth, Humana, Elevance, and Kaiser—have faced federal lawsuits alleging they inflated bills and engaged in fraudulent overdiagnosis. Furthermore, the federal Medicare Payment Advisory Commission found over $12 billion in overpayments made to Medicare Advantage plans in 2020 by the federal government.[18] Given these critiques, I do not argue for Medicare Advantage. Rather, I argue for greater accessibility to health-promoting nutrition and other measures that create health.

In this vein, Dr. Hyman exclaims in the podcast that medically tailored meals are a good example of how using an "out of the box" strategy can be more effective than the conventional medical approach. Describing an opportunity for this "out of the box" thinking in his own place of work, Dr. Hyman recalls a conversation in which the former head of Population Health at the Cleveland Clinic noted that providing housing and food to pregnant young women would dramatically reduce preterm births and neonatal costs. Although costs related to preterm birth are "literally billions and billions of dollars," Dr. Hyman emphasizes that our health care system is not set up to provide the types of resources that make the most difference (i.e., housing and food). Dr. Hyman extends his assertion to the homeless population, saying, "Providing them housing—literally paying for their apartments—reduces healthcare costs dramatically and is actually an economic benefit." With these words, Dr. Hyman essentially summarizes Dr. Atul Gawande's findings on the homeless in "The Hot Spotters," an article in the *New Yorker* that made a huge splash in 2011 (Gawande 2011). Senator Frist was already tuned in to Dr. Hyman's argument since he had worked with Dr. Gawande, who is a surgeon, and other prominent health care leaders to create United States of Care, a nonpartisan, nonprofit organization that aims to ensure all Americans have access to quality, affordable health care regardless of health status, social need, or income.

Pointing to the newly launched Cleveland Clinic Community Care approach and the Food as Medicine program, also at the Cleveland Clinic, Dr. Hyman acknowledges a recent shift in health care toward population health and, at the same time, the slow and fragmented integration of health-creating strategies into health care. He recalls a dinner conversation with the governor of Tennessee and indicates that politicians are "desperate to find the right answers" for reducing health care spending, and the answers they seek lie in addressing the social determinants that drive Medicare costs. Referring to how the nutrition focus of functional medicine could address the underlying causes of disease—and prevent the highest health care costs—if it were incorporated into mainstream medicine, Dr. Hyman analogizes himself as possessing a truck full of water while being separated by a wall of glass from patients dying of dehydration in the desert. By speaking to politicians and advocating for functional medicine in his blog, podcast, and *New York Times* best-selling books, he is engaged in a daily struggle to break the glass wall and bring chronic-disease prevention into the mainstream.

After describing his frustration, Dr. Hyman asks Senator Frist, "How do we get Congress, and the White House, and the country focused on this smoldering . . . problem?" Pointing to how state-led initiatives often dissipate when different officials are elected to office, Senator Frist asserts that grassroots efforts must inform state action; that is, civil society must educate elected officials and prompt them to act. He explains, "I think that the case just has to be made by us, like on this show, and by the American people, to get that understanding to Congress." He describes a local initiative called Nashville Health, a collaborative of 120 nonprofits and academic institutions that partners with government to address local issues, and he clarifies that the collaborative is focused on health, not health care. He asserts that 80 percent of health is determined by "things like food, and housing, and access to the Internet," so the collaborative focuses on alleviating these social deficits. Senator Frist then prompts listeners to create similar collaborations between nonprofits and government to address social inequality at the ground level.

Responding to Senator Frist, Dr. Hyman points to the communicative disconnect between those who are invested in creating health and the decision makers. He explains he does not attribute the lack of state action to politicians thinking, "I just want to keep people sick in America. I just want to maintain the status quo." Instead, he says, he wrote his book *Food Fix: How to Save Our Health, Our Economy, Our Communities, and Our Planet—One Bite at a Time* and started the Food Fix campaign "to try to create a coordinated effort . . . for the two thousand people in Washington that really need to be educated about these things." The interview concludes on an optimistic note regarding civil society's ability to inform and propel state action.

In this section, I have provided a detailed description of the interaction between Dr. Hyman and Senator Frist to explore some of the issues at stake regarding publicly funded health care. However, a question remains. Returning to the success of Medicare Advantage interventions that address social determinants of health, Dr. Hyman asks how to get private insurers to do the same. This is a question the functional medicine community has been struggling to answer, with increasing urgency.

A COMMUNITY OF FUNCTIONAL MEDICINE PRACTITIONERS

As described in the introduction and chapter 1, functional medicine is a more holistic approach to medicine, one that emerged out of conventional medicine itself and is peopled by many like-minded colleagues. Maskell recognized a need among conventionally trained doctors for consistent access to a group of such practitioners. He explains that prior to 2014, a group of doctors were already meeting monthly in Sacramento—Maskell's city of residence. These doctors told him, "We would not have had the confidence to break out of the box if we had not had two or three other doctors locally [to talk to]." Hearing of this need for community support among doctors who wanted to transition to functional medicine, Maskell set out on a mission.

Maskell explains that Evolution of Medicine, a company he cofounded, created the Functional Forum conference to give practitioners the community support they needed to practice independently of the conventional medical system, thus assuaging feelings of isolation among those transitioning to functional medicine. In his book *The Community Cure*, Maskell further explains, "In 2014, we created the Functional Forum . . . establishing a network that resulted in practitioners on six continents feeling more confident delivering a new standard of care within their communities" (2020, 24). The Functional Forum became the world's largest functional medicine conference, with monthly episodes, hundreds of podcasts, over four hundred meet-ups, two online summits, and a multicity tour.

Participants in the Functional Forum had to create their own jobs since, in the first era of functional medicine, health care institutions were not seeking to hire functional medicine doctors. This required aspiring functional medicine doctors to learn and develop a new range of skills and capabilities that they had likely not foreseen during their education. Maskell emphasizes, "Most doctors don't go into medicine to want to be an entrepreneur . . . do their own accounting, and HR, and have a private practice." Despite these obstacles, thousands of practitioners did aspire to become functional medicine doctors, and they turned to the Functional Forum for guidance and support.

In 2016, Maskell's group designed a structured program, the Practice Accelerator, to help practitioners implement their transitions to functional medicine in clinical practice. Given the difficulty of penetrating conventional health care, functional medicine practitioners initially turned to "micropractices." Maskell explains in *The Human Longevity Project*, "The truth is, right now, there's a really exciting thing happening where, for the first time in human history, you can essentially build a practice off a laptop because you don't need that much stuff—you just need real human connection."[19] The program provides a peer-to-peer community that supports doctors who are in the process of creating a functional medicine practice—sometimes after extended careers in conventional medicine.

Functional medicine is currently undergoing another transition. Maskell explains, "Our content, including my first book, *The Evolution of Medicine*, looked to 'build the army.' Since then, the focus has been on growing access to this care for everyone." During the last few years, Maskell and his colleagues have been coming up with new ways to scale up functional medicine.

In this chapter, I have explored some systemic shifts required to ensure equitable access to chronic-disease reversal. By analyzing functional medicine critiques of the pharmaceutical industry and the health insurance system, I have pointed to the inherent conflict of interest embedded in the fee-for-service model and have advocated instead for value-based care.

State-sponsored research (see Moynihan et al. 2019) and, furthermore, a reconfiguration of what constitutes legitimate science are needed to support such a shift to value-based care. While I have documented opportunities for the insertion of functional medicine into state-funded health care, in the next chapter I explore the question of how functional medicine can carve out a space in the private-payer system. Specifically, I turn to how the benefits of creating community have been reconfigured as a clinical strategy to improve health outcomes and reduce costs for patients.

CHAPTER 8
GROUP VISITS

I open this chapter with ethnographic anecdotes to explain how functional medicine providers initially adopted the use of group visits as an efficient solution for the provider problem of having too many patients and too little time. However, as emerging research in social genomics began to emphasize the importance of belonging, providers engaged the "healing power of community" as the underlying logic for group visits. Meanwhile, group visits also serve as a good strategy for attracting and retaining patient-consumers. By using group visits to maintain frequent contact with patient-consumers, functional medicine providers effectively grow their practices.

Since group visits have become more widely used, functional medicine discourse on them has shifted to explore economic benefits for multiple actors. A primary criticism of personalized functional medicine care is that it is not cost effective. Functional medicine proponents argue that group visits can solve functional medicine's high cost and inaccessibility. They argue that group visits increase access for patients and reimbursements for providers while lowering costs for the government, employers, and the self-insured. They describe the financial structures by which both in-person and online group visits can be billed to insurance or affordably paid in cash, leading them to assert that the group visit model is profitable and sustainable for a range of health organizations and a variety of medical practices.

Despite these favorable arguments, I signal several shortcomings of functional medicine group visits. In practices where the group visit structure is set up for the provider to earn a lucrative income, group visits can still represent a significant expense for patient-consumers. Meanwhile, for health organizations that seek to treat the underserved, cost constrains the personalization of functional medicine. In either case, cost is still an obstacle, and in addition, patients are often not given individualized recommendations during group visits. While group visits increase access to functional medicine providers, the care provided during group visits is not comparable to the care provided during individual functional medicine consultations.

This lack of comparability is often overlooked by functional medicine proponents, perhaps due to financial interests or due to constrained "politics of the possible"—a term Julie Guthman uses to describe how neoliberalization limits what is conceivable for activist projects because it limits "the arguable, the fundable, the organizable, and scale of effective action" (see Guthman 2008c, 1180). In essence, while group visits may allow for greater insertion of functional medicine into the mainstream, this strategy does not disrupt neoliberal ideology.

Functional medicine inadvertently perpetuates neoliberal notions of good citizenship when it promotes individuals' personal responsibility for "achieving" good health instead of underscoring structural inequality and social determinants of health. In lieu of offering logistical solutions that have been adapted to the existing neoliberal health care model, I point to untapped opportunities for challenging the neoliberal mindset and unseating the very logics that sustain unequal health care in the United States.

Ultimately, I turn to the functional medicine notion of community—a common theme in functional medicine discourse—to suggest that functional medicine proponents leverage their community-wide solidarity to engage in a politicized struggle for health justice. That is, by centering community as the motivating logic behind their actions, functional medicine proponents can begin to redefine the "politics of the possible," to address the loneliness and isolation they observe in contemporary society, and to reframe access to personalized care as an urgent matter of equity.

GROUP-DELIVERED CARE

When her physician assistant went on maternity leave, Dr. Shilpa Saxena, a family physician and functional medicine expert, found herself alone in her practice, solely responsible for seeing four thousand patients.[1] *This urgent necessity prompted Dr. Saxena to research new models of care. When she found Dr. Edward Noffsinger's Drop-In Group Medical Appointment (DIGMA) model—launched by Dr. Noffsinger in 1996—she decided to adapt the model for functional medicine. Over the next three months, she began seeing patients in groups based on shared diagnosis or likelihood of benefiting from the same information. This allowed her to spend ninety minutes with sixteen people instead of a mere five minutes with each patient in one-on-one consultations. She found that using this strategy, she saved time, she did not repeat herself to multiple patients, and she was able to dig deeper into meaningful content. Furthermore, this new way of practicing functional medicine proved profitable since she was able to bill sixteen patients' insurance companies simultaneously. Even more important, her clinical outcomes improved. Since then, Dr. Saxena has developed Group Visit Toolkit, a system that gives providers the training and resources they need to offer group visits. The Group Visit Toolkit has been monetized by the Lifestyle Matrix Resource Center, which provides resources and training for clinicians transitioning into functional medicine; the kit includes billing, teaching, and administrative resources such as visit forms, patient handouts, and multimedia education to help other doctors implement the same system.*

Dr. Saxena's approach to group visits as a strategy for increasing efficiency in the clinic is shared by many functional medicine practitioners. For example, Dr. Christopher Mote, a doctor of osteopathic medicine and chiropractor, uses group visits to deliver ninety-minute lab review classes to groups of patients.[2] *Patients complete simple but time-consuming tasks at home before the visit (e.g., recording their weight and taking their blood pressure), thus allowing Dr. Mote to devote the entire ninety minutes to educating them on their lab results. During the group visits, attendees receive their labs, learn to interpret their results, and are given a written treatment plan from Dr. Mote, along with booklets to use on their own. At the same time, group visits are a quick source of revenue for Dr. Mote's practice. He earns money from the group visits themselves and additionally he sells approximately $200 in supplements to each patient after the group visits. Calculating in his head during the webinar "Enhancing Patient Care with Virtual Group Visits," he shares, "If there are twenty patients in a class, that is $4,000." Both Dr. Saxena's and Dr. Mote's uses of group visits demonstrate how functional medicine practitioners are able to efficiently relay information and produce lots of revenue by engaging numerous patients at once during a group visit.*

Having reversed her own multiple sclerosis using diet and lifestyle treatment, Dr. Terry Wahls created the Therapeutic Lifestyle Clinic with the goal of replicating her awe-inspiring results in less privileged patients who do not have access to organic food, expensive supplements, and specialty labs, and may even be receiving food assistance.[3]

Due to an overwhelming number of new patients, Dr. Wahls began seeing patients in group visits. She witnessed how patients were more responsive to peer-to-peer suggestions than to her input—even though she also had experienced crippling disease and full recovery.

Furthermore, group lessons were more effective at helping people make and sustain behavioral changes.

Eventually, she decided to expand her delivery model into four-day events that she refers to as "group visits on steroids." During these events, Dr. Wahls and her team teach complicated functional medicine concepts to hundreds of people, thus "creating an epidemic of health." In so doing, she demonstrates that functional medicine content and methodologies can be scaled up. In November 2019, Dr. Wahls secured $2 million to conduct further research on the reproducibility of her protocol using group models.

In the first five years after the Cleveland Clinic Center for Functional Medicine (CCCFM) opened, 12,100 patients from forty-eight states and thirty-three countries had sought access to the systems-based patient care model of functional medicine.[4] Tawny Jones, CCCFM chief administrator, explains, "The math simply didn't work. We were at this critical juncture where patients were outnumbering the providers at a pace that wasn't even manageable" (Maskell 2020, 54). In 2016, nearly two thousand patients were on a twelve-to-eighteen-month waitlist to see the center's five physicians.

Around the same time, CCCFM worked with Pastor Rick Warren, founding pastor of Saddleback Church, a Baptist megachurch in Lake Forest, California, to launch the Daniel Plan, a faith-based wellness program operating in six churches in Cleveland. The program, which included 225 participants, brought small groups together weekly for six weeks. Organizers gathered biometric data from three churches and 123 individuals. This data demonstrated extraordinary results for weight loss, lowering blood pressure, and lowering cholesterol. Mean weight loss among participants was 5.6 pounds, 10 percent of obese participants went from obese to overweight, and 31 percent of hypertensive patients normalized their blood pressure. Furthermore, mean total cholesterol lowering was 13.9 points, while mean LDL-C lowering was 11.3 points. All these outcomes resulted in less dependence on medication and demonstrated the value of group-delivered health interventions to CCCFM clinicians. Fifty more churches registered for the program on November 5, 2016, at the Daniel Plan Kickoff Event at Saddleback Church.

Similar results were subsequently produced by the Healthy Choice Weight Management Initiative Program, offered by the Employee Health

Plan at the Cleveland Clinic. The program offered a series of eight one-hour Shared Nutrition Appointment (SNA) sessions facilitated by functional medicine registered dieticians and resulted in an average weight loss of 8.3 pounds.

In December 2016, CCCFM moved to a new, 17,000-square-foot space, and in 2017 it expanded to fifty-two employees. Meanwhile, the center saw steady increases in the number of new patients. One day, while driving home from work, Jones wondered, "How do we bring the essence of functional medicine to a group model and include the components of nutrition and health coaching in a way that leads to sustainable behavior change?" She wanted to deliver information to patients "in a systematic way that would teach patients to move from surviving with their chronic condition to thriving and functioning for life" (Maskell 2020, 54). This fortuitous thought process in her car led to CCCFM's launching in March 2017 Functioning for Life, a ten-week patient experience that addresses common conditions and provides participants with "this full toolbox for their health that included everything they needed and should know about self-management of their condition" (Maskell 2020, 55). The program motivates participants to address the biopsychosocial causes of their health conditions instead of relying on a provider to "fix" them.

The curriculum, which is billed to insurance, includes fourteen hours on creating a whole foods diet, the relationship between nutritional deficiencies and health, stress management through relaxation techniques, maintaining sleep patterns, and nonsedentary living. Harking back to the JAMA *study,*[5] *Jones notes, "The preliminary findings definitely demonstrate that this model of care truly improves our patients' health-related quality of life" (quoted in Maskell 2020, 57). In the first two years of the program, one thousand patients participated, with 80 percent attending every appointment.*

Jones attributes the success of the model to the functional medicine approach and the social connection that happens among patients. While she indicates that Functioning for Life unfolds at "the intersection between medical management and social connection," she goes on to assert that patients opt in "because they want that group connection. They want that support system. They want that advocacy that happens within the group model" (quoted in Maskell 2020, 57). Although patients are initially reticent about sharing health issues and feel susceptible to the social stigma associated with disease, Jones says patients become empowered, are less lonely, develop relationships, and mutually encourage each other over the course of the ten-week experience.

Dr. Hyman works at CCCFM; in fact, many patients go to the Cleveland Clinic seeking one-on-one care with him. However, completing the Functioning for Life curriculum is a prerequisite to seeing Dr. Hyman. By the time patients complete the program, approximately two-thirds have become so self-sufficient at creating and maintaining their personal healing protocol that they no longer need to see a provider.[6]

Dr. Hyman reports, "We found that, in our groups, that we see better outcomes than one-on-one doctor visits." Offering one example regarding patients with obesity, he explains that Cleveland Clinic patients who are overweight receive what he jokingly calls "a fat letter"—an invitation to enroll in the weight-loss program at CCCFM in exchange for a reduction on their health insurance premiums. He boasts that his group helps patients lose more pounds in eight weeks than the conventional medicine group loses over the course of a year. Dr. Hyman, echoing Jones, asserts that profound behavior change among patients is the result of mutual support, both in person and via an online Facebook group.[7]

Dr. Hyman indicates that, at the institutional level, CCCFM's goal is to "scale" functional medicine delivery through shared medical and nutritional appointments. This goal has been shaped by a volunteering experience Dr. Hyman had with the late Dr. Paul Farmer—a luminary medical anthropologist, physician, professor, and chair of the Department of Global Health and Social Medicine at Harvard Medical School. In 1987, Dr. Farmer cofounded Partners in Health, a Boston-based nonprofit health care organization that utilizes community-based treatment strategies to deliver quality care in resource-poor settings. In his presentation "Application of Functional Medicine in a Large Medical System (Cleveland Clinic)," Dr. Hyman includes a photo of himself with Dr. Farmer alongside the words "accompaniment and systems." Drawing inspiration from Dr. Farmer's global impact, Dr. Hyman asserts, "I think this can be really scaled around the country and the world." In this vein, he emphasizes that the group visit model "will be quite disruptive."

Dr. Hyman explains that through collaborations with other departments, the leaders of CCCFM hope it becomes an integral part of every Cleveland Clinic patient's care path.[8] *The center has participated in educational initiatives at the clinic, including grand rounds, clinical rotations, case reports, and clinician roundtables, as well as hosting lectures and CME events.*

Many functional medicine practitioners and proponents argue that the healing power of community motivates participants in group visits and renders them successful. Furthermore, the healing power of community is derived from people actively listening and supporting each other. In this vein, Maskell refers to how the act of receiving attentive care from a health professional is healing and prompts readers to consider the exponentially greater healing potential of "exquisite attention" from fifteen peers. He writes that group visits bring people together to "connect as humans in exactly the same ways we have for millennia" (2020, 22).[9] Dr. Jeffrey Geller, an integrative family medicine doctor, likewise indicates that group visits are a natural way to help patients reduce stress, lower cortisol, and feel supported. According to these interlocutors, the very act of seeking health in a group setting is a therapeutic intervention in and of itself.

However, based on my ethnographic observations, I argue that the initial motives for developing group medical visits were highly pragmatic: Dr. Saxena's clinic was understaffed and she was strapped for time; Dr. Wahls hoped to deliver cost-effective care to less privileged patients; and Jones and Dr. Hyman needed to find a way to reduce CCCFM's twelve-to-eighteen-month waitlist. Introducing the group visit model into their practices simultaneously solved multiple problems. By seeing patients "in bulk," overloaded providers could better manage large patient loads, reduce extended wait lists, and offer care at a more affordable price.

While the original motives were pragmatic and economic, social genomics were subsequently recruited to provide a fascinating argument for group-delivered care. Referring to his collaborative work with Dr. Saxena, Maskell indicates, "We saw that building community was a really important part of changing health care. We didn't really understand that there was . . . a really deep clinical component." He goes on to describe the moment when Dr. Saxena and he first became aware of social genomics, sitting side by side in the back row at the Institute for Functional Medicine's 2015 Annual International Conference. Maskell and Dr. Saxena were amazed as Dr. George Slavich, director of the Laboratory for Stress Assessment and Research and associate professor of psychiatry and behavior sciences at UCLA, took the stage and explained how social stress and isolation are the biggest underlying causes of mortality—even more so than smoking, lack of exercise, and poor nutrition. Maskell recounts how Dr. Slavich spoke about the new era of social genomics and "the impact of community, the impact of relationships on health, right down to the cellular level [and] all the way up to the macro." Maskell writes, "Dr. Saxena and I sat there in reverent silence, mixed with bursts of furious note taking" (2020, 81). Dr. Slavich's presentation described the mechanisms of action by which isolation creates disease and community creates health, thus laying out the clinical implications of conducting group visits.

Group visits have since been framed as a smart strategy for functional medicine entrepreneurs hoping to grow their practices. Josiah Bartz is the business development manager of the Lifestyle Matrix Resource Center. Bartz describes CCCFM's success in attracting patients to group-delivered care, indicating, "The Cleveland Clinic uses Dr. Mark Hyman as the carrot that they dangle out. You can't see him until you go through a ten-week group visit course." Then Bartz suggests that clinics that do not have Dr. Hyman to "dangle out" create a master class and other forms of "gated content." After the consumer has interacted with some introductory content and is interested in the clinic, Bartz recommends setting up a discovery call with the consumer to "see if our programs are right for you." His word choice evinces neoliberal logic and individualism in functional medicine business strategies, which I critique later in this chapter.

Group visits are one of many strategies functional medicine entrepreneurs use when attracting and retaining patient-consumers.[10] Not only do entrepreneurs need to convince consumers to become their patient-clients but also they must retain them. Bartz explains that much of the material produced by the Lifestyle Matrix Resource Center is meant for the phase when the provider is "dating" the patient: "A lot of the tools that we've created are really designed to be used at the very beginning—when you are meeting a patient for the first time, all the way to the follow-up visit, and through to the group visit." Referring to how multiple months ordinarily pass between one-on-one visits while patients wait for their next round of lab work, Bartz indicates, "The idea with the group visit is that it allows you to keep the patient tethered to you." Using group visits, providers are able to maintain face-to-face contact with their patients on a monthly or once-in-six-weeks basis. This strategic leveraging of group visits to attract and retain patients signals financial interests underlying the arguments that champion this clinical approach.

THE HEALTH ECONOMICS OF GROUP VISITS

Individualized functional medicine care is a time-intensive process that is not considered cost effective in many health care settings. When patients meet with functional medicine practitioners on an individual basis, their providers spend hours analyzing blood work and studying the intricacies of their cases. According to Dr. Low Dog, critics of functional medicine assert that these time-intensive techniques are only for the highly privileged "worried well." In response to critics, proponents argue that cost-effective group visits allow for functional medicine services to be covered by insurance while also rendering functional medicine more affordable to patients paying out of pocket. Pointing to how group visits produce clinical, operational, and financial benefits in multiple settings, Bartz explains, "You can get paid for it, whether you are an insurance practice or you are in a cash-based practice." While group visits save money for patients and time for providers, proponents argue that they generate equal or more revenue than the traditional one-on-one format for medical practices and health organizations. In this section, I unpack how group visits produce economic benefits for multiple actors across a range of organizations—potentially resolving different parties' conflicting interests—before turning to how financial interests may obscure shortcomings.

Patients Paying Out of Pocket

Functional medicine proponents frame group visits as an attractive option in the cash model since providers save time by avoiding the time-intensive task of billing to insurance and are thus able to provide more affordable care. Dr. Mote asserts that for patients paying out of pocket, the group visit approach is very cost effective since it is cheaper for a group of patients to split the cost of a ninety-minute class than for individual patients to each pay for a private thirty-minute lab review consult.[11] Using this logic, interlocutors like Dr. Mote argue that group visits can be used to solve the problem of functional medicine's high cost and inaccessibility for patients paying out of pocket.

Providers Seeking Insurance Reimbursements

Functional medicine interlocutors argue that changes to insurance billing (e.g., the inclusion of behavioral medicine, telemedicine, physician-led team-based care, and group-delivery models) favor the widespread delivery of functional medicine. Insurance companies have waived the physical exam requirement for group visits, thus making group visits more viable, even in a telemedicine format. As a result, practitioners who have exclusively offered their services through a cash model are now interested in transitioning to an insurance model. Rhonda Smith, director of Integrative Medicine for the

Underserved (IM4US), furthermore indicates, "Group visits [are] a way not only to enable underserved patients to get access to integrative health care but [also to enable] the clinics and providers who care for the underserved . . . to get reimbursed for those services." Her words underscore how group visits can help more providers deliver functional medicine care to patients in diverse and underserved settings by securing reimbursement for the care they provide.

Hospitals and Clinics Aiming to Increase Revenue

In comparison to the traditional model of patient care, the group visit model generates exponential revenue by billing numerous users for the same service while paying only one practitioner. In the same vein, physicians in private practice are able to earn more money by billing multiple patients' insurance at once. Thus, in the words of Maskell, group visits speak to the interests of "most American healthcare organizations—like hospitals, clinics, practice groups, and even insurance groups—[who] don't want to save money, they want to make money."

Governments, Employers, and the Self-Insured

Functional medicine proponents argue that group visits lower health care costs for governments, employers, and the self-insured. Through efforts such as giving a TEDMED talk; participating in Morgan Health (a business unit that invests JP Morgan Chase & Co. capital to accelerate the adoption of new and innovative care delivery approaches that improve health outcomes, quality, affordability, accountability, and equity); and hosting a daily livecast, *The Rogue Health Economist*, Maskell hopes to "connect our movement to the decision makers that can take this care to everyone in their organizations through group visits." Maskell speaks to the interests of decision makers when he writes, "Group-delivered services have saved significant amounts of money for organizations when compared to one-on-one care" (2020, 62). He further asserts that the group visit model appeals to health organizations serving Medicaid and Medicare patients since it saves money by keeping patients out of the emergency room, weaning patients off medication, and ultimately "creating self-efficacy" in patients. Maskell's assertion is supported by Duke Center for Integrative Medicine director Dr. Tracy Gaudet, who, referring to data from the Department of Veterans Affairs, explains that as people do more "self-care," health care costs go down.[12] Veterans Affairs data supports functional medicine proponents' argument that group visits reduce health care costs for entities that approach saving money as an economic imperative.

Functional medicine proponents argue that group visits are both accessible *and* profitable because they focus on value *and* volume—they save money for patients, employers, and governments while making money for providers, clinics, hospitals, and insurance companies. These interlocutors emphasize that financial structures are now in place to support online and in-person group visits, making group visits financially advantageous in both insurance and cash models. However, as a consumer seeking cost-effective content and aiming to reduce expensive one-on-one care from a functional medicine provider, I found that even group-delivered content can represent a significant expense for many consumers, and it can be prohibitively priced for lower-income Americans.

For example, the Wahls Protocol Seminar, offered by Dr. Wahls from May 10 to July 15, 2020, was priced at $1,097.[13] The virtual experience included Sunday support calls lasting two and a half hours and Wednesday support calls lasting one hour most weeks, for a total of seventeen and a half hours of group calls with Dr. Wahls via Zoom. The price of the seminar pales in comparison to Dr. Wahls's Health Optimization Program, which, in 2020, was priced at $7,997.[14] The program included an initial three-hour functional medicine consultation with Dr. Wahls, six group coaching calls with Dr. Wahls, three health coaching calls with a Functional Medicine Coaching Academy apprentice or certified health coach, and access to online content (e.g., digital modules, menus, shopping lists, and recipes). In both the Wahls Protocol Seminar and the Health Optimization Program, Dr. Wahls maintains a lucrative hourly income.

Using a comparative lens, the Wahls Protocol Seminar can be seen as Dr. Wahls's effort to make herself more accessible to less privileged patients. Unfortunately, the $1,097 sticker for the relatively "affordable" option continues to be an obstacle for many people seeking to reverse chronic disease using functional medicine. Those who are unable to afford this "modest investment" may follow Dr. Wahls's advice to stay positive, use the library, and "let go of what you cannot do or access" instead of "obsess[ing] over whether you can afford functional medicine;"[15] however, doing so does not help them gain access to personalized recommendations from a functional medicine provider.[16]

Functional medicine proponents are acutely aware of the problem of unequal access to their healing approach. In fact, Maskell considers it his "life's work to ensure [the functional medicine] caliber of care is accessible for everyone" (2020, 24). Likewise, Dr. Low Dog indicates she would not want to take part in a medicine that could not serve everyone, across the socioeconomic and "racial" spectrum. She especially admires IM4US and other organizations that are working to bring functional and integrative medicine to those who can benefit the most. However, I argue that while many functional medicine practitioners are turning to group visits to make functional medicine more accessible, group visits are not equivalent to one-on-one care.

Dr. Geller, founding member and past president of IM4US, laments that costs constrain the work he is able to do in the organization: "We don't do the full-on functional medicine analysis . . . that would be even more helpful in discerning [the patient's health status], but we try to get the low-hanging fruit." He explains that in his functional medicine group visits, they focus on food, exercise, sleep patterns, and ways to avoid using medications. Dr. Geller's comments indicate that group visits are "cost effective" in the sense that they are comparatively more affordable than one-on-one care with a functional medicine provider. However, they are not a replacement for functional medicine treatment in a one-on-one setting.

Functional medicine proponents may overlook the lack of comparability between group visits and one-on-one care because group visits speak to multiple actors' financial interests. Given that individual practitioners can conduct group visits "off a laptop" with no additional infrastructure, group visits allow practitioners to turn a greater profit with less investment of time and resources. At the same time, group visits may be attractive to clinics, hospitals, and insurance groups.

However, the lack of comparability may also be overlooked by functional medicine proponents due to constrained "politics of the possible" (see Guthman 2008c).[17] Functional medicine proponents pursue group visits as a strategy because they consider them the only way to scale up and deliver functional medicine to the masses. For example, Maskell argues that group visits are uniquely positioned to solve the conundrum of how to get functional medicine to the masses since they are more affordable for patient-clients while also being extremely lucrative for providers. As a group, proponents are acting on the assumption that delivering one-on-one functional medicine at the level of primary care is not financially feasible because it will not be reimbursed by health insurance. This assumption may or may not be true, depending on whether decision makers can be convinced that investing in personalized primary care can reduce downstream costs of chronic-disease management and treatment with specialists—and whether reducing costs is an economic imperative for those decision makers. However, leading with this assumption inadvertently places too much emphasis on group visits as a lucrative alternative and too little focus on the circumstances of those who cannot access needed one-on-one care, thus obscuring injustice in the health care system.

In essence, group visits may allow for greater insertion of functional medicine into the "mainstream" because they fit neatly into existing health care structures; however, they do not disrupt neoliberal ideology. Group visits oppose the outcomes of neoliberal market orthodoxy (i.e., unequal access to functional medicine) without explicitly rejecting neoliberal governance itself. In essence, the group visit approach does not challenge the incentives structure of health care and, as a profit-driven enterprise, evinces neoliberal logics. By failing to challenge the neoliberal worldview shaping health care structures to begin with, functional medicine proponents are missing an opportunity to push for health care reforms that would increase health justice.

FUNCTIONAL MEDICINE AND NEOLIBERAL IDEOLOGY

Neoliberalism is the principle behind free trade and austerity. Its components include deregulation, trade liberalization, and the privatization of state enterprises and public services. The term "neoliberalism" is often associated with the World Bank's and the International Monetary Fund's efforts to encourage the free flow of capital, pressure governments to eliminate taxes and tariffs, and remove public assistance. As political economic philosophy, neoliberalism asserts that human well-being is best achieved in the so-called free market without intervention from the state (Harvey 2005, 2). Neoliberal approaches assume market solutions are superior to those offered by the public sector and civil society. In practice, neoliberalism involves the development of new regulatory mechanisms to shore up corporate profitability (Harvey 2010; Mann 2013). Meanwhile, social benefits are expected to somehow "trickle down."

I argue that functional medicine is unwittingly steeped in neoliberal ideology. Functional medicine proponents have focused on training practitioners to be effective entrepreneurs.[18] At the same time, functional medicine encourages patients to be informed consumers who take personal responsibility for their health and embrace their bioindividuality.[19] In so doing, functional medicine inadvertently perpetuates neoliberal notions of good citizenship, casts health as a consumer item for purchase in private markets, and promotes individual responsibility at the expense of true social solidarity.

One of the key principles of neoliberalism is individualism (see McGregor 2008), a principle to which functional medicine fervently adheres. As I have described in chapters 2 through 4, a great portion of functional medicine discourse is presented as the hero's journey. Patients become the heroes in their own recovery as they position themselves as the doctors of the future. At the same time, providers are the heroes of their healing journeys when they position themselves as wounded healers. Maskell explains that within the context of a therapeutic relationship, patients are heroes and practitioners are "the Yoda."[20] Dr. Zach Bush's web page on the Intrinsic Health Coaching Program notes how the whole team has "learned through thousands of client journeys that healing comes from within the individual, rather than an external educator, physician, product, or technology."[21] The coaching program aims to empower individuals' unique path to health by sharpening their intuition and self-awareness. These examples demonstrate the discursive tendency to place the patient at the center of their unique hero's journey—a tendency that reinforces individualism and thus inadvertently reproduces neoliberalism.

This discourse is rooted in the very nature of personalized medicine, which, in turn, is undergirded by technological advances in the era of Big Data.[22] Advances in technology have increased consumers' access to genetic information and biometric tracking—the building blocks of personalized medicine.[23] As a self-styled "rogue health economist," Maskell "put his ear to the ground" in Silicon Valley to learn about personalized medicine. The experience led him to assert that functional medicine, not increasingly narrow pharmaceutical interventions, is the most effective operating system for delivering P4 (predictive, precise, personalized, and participatory) medicine. He further elaborated that functional medicine can scale up P4 medicine by making it "available to every American, or everyone around the world." So far, however, the high costs of personalized medicine—described by President Barack Obama as "delivering the right treatments, at the right time, every time to the right person" (Office of the Press Secretary 2015)—have rendered this type of care inaccessible to most American consumers.

However, Maskell argues that the way to make personalized medicine available to the masses is through group visits. He writes, "Personalized medicine and group-delivered care are not mutually exclusive; they are both necessary to actualize an emerging vision of 'precision public health'" (2020,

69). Maskell further explains that while precision medicine was "previously too time intensive or costly for most physicians, [it] can be elegantly executed in a group format" (2020, 69–70). Maskell's words point to a paradox: given financial constraints presented by the current health care system, functional medicine proponents are championing a group format for the delivery of personalized medicine. I have already offered Dr. Geller's functional medicine group at IM4US as an example of how cost constrains personalized, precision medicine in underserved settings; here, I furthermore note that even when individuals meet as a group, emphasis continues to be placed on the individual.

The problem with individualism is that it legitimizes "personal responsibility" for health, which, in turn, runs the risk of blaming the victim.[24] As Maskell describes it, "It's not really about doctors doing things to you, it's about you taking responsibility to build a healthy life, and that includes the lifestyle factors like sleep and nutrition and exercises." Kresser expands, "We need to train people to understand that they are primarily responsible for maintaining and improving their own health." By including recovery stories in the online conference he hosts, Alex Howard hopes to inspire listeners to take personal responsibility for their health, opining, "There is a place [for] the patient taking a level of personal responsibility that I think is crucial to be effective on a healing path." In the same vein, Jones says CCCFM's goal "is to truly transform health care by empowering patients to take control of their health." I argue that by beaming a spotlight onto patients' personal responsibility for their health, functional medicine interlocutors unwittingly obscure issues of structural inequality.

When functional medicine interlocutors fail to explicitly acknowledge how socioeconomic and "racial" inequalities structure access to health-sustaining resources, they can be (mis)read as asserting that those who have ill health are personally responsible for their poor health outcomes. That is, by focusing on diet and "lifestyle," functional medicine lapses into what Lara Zakaria, a nutritionist, pharmacist, public health professional, and Institute for Functional Medicine certified practitioner, calls the "should phenomenon" (i.e., "you should eat better" and "you should exercise more"). Jessica Mulligan has made similar observations in distinct contexts. She argues that the Affordable Care Act uses "financial techniques . . . [to] 'unpool' risk by devolving financial and moral responsibility for health care onto individual consumers" and points to how contemporary choice rhetoric uses consumer choice as a justification for exclusionary health care in the United States (2016, 37; 2017). Similarly, I argue functional medicine discourse inadvertently promotes a well-being meritocracy that conceals social determinants of health. The notion that good health is an "achievement" ignores how patients' so-called choices are influenced by their access to stable employment, nutritious food, a nontoxic environment, and quality health care (see Mulligan 2017, 34).

My argument is substantiated by how many functional medicine practitioners and proponents use the terms "personal responsibility" and "ownership" interchangeably. The word "ownership" begs the question, who can afford to be an owner? For example, Tom Blue indicates, "The topic of responsibility and ownership for health, I think, is one that is ready to really be revisited in a profound way." Blue argues that, as a society, we need to "upgrade" our understanding of health, how it is produced, and why it is appropriate for individuals to take ownership. Pushing back against assumptions that disease is the result of bad luck, "punishment from God," and unfortunate genetics, Blue explains that it is important for individual patients to act as stewards of their own health and of health resources. Although Blue addresses the perspective of a financier, he does not address how socioeconomic inequality shapes stewardship.

I argue that functional medicine proponents often overlook socioeconomic inequality—a tendency I call "structural myopia"—and I suggest that this tendency may be linked to their own socioeconomic privilege.[25] As Andrea Nakayama explains, "I live in a bubble where the population that comes to me wants to take ownership." Nakayama describes how, in her bubble, children attend Waldorf School, drink green smoothies, and assist in their families' organic gardens—all markers of affluence. In contrast, she indicates that, in the population at large, a lot of people are "buying into" the "pill-for-every-ill" mentality. I note that less privileged people do not have access to the "bubble" Nakayama describes. They simply cannot afford to *buy into* (double meaning intended) a neighborhood and lifestyle like hers.

Functional medicine interlocutors' perspectives on the circumstances patients face are largely shaped by their interactions with individuals who are already seeking functional medicine (and can, therefore, afford to pay out of pocket for functional medicine services) and by their own experiences as wounded healers.[26] This partial perspective (Haraway 1988) leads functional medicine proponents to frame the solution to widespread autoimmunity as, in Nakayama's words, "really understanding what is true for ourselves . . . and being able to mitigate that by taking ownership . . . and assembling a team that really sees the whole individual." In response, I assert that understanding "what is true for ourselves" (read: individualism) and "taking ownership" is possible only for privileged patient-consumers who can afford to "assemble a team." I am among them, and I recognize and call out my own privilege.

I point to the role of socioeconomic inequality, along with many other types of social inequality, in determining whether patient-provider relationships will be successful. Cheryl Mattingly writes, "The ability of professionals and families to recognize, acknowledge, and build upon commonalities that cross race, class, and culture is an important and undertheorized aspect of clinical work" (2010, 141). With these words, Mattingly indicates that the relational quality of clinical encounters is shaped by the degree of similarity or difference between the patient's and the provider's positionalities in society. One's positionality is intersectional in nature (Crenshaw 2014); thus, while Mattingly mentions "race," class, and culture, I would add other axes of social inequality such as gender, age, religion, and sexual orientation. My having obtained an intermediate education in the health sciences played a huge role in shaping how I interacted with my providers. While I was able to use this cultural capital (Bourdieu 1984) to relate with my functional medicine team, I was simultaneously unable to relate with all of my providers on the basis of "race" and, in the case of my functional medicine doctor, gender.

Thus, my goal is not to indict myself, individual functional medicine proponents, or other functional medicine patients, but, rather, to argue for a critical and nuanced examination of privilege. As demonstrated throughout this book, class privilege, Whiteness, and neoliberalism have constrained access to functional medicine (see also Vega 2023). Moving forward, I hope for "racial" and socioeconomic equity in access to quality care.[27] However, functional medicine proponents must recognize how their approach has thus far been embedded within neoliberal ideology in order to facilitate the emergence of a multi-"racial," class-inflected movement that can transform health care.

In so doing, I ask functional medicine proponents to explore their own potential as health justice advocates who engage in a politicized struggle that challenges the neoliberal mindset and unseats the very logics that sustain unequal health care in the United States. By suggesting that "group visits can dynamically solve the social determinants of health for some of the poorest and most vulnerable members of our society" (Maskell 2020, 22), functional medicine proponents often neglect other resources (e.g., food, housing, one-on-one health care) that patients also need to be well. Ultimately, I argue for a deeper and broader commitment to social justice. In the next section, I utilize the functional medicine notion of "community" as a springboard for my argument.

(COMM)UNITY: COMMITMENT TO COMMUNITY

Maskell has frequently explained, on multiple platforms and across many years, that community is the theme undergirding all of his work. He says, "Building local communities of integrative practitioners around the world is the most important next step for the evolution of medicine." Maskell describes his organization in an email newsletter, writing, "At Evolution of Medicine, our efforts have always been about community and bringing people together." In the newsletter, he refers to building functional medicine communities among practitioners as going "back to our roots" before introducing Evolution of Medicine's Community Builder of the Year Award. Turning to how "our roots" must inform the future, Maskell continues, "Many have thrived, some have burned out, many need a little more guidance and support." With these words, Maskell calls on functional medicine practitioners to strengthen the paradigm through ongoing support for one another. His Practice Accelerator program provides a space and a structure within which practitioners transitioning to functional medicine can mutually support one another as they build their own "micropractices."

More recently, Maskell's focus on "community" has been aimed at patient communities. Maskell hosted a thirteen-part group visit series on FunctionalForum.com from April 2019 to March 2020. The series dovetailed with the "2020 Group Visit Challenge"—a free, five-day training in which Functional Forum listeners could participate by joining the Facebook community. Maskell designed the challenge to help participants "map out a plan based on your practice structure and [to] support you as you create a clear path to billing, building presentations and handouts, picking topics and effectively promoting and enrolling patients into groups." The framework of the challenge points to how functional medicine practitioners harness community among themselves to create community among patients. In his book, Maskell furthermore writes that group visits facilitate "collective group creativity" and individual patient agency, thus allowing participants to leave behind shame, guilt, and pain while finding trust, companionship, and self-efficacy (Maskell 2020, 22).

While functional medicine proponents have tapped into the concept of community to emphasize the need for mutual support among functional medicine practitioners and the innovative power of group visits, I argue a commitment to community can be put to work in even more transformative ways. Thus, by pointing out how social genomics was inserted as a justification for the group visit model after the fact, I do not mean to delegitimatize group visits as a social genomic strategy. Instead, my intention is to signal how the social genomics approach has been *underutilized.*

A commitment to community can begin to decenter neoliberal ideology—and especially its individualistic underpinnings—by framing health as a matter of social justice. From this perspective, health is not the sole responsibility of the individual, but something that is created by the individual, together with their provider, and in the context of their community. Dr. Susan Prescott, a physician, artist, and author, hints at the type of community I imagine when she describes "community immunity" and "resilient societies" based upon "mutualistic collaboration" in the context of the COVID-19 pandemic. In this book, I argue that the actions of the community (read: the social environment) are also inscribed on the health of the individual—this is the very essence of social genomics.

From this point forward, I will use the parenthetical term (comm)unity to embed *comm*-itment into *comm*-unity. I illustrate how functional medicine proponents have described community and indicate how more work can be done through (comm)unity. Instead of merely gathering people in groups to build community, I am signaling the need for radical change in the health care system through (comm)unity. In so doing, I am arguing for proactive disassembly of intersectional inequalities (Crenshaw 2014), community-wide responsibility for the health of individuals, the equal valuation of life, and, ultimately, social justice.

I must further clarify that, by arguing for (comm)unity, I am explicitly not dichotomizing community and the state. Maskell writes, "We are constantly looking to the economy, the market, the state, or the government to solve our problems" (2020, 18). He is critical of how our "myopic view of the world" causes us to consider the market and government as our only two options for health care and suggests community as an alternative. Like Maskell, I reject market-based solutions—strategies pursued through the market are, by definition, less accessible to low-income people. However, my framing of (comm)unity differs from Maskell's argument for "communities" since Maskell is carving out a space for functional medicine to operate alongside existing health care structures instead of suggesting that patients turn to the state to pursue change. In contrast, I insist the state should be beholden to the (comm)unity. Stated simply, the commitment is also from the state to the community.

My notion of (comm)unity builds upon Dr. Gaudet's vision of "system strategies" for improving health. Dr. Gaudet's perspective starts out very similar to Maskell's but quickly expands in a way that resists and challenges neoliberalism. She asserted at the Institute for Functional Medicine's 2020 Annual International Conference (IFM 2020 AIC), "If the community can get on board with addressing health and supporting the community, lots of things can change." Her assertion provoked me, as a conference attendee, to write down: "I argue that poor, disenfranchised communities should not be made responsible for changing their plight. This is blaming the victim. What about the role of the state?" As if responding to my query, Dr. Gaudet navigated to a slide that positioned "communities" as merely the first of thirteen strategies. Other strategies included upgrading health care delivery systems, transforming medical school education, regulating Big Pharma and biotech industries, and restructuring health sector finance and policy—perhaps by leaning into the financial interests of employers and the self-insured. Importantly, she pointed to the role of governments at the federal, state, and local levels and argued that population health depends on changes to the food industry. In a similar vein, Dr. Patrick Hanaway—a board-certified family physician, the past president of the American Board of Integrative Holistic Medicine, the chief medical education officer at the Institute for Functional Medicine, and the founding medical director of the Cleveland Clinic—argued at the IFM 2020 AIC for giving food to people, regardless of whether they have health insurance, as a form of prevention.

I agree with Dr. Gaudet's and Dr. Hanaway's "system strategies" and offer (comm)unity as a container for this multipronged approach to health justice. Furthermore, when describing (comm)unity, it is important that I simultaneously offer an analytic for thinking about the absence of (comm) unity. Based on Dr. Slavich's research, Maskell asserts, "Loneliness is the biggest driver of chronic disease and death." He points to a 2018 survey that found that half of Americans feel isolated and identified Millennials and Generation Z as the loneliest generations ever (Maskell 2020, 15). In response to Maskell, I argue the isolation he diagnoses is a symptom of neoliberal individualism. Therefore, I put the *I* in "isolation." By using the term with the *I* in parentheses, "(I)solation," I point to how neoliberal individualism is the scaffolding upon which epidemic loneliness rests.

To understand the emergence of loneliness, Maskell turns to the work of Raghuram Rajan, an Indian economist, the Katherine Dusak Miller Distinguished Service Professor of Finance at the University of Chicago Booth School of Business, and former chief economist of the International Monetary Fund. In Maskell's words, "Raghuram Rajan chronicles our collective history right back to the Dark Ages," documenting how the acceleration of technology during the industrial revolution and the subsequent information technology revolution have "ripped apart the fabric of traditional communities" (2020, 17). While historically, many people lived in multigenerational homes and interdependent communities, "the invention of the automobile allowed people to move into the suburbs and live in isolated single family homes. . . . Now, the majority of goods we purchase or consume are sourced from individuals we don't know" (2020, 17). Over the course of a few decades, downtown stores were superseded by shopping centers, which in turn were replaced by internet sites. Maskell, further revealing his training in economics, then turns to Charles Eisenstein's (2011) seminal work *Sacred Economics*.[28] Maskell explains, "We've shifted from the gift economy into an age of separation, one in which we are 'helplessly independent.' We're self-sufficient to the people we know, but totally dependent on strangers living miles, if not oceans, away" (2020, 17). He describes what I call "the outsourcing of care"—how, in the absence of family and community support, consumers turn to commodified forms of care such as babysitters, counselors, and eldercare.

In essence, Maskell's descriptions point to a lack of (comm)unity and widespread (I)solation. Turning to "targeted social rejection"—a concept used by Dr. Slavich to signal the noxious genomic effects of social suffering—Maskell signals that there is a fundamental difference between experiencing a difficult life event as part of a group (e.g., when an entire team of employees are simultaneously fired) versus experiencing "targeted rejection" (e.g., when only one individual is fired). He explains, "There's something . . . about our own instinct . . . and the way that we lived in community [where] targeted social rejection comes with significant health issues for the person rejected." From my perspective, feelings of targeted social rejection are folded into (I)solation; that is, feelings of rejection are refracted through neoliberal structures and "I"-oriented landscapes.

The answer to this problem, in Maskell's view, is a return to community. Maskell idealizes the Blue Zones, discussed in chapter 6, and asserts that healthy behaviors are built into these communities. He indicates that the longevity among populations that live to one hundred is not owed to increased access to medical care. Rather, "it's because the environment is created, and the social structures are created, where community built around healthy behaviors [is] just the norm." From his perspective, he and his colleagues are "advocating for . . . a movement toward those principles" through group visits and "participatory medicine for the masses." Maskell argues that in one fell swoop, group visits promote healthy habits, satiate cravings for community among lonely patients, and create a deep sense of purpose for practitioners.

In response to Maskell, Howard describes how group visits could help alleviate the isolation experienced by many chronic fatigue patients. He shares, "It's not just that people haven't got contact with people who have a similar condition and are on a similar healing trajectory, it's also that people are just isolated from the world as a whole." Howard explains that when individuals begin to physically recover after an extended period in isolation, they may face difficulty reinserting themselves socially into the world. His words signal how disease can be a totalizing form of social exclusion. For Howard, group visits are a supportive therapeutic context where chronic fatigue patients can learn to reconnect and have human contact.

Functional medicine proponents argue that online support groups can also serve as spaces for the healing power of community. Ari Whitten describes the private online community he hosts, saying, "I know that even just that online engagement, not even having the in-person interaction, is hugely healing for so many people." In a similar vein, Maskell points out how sometimes community is created by a practitioner in their clinic, and at other times community emerges online through websites such as Facebook. Maskell has asserted in multiple venues that online communities are helpful—especially in the context of COVID-19 sheltering in place; however, they are not a replacement for in-person connection. He writes, "We can start fixing it today, using online tools to create offline connections, and unleashing the power of community to transform health outcomes together" (2020, 195). I agree with Maskell's point, but I push the issue even further.

Delivering care in a group setting is not enough to unseat (I)solation since it does not dismantle the neoliberal ideology of personal responsibility upon which functional medicine largely rests. The philosophy of group visits suggests that everyday people can empower one another to solve health problems and reverse chronic disease. While functional medicine's focus on "community" is beneficial in many ways, it also reinforces the notion that individuals—operating in communities—are responsible for addressing problems that are structural in nature. This focus is depoliticizing, sidesteps the role of government policy to ensure the human right to health, and inadvertently lets the state off the hook. Thus, (comm)unity is not created by a practitioner in their clinic, or by a social media platform, but, rather, by society-wide contributions to ensuring equity and social justice.

This is not to say that group visits are not valuable—I acknowledge group visits may improve accessibility of functional medicine within the existing neoliberal health care system. However, my critique points to how group visits may also constrain the "politics of the possible" (see Guthman 2008c) by eclipsing our collective imaginaries of how health justice might be achieved through political action. By offering group visits as a viable alternative to one-on-one care, functional medicine proponents implicitly suggest that it is impossible to confront the state in the interest of human health. A deeper (comm)unity is required.

Dr. Hyman's descriptions of community edge toward the (comm)unity I would like to see from functional medicine. His perspective is informed by his experience with physician-anthropologist Dr. Paul Farmer, as discussed earlier in this chapter. Dr. Hyman describes how he volunteered in Haiti after the 2010 earthquake and "was one of the first on the ground" there. He traveled with Dr. Farmer, who, in Dr. Hyman's words, "created [an organization] called Partners in Health where the core philosophy is something called accompaniment, that we accompany each other to health." Dr. Farmer's model of accompaniment assembles a team of community health workers—comprised of neighbors and peers, not medical experts—to support patients with tuberculosis and AIDS. This model applies anthropological thinking to diseased populations in low-resource settings (see Harvard News Office 2011).

Witnessing how effective the accompaniment model was for infectious disease, Dr. Hyman began thinking about how this model might be applied to chronic disease. He explains, "I realized, and this was my big insight, that [although] chronic disease is called noncommunicable disease . . . it's actually very communicable. It's infectious in the sense that it's contagious." Turning to Nicholas A. Christakis's work at Harvard on social genomics,[29] Dr. Hyman indicates that if your friends are obese, you are more likely to be obese than if your family is obese, noting, "You're more likely to have the social threads and connections determine your health than your genetic threads." In the same vein, Maskell indicates that referring to obesity as a "social disease . . . reframe[s] the understanding of how you actually get diseases in the modern era." He asserts that while thinking of so-called lifestyle diseases as "contagious" may be "mentally offensive," there is increasing evidence that the health of our community is increased through social genomic means onto individual health outcomes.

The idea that "lifestyle" is "contagious" has already shaped Dr. Hyman's approach to health care. Dr. Hyman says he asked himself, "Well, if diabetes and obesity and heart disease are contagious, then how do we use the same model of behavior change?" He recounts how, at this point in his thought process, Pastor Warren fortuitously walked into his office. Warren asked Dr. Hyman for help losing weight and "getting healthy." The two agreed to have dinner, and later that night, Warren told Dr. Hyman that he leads a church, Saddleback Church, with thirty thousand congregants. Warren explained,

"Well, we've got, you know, five thousand small groups that meet every week to help support each other with better lives." Hearing this, Dr. Hyman proposed a collaboration to bring a healthy lifestyle program to the church. To this, Warren responded, "Great, 'cause we're a very fat church, and I'm fat, and we should do this."

As noted above, CCCFM provided the content for the wellness program, the Daniel Plan, which focused on a "functional medicine way of eating and living." Dr. Hyman recounts, "We had fifteen thousand people sign up. They lost a quarter of a million pounds in a year." Instead of relying on "expert care," the small group setting "infused Bible studies with healthy behavior" and created accountability through feedback and support. Maskell elaborates, "You end up with a situation where now you have people working, being accountable to each other, changing behaviors, cooking together, eating, creating health together, and you see ridiculous results." Given the program's astounding success, the model has been adopted and replicated by dozens of churches in Cleveland and beyond. This experience has led Dr. Hyman to believe that the way to change behavior is "through the power of each other." He explains that, ultimately, people need to be on "the love diet—essentially, the power of love and community and connection"—and the key to success is "friend power, not willpower."

Dr. Hyman's assertions about the communicability of behavior (and, therefore, chronic disease and health) are supported by emerging studies on the human microbiome.[30] Maskell indicates, "You're in a group of people and you're sharing bacteria back and forth. Here's a mechanism that we never really understood." Underscoring the negative effects of (I)solation, he says, "There could be a lot of healthy people together keeping themselves healthy. Unhealthy people are isolated [and] not connected with other people." Maskell posits that our community of bacteria thrives only when humans live in community. I extend the mechanism and outcomes of Maskell's hypothesis by arguing that community-wide health unfolds through living in (comm)unity—through a lived commitment to the equal valuation of life and social justice.

In an email newsletter, Maskell takes a giant leap toward the (comm) unity I envision. He references how Frome, a small English village two and a half hours southwest of London, has "seen a significant drop in both chronic illness and acute care, and is being hailed for making health care more cohesive and human."[31] In his description of Frome, Maskell indicates that the "community's commitment to each other has directly affected healthcare costs and office visits." He clarifies that the lower health care costs are not due to improved health services but, rather, to the community-wide feeling that everyone has access to meals, rides, compassion, and support. I appreciate Maskell's emphasis on the ways Frome enacts (comm)unity through the provision of specific, needed resources to community members. However, I am wary of how Maskell's romanticization of Frome—like his celebration of the Daniel Plan's success at Saddleback Church—sidesteps the state's obligation to its people by asserting that the town is "curing loneliness." In contrast, I argue for a community-wide responsibility for the health of individuals that is openly premised on social justice.

Before functional medicine proponents can take up the flag of social justice, they must first redefine the "politics of the possible" (see Guthman 2008c). During the lunch break at the Advances in Mitochondrial Medicine Symposium in 2019, Maskell took the stage and said, "If there is anyone out there that wants to deliver medicine to the seventy percent, not just the thirty percent, come see me." As a member of the audience, I detected a mixture of hope and frustration in his voice. Less than a year later, at the Integrative Medicine for the Underserved Conference, Maskell described, in awe, the potential for functional medicine practitioners to deliver care to the underserved. He explained that functional medicine has lost its moral authority by focusing on delivering functional medicine "mainly for cash, and mainly to rich people," and asserted that, as a community, functional medicine practitioners can seize back moral authority by transforming the standard of care through "an operating system within medicine to get people healthy, off medication, and to create self-efficacy in humans." I am encouraged by Maskell's assertions.

I hope this book will serve to inspire functional medicine providers, proponents, patients, and those interested in functional medicine to reimagine functional medicine as a tool for achieving greater health justice through (comm)unity-focused public policy. As someone who used functional medicine to reverse chronic disease, I urge functional medicine practitioners to continue reenvisioning personalized medicine as health care for the masses and not just the privileged. Through (comm)unity, functional medicine can begin to decenter neoliberal ideology and its individualistic underpinnings, thus championing health as a matter of health justice. This would require functional medicine advocates to focus not only on increased access through group-delivered care but also on reimbursement for one-on-one care. In the fight for health justice, the functional medicine movement must be guided by social solidarity and impassioned desire to ensure that everyone has the resources to create health.

In the lead-up to the COVID-19 pandemic, a number of functional medicine interlocutors argued that group medicine could be harnessed to transform functional health care delivery, build patient communities, improve accessibility, and meet providers' needs. At the time, these group visits were primarily delivered in person. However, when the pandemic began, functional medicine providers were forced to pivot and reenvision group-delivered care as unfolding online. This was a natural transition since, even before the COVID-19 pandemic began, many functional medicine practitioners used telecommunication technologies to provide "telemedicine/education consultations" to patients around the world. Dr. Kara Fitzgerald commented after COVID-19 began on how virtual group visits were becoming an integral part of functional medicine due to self-isolation during the pandemic, writing, "And it works—in insurance, self-pay, and even Medicare. . . . The promise of functional medicine and the accessibility of functional medicine for all—is timely, inspiring, and essential." Echoing Dr. Fitzgerald, in his presentation for the IFM 2020 AIC, Dr. Jeffrey Bland signaled that the pandemic created the conditions for reimbursement for telemedicine, health coaching, and group medical visits.

In the conclusion, I turn to how COVID-19 thrust issues of "racial" equity and health justice into stark relief and how the functional medicine community is responding. I will continue to argue that while group visits can, indeed, improve accessibility to some forms of functional medicine care, more is required. Furthermore, I will point to the potential role of medical anthropologists in helping functional medicine interlocutors move past debates on "cultural competency" to implementation of health justice.

CONCLUSION

LOOKING FORWARD: OPPORTUNITIES FOR HEALTH JUSTICE

During my ethnographic research, I found that functional medicine was delivered by predominantly White providers to mostly White and socioeconomically privileged patients. Functional medicine discourse has often avoided the question of "race," thus ignoring how functional medicine practitioners can ensure that their approach is adapted to and equitably reaches people of all "racial" and ethnic backgrounds. Black Lives Matter protests in 2020 and disparities in COVID-19 death rates brought the topic of "race" and health equity to the fore among functional medicine interlocutors. In this context, they are beginning to reject uncritical notions of "choice" and problematize "lifestyle" changes as the path to good health.

In response to this discursive shift, I critique how the concept of "cultural competency" has been applied in clinical settings (see Kleinman and Benson 2006) and instead make a case for "community engagement" (see Briggs and Mantini-Briggs 2008; Tuhiwai Smith 2012; Boston et al. 2015). Well-meaning functional medicine interlocutors have taken up the flag of cultural competency in their efforts to make functional medicine broadly accessible. Unfortunately, focusing on "culture" again creates a potential slippage—characterizing communities with poor health outcomes as having a unique "culture" can inadvertently lapse into blaming the victim and racializing Others (see Lee and Farrell 2006; Pon 2009). I take a historicized perspective to argue that "cultures" that are deemed "distrusting" are, in fact, communities that have faced egregious human rights violations in the past. Ultimately, I argue that equitable engagement with these communities is needed to address dire health disparities that are not attributed to "culture" but, rather, to a history of "racial" violence.

Despite well-intentioned efforts to insert functional medicine into the "mainstream," the movement for social justice in access to functional medicine has quite a long way to go. I thus ask the following questions: How have doctors, social epidemiologists, and medical anthropologists characterized health disparities? Whose responsibility is it to ensure health, including access to techniques and strategies that reverse chronic disease—the government, the whole of society, or, as Tom Blue puts it, "legions" of individual bioconsumers? At stake is the question of health as a citizenship-based right versus an individual goal.

I argue that health is a matter of social justice that therefore calls for a health system that not only is effective at preventing and reversing chronic disease but also responds to "racial" and economic disparities. I examine citizens' relationships to the state and argue for "health justice"—the removal of racism, exploitation, and oppression in the health care system and the provision of equitable access to health-promoting resources. Ultimately, I call on functional medicine proponents to engage in a politicized struggle for health as a citizenship-based right.

THE FAILURE OF FUNCTIONAL MEDICINE TO ADEQUATELY ADDRESS SOCIAL AND "RACIAL" INEQUALITY

Prior to May 2020, the functional medicine community largely remained silent on issues related to inequality, and when inequality *was* mentioned by well-meaning interlocutors, the discussion was often inadequate and incomplete. For example, in his book *The Community Cure*, published in January 2020, Maskell includes a graphic that emphasizes how socioeconomic factors play the largest role in determining health. Noting the dire health statistics for Black men when compared to their White counterparts, Maskell notes that "these individuals often don't have the same access to information, education, healthy foods, or reliable health care" (2020, 138–139). However, his section "Transforming Care for Minorities"—a rare endeavor to investigate how functional medicine can ameliorate racialized inequality—is a mere four paragraphs long. Over the course of my ethnographic research, I found functional medicine discourse often lacked in-depth engagement with issues of inequality, thus failing to interrogate the underlying logics that reproduce social and "racial" health disparities.

In the same publication, Maskell describes unique efforts at CCCFM to create a Functioning for Life program specifically for minority men.

In 2003, Dr. Charles Modlin—physician lead for public health, executive director of minority health, and founder and director of the Minority Men's Health Center (MMHC) at the Cleveland Clinic—established the Cleveland Clinic's Annual Minority Men's Health Fair. Maskell quotes Dr. Modlin, who described the MMHC as a "friendly point of entry to the Cleveland Clinic's network of care for populations who do not frequently receive medical attention—either due to financial burdens, misconceptions, or general distrust" (2020, 139). However, Maskell does not provide a detailed explanation regarding the historical underpinnings of so-called misconceptions and general distrust. In the absence of this necessary explanation, Maskell runs the risk of blaming racialized victims by inadvertently casting minorities as ignorant and distrusting. Maskell furthermore comments, "The men who go through the program are able to bring the information back to their friends, family, and communities" (2020, 139). This wording reinforces notions of the lives of people in minority groups as unfolding at a distance from predominantly White functional medicine.

By using Maskell as an example, I am pointing to the functional medicine community's inadequate engagement with issues of inequality prior to May 2020. Having observed Maskell's work through in-person ethnography, as a listener of his podcast and a reader of his books, I am convinced his intention is to make functional medicine accessible to as many people as possible—thus, my intention is not to personally criticize Maskell. Furthermore, I am not denying that there is unequal access to health care and education for minority populations. I strongly agree with Maskell regarding racialized inequalities in access to information, education, nutrition, and health care. Instead, I am suggesting that functional medicine providers and proponents critically analyze their discursive practices to prevent reinscribing difference.

Critical analysis can begin with media representations of minority patients. The September 2019 Functional Forum was held at the Integrative Medicine for the Underserved (IM4US) Conference in Santa Clara, California, and video footage of the forum was later archived on YouTube. When watching this footage, I noticed that the hour-long YouTube video included only one patient. Everyone else featured in the video from that conference was a provider or health professional of some kind. The sole patient, Jerry Fusilier, was a Black man wearing a beanie cap. In his interview clip, Fusilier slowly introduces himself and explains that joining Open Source Wellness—a community-based "behavioral pharmacy" cofounded by a primary care health psychologist—has left a lasting effect on his life, saying, "I continue to trust people, where at one time, I didn't trust anybody. . . . I'm not embarrassed anymore. I'm not scared to be vulnerable. It's really helped me." I wonder why Fusilier was selected to be the only patient interviewee in the video. If other patients were also present at the conference, why were they not interviewed, or why were their interviews not shown? If no other patients were present, why was Fusilier the sole patient in attendance? Was he uniquely invited to the conference, and, if so, by whom and for what purpose?[1]

Fusilier's interview clip speaks clearly to the perspective that Black men avoid medical care due to what some in health care consider their "misconceptions" and "general distrust." However, in the absence of a historicized explanation, Fusilier's comments about fear of being vulnerable can be (mis)interpreted as a personal shortcoming to be overcome by the individual (i.e., Fusilier and other Black men like him). While Fusilier's interview indicates group visits are effective in helping Black men be more vulnerable, I am acutely attuned to how specific narratives are selectively positioned to support racializing logics and how these, in turn, can obscure discrimination in health care provision. In essence, the uncritical positioning of a token Black patient underscores difference while failing to examine the structural violence that underpins "race"-based health disparities (Farmer et al. 2006). Engaging Farmer (2001), I argue that we cannot claim that cultural beliefs and personal motivations determine the efficacy of medical interventions when we can readily document how logistical and economic barriers to access play a major role in health care delivery.

While I argue that minority populations must be engaged as equals, well-intentioned functional medicine interlocutors and practitioners sometimes unwittingly otherize minority patients. For example, Marena Burnett, senior director of Health Care Engagement and Innovation at the Centering Health Institute in Boston, addresses the question of how to improve pregnancy outcomes in African American women by explaining that these women are greatly comforted by participating in a group of people who look like them and may even live in the same neighborhood. Burnett says, "If you are a patient and you have a one-on-one experience with a provider, sometimes you don't have the same level of trust with that provider, particularly if they don't share your lived experience." From Burnett's perspective, the sense of trust and belonging that occurs in a group setting is simply not present in patient-provider interactions. Her perspective is aligned with Maskell's assertion that group visits are a "universally culturally appropriate" way to reverse chronic disease without medication.[2] In contrast, I highlight how group medicine may inadvertently homogenize racialized individuals while simultaneously essentializing them as "Others" to the provider.

I admire Burnett's and Maskell's positive intentions of providing comfort and a sense of trust to minority and underserved individuals; however, I am attentive to how grouping patients based on similar appearance, co-residence in the same neighborhood, and "shared lived experience" may unintentionally widen the distance between underserved patients and class-privileged, often White providers. My fear is that "race"-segregated groups may be held out as infusing patient care for underserved populations with a "personal touch," leading providers to think they are unable to or do not need to do this themselves. These groups may naturalize the idea that patients and providers cannot build trusting relationships that bridge "racial" and socioeconomic differences.

I am also wary of how changing behavior has been framed as a solution to systemic problems within functional medicine discourse. Mary Purdy, a nurse and registered dietitian nutritionist, indicates that people may lack access to healthy food "for a variety of reasons, including policy, poverty, racism, climate change, all of the above." Her opening statement at the September 2019 Functional Forum suggests that her comments will unfold along the same lines as those of Maskell, who, highlighting obstacles to behavior change in low-income communities, wrote, "There might not be access to stable, reliable housing, or a grocery store with access to healthy food. Facilities for mental health and wellness might not exist or be financially accessible" (2020, 91). But Purdy goes on to state, "I love working with people around their diet, especially when people don't have access to food. . . . We as dieticians can take hold of this issue and . . . we can work with them in so many other ways." Specifically, Purdy signals that dieticians can "convene with" food-insecure individuals around mindful eating practices; about how sleep and stress affect "food choices" and vice versa; and about how cultural practices shape one's relationship with food. She concludes that underserved individuals who lack access to healthy food "can still have an amazing relationship with food that will help them to have a more well-balanced life and a healthier body." Purdy's approach individualizes systemic problems, thus normalizing the idea that individuals may not have access to healthy food due to structural inequality.

These examples point to a larger trend I observed among functional medicine interlocutors; that is, the functional medicine approach to health creation often attempted to change individuals' "lifestyle" without a nuanced understanding of the structural factors shaping so-called choices and behaviors (see Bourdieu 1984). This was especially problematic when class-privileged, mostly White providers targeted the "culture" and "choices" of low-income and racialized individuals. I strongly disagree with Purdy's statements that the solutions are "convening with them around what their relationship is to food" and "identifying cultural practices that connect them with food." *The solution is to address structural inequality.* In this vein, I urge the entire functional medicine community to make a focused commitment to achieving equity in how functional medicine is delivered.

In the next section, I turn to functional medicine discourse that unfolded during the 2020 Black Lives Matter movement and the COVID-19 pandemic. This discourse suggests that the needed commitment to equity I have identified may just be underway.

2020: COVID-19 AND BLACK LIVES MATTER

The year 2020 marked a massive shift in functional medicine discourse, largely due to the resurgence of the Black Lives Matter movement and the beginning of the COVID-19 pandemic. In a June 29, 2020, article posted on the Institute for Functional Medicine (IFM) website, "Expanding Access to Functional Medicine in Vulnerable Communities," IFM CEO Amy R. Mack described COVID-19 and Black Lives Matter as two "cataclysmic events" that propelled IFM's thinking forward. Dr. Mack indicated that while flaws in health care have been apparent for decades and change is long overdue, inequities to access were amplified in the context of COVID: "The system is irrevocably broken, and in today's environment, the cracks and the fissures are bigger than ever." She argued that it was time to "be bold" and "take decisive action" to ensure that health is not determined by one's zip code, accumulation of wealth, or skin color. Dr. Mack indicated that for the first time, disparities between health, wealth, and "race" would inform the work of the IFM. Indeed, according to the IFM's website, the 2021 Annual International Conference aimed to enable functional medicine practitioners to "fulfill their role in reducing health disparities" while building a healthier world.

As I will discuss further below, functional medicine practitioners, like those in conventional medicine circles, turned their attention to the physiological underpinnings of COVID-19; however, they framed the pandemic as a call to focus on the social determinants of disease and the public health crisis of racism that disparate COVID outcomes were quickly laying bare. Dr. Fitzgerald noted these reported COVID outcome disparities, including hospitalization and mortality rates, among multiple Black, Asian, and other minority ethnic groups. Dr. Mack explained that people of color are less likely to receive preventive health services and more likely to experience poorer-quality medical care when compared to Whites, thus resulting in a higher level of chronic-disease burden beginning at a younger age. She wrote, "In medicine, racial and economic differences determine both the quality and the type of health care an individual receives, and the disparities in health outcomes between Whites and people of color are exceedingly stark." Pointing to the effects of intersectionality, she indicated that impoverished adults experience poor health at a rate that is multiple times higher than their privileged counterparts. Dr. Mack emphasized that "racial" and economic inequality in health care is true from "conventional medicine to Functional Medicine and beyond" and asserted, "It is true, and it is unacceptable."

As a community, functional medicine interlocutors began pointing to what they termed a "pandemic within a pandemic." Dr. Susan Prescott referred to COVID as a "lifestyle disease" during her presentation at the IFM's 2020 Annual International Conference and pointed out that the spread of the virus is linked to social inequality and poverty. As a co-presenter in the same conference module, Dr. Bland similarly pointed to the "sociobiological interrelationship" between the COVID virus and the social, political, and economic factors shaping its spread.[3] Dr. Mack went on to explain there were higher rates of infection among minorities because these populations disproportionally make up essential workers in the United States. She noted that essential workers—grocery store and restaurant staff, health care practitioners, delivery drivers, factory and farm workers—cannot distance themselves from the public and therefore risk themselves and their families to protect and bring comfort to others. Meanwhile, essential workers are also often among the most susceptible to COVID because they have higher proportions of chronic diseases.

This situation is an example of what Sharrelle Barber (2020) calls "death by racism." However, "death by racism" is certainly not unique to the COVID pandemic. Kaya Purohit, chief content officer for Hyman Digital (Dr. Hyman's private company), emphasized that Black, Indigenous, and people of color are much more likely to succumb to the ten leading causes of death due to "lack of access and the cascading effects of racism, prejudice, stereotyping, and unconscious bias on minority health." Linking preexisting conditions back to fatal COVID outcomes among minority groups, Dr. Fitzgerald clarified, "Comorbidities including diabetes, hypertension and obesity are associated with much worse COVID outcome. And in the United States, Black people are far more likely to suffer with these comorbidities and thus COVID mortality rates are higher with people of color." In essence, preexisting chronic conditions among people of color, combined with long-standing "racial" discrimination, make them more vulnerable to the COVID virus.

At the same time as "race"-based disparities in COVID outcomes were sparking conversations among functional medicine interlocutors about "racial" injustice, the May 25, 2020, brutal killing of George Floyd in Minneapolis emphasized the dire need for action. In a June 2020 email newsletter describing her upcoming webinar "Functional Medicine, COVID-19 and Racial Disparities, Bridging the Gap," Dr. Fitzgerald asserted, "Functional medicine is not (yet) adequately addressing the profound racial disparity in medicine." Dr. Fitzgerald prefaced Dr. Mack's comments, which appeared less than a week later: "For certain, those who need functional medicine the most are not receiving this care." Functional medicine practitioners agreed that while "racial" disparities exist in both functional and conventional medicine,[4] functional medicine was best positioned to address the disparate outcomes of COVID and chronic disease. From this perspective, ongoing "racial" disparities signal that functional medicine has not yet lived up to its potential.

Framing the presentations from experts in Dr. Fitzgerald's webinar, Lara Zakaria, a member of Dr. Fitzgerald's team, presented a "social inequality and change road map." The four-phased approach began with seeking input from experts to identify shortfalls and recommendations, which also typified Dr. Mack's instructions to listen to "the clinical experts and visionaries who are already on the path to transforming health care in America." The road map continued with developing and implementing an action plan to address structural racism within providers' own spheres of influence, assessing progress to ensure accountability, and ultimately creating lasting change. Zakaria indicated that Dr. Fitzgerald's team wanted to be part of the solution for Black individuals and other oppressed groups.

Dr. Alauna Curry, the first expert presenter in Dr. Fitzgerald's webinar, began outlining what she sees as the solution by encouraging her colleagues to identify how biomedicine's situated knowledge (see Haraway 1988) results in "shitty thinking." She called out racism and offered "L.O.V.E." as an alternative—an acronym that instructs individuals to *L*isten and *L*ook with suspended judgment, *O*bserve the emotions of all involved parties, *V*alidate the different perspectives, and *E*xpress your Self skillfully. Dr. Curry defined empathy as one's ability to skillfully put L.O.V.E. into action.

During her presentation in the webinar, Dr. Safiya McCarter reiterated Dr. Mack's descriptions of racism as a public health crisis, COVID shining a bright light on health disparities, and the problematic relationship between "race" and quality health care in the COVID era. However, she also incorporated the medical anthropology concept of a "syndemic" (Singer 2009)—that is, how co-occurring diseases interact synergistically to produce excess burden of disease when nested in certain social, economic, and political contexts—and argued that the comorbidities that make people more susceptible to COVID are best addressed by functional medicine.[5] Dr. McCarter went on to describe sociologist and civil rights activist W. E. B. Du Bois's critique of "scientific racism" and to ask her colleagues to follow his lead by naming racism in the natural health sciences. Offering an example of intersectionality (see Crenshaw 2014), she noted that most people do not know what it feels like to be the only woman of color trying to obtain tenure. According to Dr. McCarter, it is imperative that we uncover underrepresented perspectives by bringing individuals affected by intersectionality, racism, and syndemics to the table as interlocutors. She applied these interrelated arguments to COVID when she opined that turning the pandemic into an opportunity for facing racism head-on is dependent on health care professionals "learning to ask" (see Briggs and Mantini-Briggs 1986). Dr. McCarter's presentation demonstrated a welcome engagement with concepts originating in anthropology and sociology.[6]

Dr. Bland, the final presenter in the webinar, began his presentation by "addressing the obvious"—as "an old White male" presenting alongside two African American women, he said he was painfully aware of his own privilege. Dr. Bland went on to recount his experience taking a class on "the culture of marginalization" as a college student. He has since applied what he learned to emerging science; for example, he asked the audience to consider the epigenetics of both fear and privilege. Responding to Dr. McCarter's description of syndemics, Dr. Bland debunked comorbidity and instead argued for a biopsychosocial model—what he described as "a pandemic within a pandemic within a pandemic." He concluded by presenting his three-part manifesto: a commitment to call out others when he detects racism, acknowledge his own privilege, and always be willing to learn.

As a webinar attendee, I found Dr. Bland's manifesto to be very inspiring; however, I was struck by how the entire discussion on "racial disparities" was mostly framed in terms of Black vs. White. Blacks have uniquely suffered egregious human rights violations in the form of slavery, unethical medical experiments, and police brutality (to name a few forms). At the same time, I wondered why members of other minority groups were not included in the discussion.[7] Apparently, other viewers had the same question. In the chat box, one viewer asked about the potential inclusion of Indigenous approaches. Dr. McCarter responded to this question by indicating that medical professionals cannot know what communities need if they are not connected to those communities. She instructed her colleagues to "invite folks that we intend to serve to the table." I could not agree more.

The questions posed by the audience seemed to inform some of the commitments Dr. Mack made the following week. An audience member asked, "How do FM practitioners self-educate about racial differences in medicine? Second, how do you get an affordable form of that critical chronic-medicine care to the communities that need it most?" Dr. Mack did not have answers to these questions. Instead, she acknowledged that functional medicine is delivered by predominantly White providers to mostly White and socioeconomically privileged patients, and she pointed to how these inequities require further interrogation. She noted, "We will ask questions about why clinicians of color are not attending our courses." Furthermore, she indicated the IFM's determination to increase diversity among functional medicine patients, writing, "We will uncover the reasons why the population who could benefit the most from a Functional Medicine approach, including essential workers and their families, aren't aware of or aren't able to access this kind of care." Dr. Mack's readiness to acknowledge functional medicine's existing shortcomings paves the way for the IFM's first steps toward achieving social justice.

However, I simultaneously emphasize that training more clinicians of color in functional medicine may encourage greater diversity among functional medicine patients, but it will not directly translate to it. Furthermore, in the words of Purohit, "Educating healthcare providers on the historical and current-day practices that exacerbate racial health disparities is an important step in creating a healthier population overall." While working alongside clinicians of color may expose White functional medicine practitioners to some of the issues at stake, direct education and training about "race"-based determinants of health are needed for all practitioners.

The integrative medicine program at the George Washington University School of Medicine and Health Sciences, under the direction of Dr. Andrew Heyman, was quick to respond to the IFM's call for action. A July 10, 2020, *GW Whole Health* newsletter article titled "Integrative Medicine, COVID-19, and Health Equity" reiterated that while "racial" and ethnic minorities have experienced health inequities for decades, the novel coronavirus had demonstrated the extent to which this is the case. The newsletter advertised the Health Equity Series, designed by Dr. Maranda Ward, assistant professor of clinical research and leadership at George Washington's medical school. Lectures in the series defined health equity and outlined contemporary challenges, explained social determinants of health, recognized vulnerable and socially disadvantaged US populations, and argued for cultural humility during difficult discussions. This series is just one example of how functional medicine interlocutors are beginning to address the urgent need among health care providers for education and training to ensure that they understand patients' health problems in a wider context (read: social determinants of health).

In essence, functional medicine interlocutors saw the COVID pandemic and the Black Lives Matter movement as, in Dr. Mack's words, a "global tipping point" and an "enormous opportunity for change." During "Telehealth: Navigating the Changing Landscape of Medicine," a June 2020 webinar for Fullscript, an online supplement dispensary, Dr. Low Dog indicated to Maskell that the "racial" injustice evinced by George Floyd's death could spark a movement toward more care. She said she hoped that patients would demand care that focuses on wellness and healing beyond managing disease with more and more pharmaceuticals. In the context of the pandemic, Dr. Bland argued during his presentation at the IFM's 2020 Annual International Conference that functional medicine is uniquely positioned to focus on the immune system as a target for preventive medicine.[8] Similarly, Dr. Fitzgerald wrote in her June 23, 2020, email newsletter, "Functional medicine is well positioned to address the pandemic of chronic disease," which would reduce many of the risks associated with poor COVID outcomes. These practitioners all point to functional medicine's potential for reducing health disparities by addressing and preventing chronic disease if functional medicine were more accessible to the underserved populations who need it most.

As a result of functional medicine's distinct strengths, Dr. Tracy Gaudet indicated that, although functional medicine has thus far been an "adjunct" or "garnish" to conventional medicine, the COVID pandemic could open the door to the widespread incorporation of functional medicine into the health care system. She opined that the conventional medicine paradigm was "massively breaking down" during the pandemic, allowing functional medicine practitioners to take the lead toward an enormous breakthrough. She emphasized to her colleagues, "Breakdowns lead to breakthroughs, and you are needed now more than ever." Dr. Gaudet suggested that functional medicine practitioners are the ones who can create radical change in health care delivery because they "walk the walk" in their clinics and see transformations every day among their patients.[9]

Dr. Gaudet's assertions reflect IFM's mission to ensure the widespread adoption of functional medicine. However, Dr. Mack explicitly clarified that this mission "does not mean to ensure the adoption of Functional Medicine for those who can afford it; it does not mean Functional Medicine for the elite or those who have been born with a certain skin color." Instead, she explained that IFM's mission is all encompassing—to ensure the widespread adoption of functional medicine for all. Maskell agreed with Dr. Mack's perspective, writing, "Our work must be to bring [health and resilience] to everyone, but particularly those who need it the most, who have suffered disproportionately historically." In his view, the functional medicine community is "stepping up" by assuming a leadership role and working to transform the existing health care system. Dr. Gaudet concluded that COVID had brought the future into the present and argued, "If there was ever a time for hope, it's now."

PROBLEMATIZING "LIFESTYLE" AND "BEHAVIOR"

Functional medicine interlocutors' heightened attention to "racial" disparities in health outcomes during the pandemic resulted in much-needed problematization of so-called lifestyle and behavior concerns. In May 2020, as host of the webinar "Enhancing Patient Care with Virtual Group Visits," Maskell indicated that living in a food desert is not a lifestyle that individuals choose. He explained, "What we call 'lifestyle' is really an environment that people can't afford to get out of." One month later, in his June 6, 2020, email newsletter, he further critiqued how functional medicine interlocutors often talk about "lifestyle diseases" and "lifestyle choices." He clarified that while behavioral medicine is incredibly important, "the reality is, sometimes 'lifestyle' is not a choice." Building upon his perspective from the webinar, Maskell indicated that racism, trauma, and systemic oppression are among the environmental issues that individuals are unable to escape because of their socioeconomic disadvantage—a sentiment he further emphasized to listeners of the Fullscript webinar "Expert Insight on Telehealth" that same week.

Maskell's email newsletter was circulated and his webinar was posted seventeen days before Dr. McCarter unpacked systemic racism for the audience of Dr. Fitzgerald's webinar "Functional Medicine, COVID-19 and Racial Disparities, Bridging the Gap" and rejected uncritical notions of "choice." In the same webinar, Dr. Curry explained, "It's hard to exercise in the hood when you are running and getting shot." During the discussion portion of the webinar, Dr. Patrick Hanaway argued for increased awareness about adverse "racial" trauma among health care providers. Six days later, Dr. Mack wrote, "We know that the disparities seen in health and health care are not the result of personal health and lifestyle choices alone." While it is too soon to tell, I am hopeful that this problematization of "lifestyle" marks the beginning of a new era in functional medicine.

Some functional medicine proponents are beginning to acknowledge that they should focus not only on increasing access to functional medicine services but also on securing other resources necessary for health. In a different newsletter, Maskell pointed to the need for food security, "racial" equality, and environmental justice, writing, "We have much work to do on this front, but there is immense opportunity for leadership here." At the same time, however, functional medicine interlocutors continue to occasionally lapse into a neoliberal mindset. For example, at the IM4US Conference, Maskell admired how "racially diverse people [support] each other to live healthy lives in spite of their environment." I likewise value mutual support within communities, but instead of celebrating resilience in the face of discriminatory environmental factors, I argue that these factors must be eliminated by society as a whole.

Dr. Gaudet takes a step in the right direction with her concept of "whole health," which, she indicates, empowers *and* equips patients to take charge of their health and well-being. She explains that the health care system is not designed to do either of these activities, but she argues that both are necessary for creating "whole health." She emphasizes that "empowering" patients without including practical skill building and teaching new habits will not result in success. I add that "equipping" patients should not refer merely to strategies that engender behavior change, since this can reproduce a neoliberal emphasis on personal responsibility and neglect tangible, material resources that are necessary for creating and sustaining health (e.g., nutritious food, a clean environment, and safe housing).[10]

PROBLEMATIZING "CULTURAL COMPETENCY"

Functional medicine interlocutors frame "cultural competency" as key to creating a healthy population. According to Dr. Mack, culturally sensitive functional medicine training is needed to expand access to functional medicine in vulnerable communities. At CCCFM, Dr. Hyman and his colleagues are attempting to provide culturally competent care to underserved communities in the Cleveland area. Dr. Modlin affirms that providers must be culturally competent to establish a relationship with the community: "You have to be able to resonate with the community. Nobody cares how much you know until they know how much you care." Tawny Jones, chief administrator of the CCCFM, agrees. She explains that being "racially" and culturally sensitive is her initial step when creating programs at the Cleveland Clinic. These functional medicine interlocutors readily acknowledge obstacles to accessing functional medicine in low-income communities and communities of color, and—while I argue that cost is the primary obstacle to functional medicine on a national scale—these interlocutors have offered "cultural competency" among practitioners as a way to bridge the communication gap between functional medicine practitioners and the communities who need chronic-disease reversal the most.

Despite these positive aims, I am apprehensive of how the implementation of "cultural competency" and its derivatives (e.g., "cultural sensitivity") can reduce "cultures" to homogeneous, bounded units, thus creating a caricature of what it means to be Hispanic, Black, Asian, etc. (see Kleinman and Benson 2006). While "race"-segregated group visits and health centers are meant to ensure "culturally appropriate care," they also inadvertently reinscribe racialized narratives and reproduce difference. In fact, while S. Agnes Lee and Michelle Farrell (2006) ask if cultural competency is the back door to racism, Gordon Pon (2009) goes as far as to characterize cultural competency as "new racism." Thus, instead of examining "race"-based inequalities through the lens of "culture"—a move that risks blaming racialized victims—I suggest functional medicine providers focus on "race"-based inequalities in access to quality care. Words matter because they shape frameworks that, in turn, inform action. Therefore, rather than "cultural competency" and "cultural sensitivity," I argue for "community-engaged" work—work that includes community members in its design, implementation, assessment, and, if applicable, financial earnings (Briggs and Mantini-Briggs 2008; Tuhiwai Smith 2012; Boston et al. 2015).

Failing to actively and equitably engage communities in health education, clinical interventions, and medical research leads to justified distrust. A video compilation of interviews from *The Doctor's Farmacy* posted on July 31, 2020, provides essential historical context behind the Black community's fear of the health establishment. Harriet A. Washington, a medical ethicist and award-winning author of *Medical Apartheid: The Dark History of Medical Experimentation on Black Americans from Colonial Times to the Present*, indicates in one interview, "A lot of people have justified trust issues with the health establishment and frankly want to avoid it as long as they can." Dr. Modlin similarly asserts, "A lot of people in the Black community are really fearful of going to the doctor and they are fearful that the doctor is going to use them as a guinea pig." From this perspective, lack of engagement with medicine contributes to health disparities among the Black community.

Both Dr. Modlin and Washington point to a complex history of medical experimentation on African Americans. Dr. Modlin signals that distrust in medicine and doctors among African Americans can be traced to the Tuskegee syphilis experiment—a forty-year experiment started in 1932 in which African American men with syphilis were intentionally denied treatment, without their knowledge, to allow researchers to observe the progression of the disease at all stages. While the Tuskegee syphilis experiment is the most well-known example, Washington documents medical experiments on African Americans ranging from the middle of the eighteenth century to the present day. Responding to Dr. Hyman's assumption about the primacy of Tuskegee, Washington explains, "The other studies were actually much worse and very dense. I have fifteen whole chapters and only one of them mentions Tuskegee. And not only in the past, but in the present." Then, describing a present-day study in Baltimore, she notes, "We have young Black men being actively recruited into studies without their knowledge where they are going to be forced into hypothermia as treatment for gunshot wounds." A long-standing history of human rights violations, inflicted upon African Americans in the name of medical experimentation, informs African American individuals' distrust of the medical establishment.

Furthermore, Black patients' attitudes toward medicine have been shaped by diverse forms of "racial" discrimination within health care. Dr. Modlin adds that while Blacks have been the targets of unethical medical experiments, they are simultaneously excluded from the type of research that would benefit their health. He explains, "A lot of the medications on the market have been developed and designed and tested especially just in White men."[11] The combined experience of violence and exclusion has prompted many African Americans to focus on nutritious food as a way to stay healthy and steer clear of medicine. Pointing to how African Americans' meticulous concern with food typically is not addressed in the news media, Washington says, "I'll leave you to speculate why that would be, but . . . you have to be in the community to see and hear this." Her words emphasize the importance of community-engaged work.

Well-meaning functional medicine interlocutors may assume that "cultural competency" and "community engagement" are synonymous, or interrelated to such a degree that the former necessarily engenders the latter; however, I argue that "cultural competency" is a poor proxy for "community engagement" and that, furthermore, relying on "cultural competency" as an explanatory framework can unwittingly bolster racializing logics. In practice, "cultural competency" is often approached as a series of concrete "culturally appropriate" or "culturally sensitive" modifications to how health care and health information are delivered to patients of a given ethnic background (see Kleinman and Benson 2006, referring to Betancourt 2004), while "community engagement" is a multipronged commitment to community embeddedness that unseats existing power differentials and restructures financial streams by incorporating community actors as leaders.

Over the course of my ethnographic research, I noted how the term "cultural competency" was conflated with presenting information in an accessible way. For example, Jones explained, "We are not using terminology that would be offensive to them. We are not putting information in front of them, you know, ten-syllable words that they would have no idea." Jones indicated that community members are often unfamiliar with medical terminology but are hesitant to ask questions because they do not want to be judged or stigmatized. As a result, she designs health education programs that assume everyone is starting from square one. Health educators unpack terms like "hemoglobin A1C" and "lipid panel" when explaining laboratory test results. Imitating the reaction of someone receiving these explanations for the first time, Jones said, "For years, I've been wondering what a lipid panel [is]. That's what that means!" She indicated that as a result of this approach, individuals are immersed in the conversation. I argue that using the term "cultural competency" for providers in this circumstance obscures a history of limited access to upper education in a shroud of so-called culture. Although I know this is not Jones's intention, she and other functional medicine interlocutors can be (mis)read as affirming that limited health literacy is a "cultural" deficit among lower-income Blacks. Instead, I suggest that functional medicine interlocutors engage the communities they aim to serve as equals, while acknowledging the historical—not "cultural"—challenges they have faced.

As part of their efforts to deliver "culturally competent" care, functional medicine proponents have focused on selecting accessible physical locations for the delivery of health education. For example, Jones asserts that in order to help people "reclaim their life," health education programs must take place where community members feel comfortable. She critiques how health professionals have tended to host health fairs, thus creating sporadic contact with members of the community. Instead, she suggests health professionals make an ongoing, concerted effort to bring the community into the conversation. Specifically, she recommends, "There should be weekly meetings, whether it's at the church, whether it's at the community center, in a space where they feel comfortable going to." Jones indicates that Black community members readily commit to a ten-week health education program at the Langston Hughes Community Health and Education Center because Cleveland Clinic employees have removed barriers that would prevent them from learning. Pointing to the program's success, she positions it as a template for health education programs in other contexts. While functional medicine interlocutors should remain wary of the potential slippage between space segregation and "racial" segregation, steady attendance at the Langston Hughes center suggests that this is an effective location for community engagement.

In this section, I have pointed to the need for explicit and intentional efforts among functional medicine proponents to activate community-engaged work as an integral part of their overarching goal to make functional medicine accessible to the masses. In the next section, I turn to how perspectives from epidemiology and medical anthropology can inform their work.

FIXING HEALTH DISPARITIES FROM THE PERSPECTIVES OF MEDICAL ANTHROPOLOGY AND SOCIAL EPIDEMIOLOGY

Functional medicine interlocutors have much to learn from medical anthropology and social epidemiology perspectives on health and disease. The medical anthropologist Dr. Paul Farmer argues that we must examine the role of social inequalities in health care delivery (see Farmer 2001). In a similar vein, Michael Marmot, a renowned social epidemiologist, contends that "social gradients" are the underlying cause of health disparities (2015). Marmot's suggestion—addressing the root cause—sounds a lot like the arguments made by functional medicine practitioners.[12] However, there is one vital difference: Marmot unequivocally identifies the root cause to be *social* in nature. Meanwhile, functional medicine practitioners, at least prior to 2020, tended to (over)emphasize systems biology and neglect social factors.

Both Farmer and Marmot, drawing from transnational perspectives, argue that social inequality plays a greater role in determining health than the mere existence of effective therapies—albeit in different ways. Much of Farmer's lifework unfolded in rural, underdeveloped settings where the fatal effects of infectious diseases such as HIV/AIDS, malaria, and tuberculosis loom large. Farmer thus examined how social inequality structures access to effective therapies for infectious diseases, deepening the divide between the haves and the have-nots. In his view, the better the therapy, the more injustice for the untreated. In contrast, Marmot's work places greater emphasis on urban and developed settings. Marmot reminds his readers that the United States ranks fiftieth in male "adult mortality" (the likelihood of living to age sixty), arguing it is not the availability of medical care or even public health that shapes individual health. Signaling how the high mortality rate of young men is attributed to "homicide, suicide, car crashes, other accidents, drugs, alcohol and some other disorders" (2015, 34), Marmot argues that society should address the social causes of these deaths instead of erroneously pinning high mortality rates on lack of medical care. As a medical anthropologist and social epidemiologist, I appreciate both Farmer's and Marmot's points and advocate for transdisciplinary research—a biosocial framework that spans biomedical and social sciences (see Farmer 2001).

I argue that to remove existing health disparities, health professionals must recognize disease as processual by using conceptual tools that are historically deep. To do so, policymakers and health care providers must educate themselves about how structural violence is unleashed at the intersection of poverty, racism, and gender inequality. At the same time, I signal that neither Farmer's nor Marmot's respective arguments regarding infectious disease and violent deaths address the pressing problem of chronic disease in America. Rapid increases in chronic disease resemble the infectious disease "pandemics" Farmer describes (2001; see also Terzic and Waldman 2011) since intersectionally vulnerable individuals are those least likely to have access to "effective therapies" for chronic-disease reversal.[13] At the same time, the answer to this problem is not simply more pharmaceuticalized medicine; instead, the growing burden of chronic disease must be met by equitable access to therapies that address the root biological cause while also addressing social causes. The first step is ensuring access to health care, while also shifting the very meanings of "health care" from treating disease to creating health.[14]

Looking to the future, I suggest that functional medicine interlocutors expand their perspective on health disparities. Although the term "health disparities" is commonly used as a signifier for "race"-based differences in health outcomes, health disparities are, in fact, structured by intersectional logics of inclusion and exclusion—not by "race" alone (Crenshaw 2014). Among other intersectional axes are socioeconomic class and gender. Furthermore, "race" does not refer merely to differences between Blacks and Whites. Other minority groups also face health disparities, and their needs must be addressed in the next era of functional medicine.

Some functional medicine interlocutors are already aware of the striking effect of socioeconomic class on life expectancy. When speaking to Dr. Hyman, Dr. Anand Parekh, the Bipartisan Policy Center's chief medical advisor, points to a fourteen-year life expectancy difference for men and a ten-year life expectancy difference for women when comparing the wealthiest 1 percent of Americans to the poorest 1 percent. His comparison is reminiscent of Marmot's observations in different cities around the world with extreme health disparities. In Glasgow, Marmot points out, a twenty-eight-year gap in life expectancy means men living in the Calton district—a neighborhood marked by violence, drugs, alcohol, and prostitution—can expect to live shorter lives than men living in India (2015, 25). Marmot furthermore notes cumulative differences in life expectancy for every mile traveled on the Washington Metro between downtown Washington, DC, and Montgomery County, Maryland, and for every stop east from Westminster on London's Jubilee Underground line (2015, 27). These latter examples demonstrate how differences in life expectancy can be greater *within* nations (comparing the richest individuals to the poorest) than *between* so-called developed and underdeveloped nations, which points to the importance of individual wealth over national wealth in determining health.

At the same time, income inequality does not operate in a vacuum, it unfolds together with racialized inequality. Dr. Parekh goes on to acknowledge the importance of intersectionality by emphasizing that although infant mortality has decreased, the United States still trails behind other nations. He attributes relatively high rates of infant mortality to disparities based on "race" and ethnicity, saying, "African American populations [and] American Indian populations have significantly higher infant mortality rates than other subgroups. So, race is also important." Also speaking to the concept of intersectionality—what Marmot calls "social status"—Marmot argues that huge gaps in life expectancy within US cities like Baltimore and Washington, DC, cannot be attributed solely to "race." He argues we must go beyond simple categories like "race" and social class to fully understand health inequality. It is not just "race" or just "class." Instead, what individuals with poor health outcomes have in common is disempowerment and different forms of social exclusion.

In the absence of adequate social programs and services, the health care system in the United States is sometimes used as a social safety net. Dr. Parekh celebrates this as "health care without walls" and explains, "Health care is getting into the business of social needs because they see it as connected to the value proposition of improving outcomes and potentially reducing preventable health care costs." In contrast, according to Dr. Anna Lembke, a professor at the Stanford University School of Medicine, this (mis)use of the health care system has led to the medicalization of poverty. Dr. Lembke specifically points to how individuals who are jobless, homeless, and suffering from intergenerational trauma are prescribed medication for social, not biological, problems. Her perspective incorporates Marmot's assertion that social gradients share a direct relationship not only with life expectancy but also with the likelihood of disability. Building upon Marmot's perspective that doctors should not treat illness in homeless patients without working to address homelessness, Dr. Parekh and Dr. Lembke ultimately both believe that if doctors are expected to play safety-net roles, they must be given the proper resources and training to deal with nonbiological problems.

I applaud functional medicine interlocutors' advocacy for meeting patients' social needs; however, I signal how "healthcare without walls" runs the risk of legitimizing the absence of social programs and services while inadvertently medicalizing social inequality. Instead, I argue for biosocial training in medical education (thus providing doctors with the skills to diagnose how biological problems are nested in social context),[15] while also maintaining that the health care system (and, specifically, pharmaceuticalized medicine) is not a replacement for robust social programs and services. However, I do believe that "clinical-community linkages"—connecting patients to existing social services—are important for reinforcing clinical efforts. In the next section, I offer the term "health justice" to frame my arguments.

HEALTH JUSTICE: A NEW FRAMEWORK FOR ACHIEVING HEALTH AND SOCIAL JUSTICE

Health is a matter of social justice. Social justice has been notably absent from functional medicine discourse, as evidenced by Maskell's observation during the September 2019 Functional Forum, which was held at the IM4US Conference: "This conference has the theme of social justice, and this is the first time that I have been to a medical conference with anything like that theme." Maskell then asks Rhonda Smith, IM4US director, about the conference theme, to which Smith responds, "Our health care, especially for the underserved, is under threat." She explains that, as a relatively privileged woman, she is concerned about being insured and having access to quality care. In comparison, individuals who are underserved are at a greater risk for not having access to any form of health care, let alone quality health care. She explains that for those who are concerned about social justice and equity, "It is important that everyone have access to quality care, whole person care, and integrative health care—regardless of who they are, what they look like, where they live, how much money they make, and who they are friends with, even." Smith and her colleagues at IM4US were actively engaging the topic of social justice well before 2020; however, their work was unfolding at the periphery of functional medicine discourse. During the COVID-19 pandemic and the resurgence of the Black Lives Matter movement, messages like hers took center stage.

Ultimately, the key question of this book is, whose responsibility is it to ensure health? At stake is the distinction between health as a bioconsumer item that can be purchased through private markets versus health as a citizenship-based right and a public good. The answer to this question reveals the nature of citizens' relationships to the state and illuminates the very issue of how we govern ourselves.

In responding to this question, I call for collective action to denounce inequalities and advance the project of social justice in health care delivery. In so doing, I propose the term "health justice," meaning the goal of the struggle against racism, exploitation, and oppression taking place within the health care system, to be achieved by addressing inequality's root causes, which lie both within and beyond this system. My notion of health justice critiques deeply entrenched inequality in conventional medicine. At the same time, health justice is something to be sought in response to the privilege and Whiteness I have observed among functional medicine patients and providers (myself included). Health justice must ensure access to functional and preventive medicine to achieve the goals of economic sustainability and social equity. I have chosen the term "health justice" instead of "health care justice" since, in the same vein as functional medicine practitioners who contrast "disease care" with "health creation," I am emphasizing the need for equitable access to the resources needed to create health (e.g., nutritious diet, safe housing, and clean environment).

The lack of universal health insurance in the United States, when compared to other high-income countries, is evidence of how health in America is treated as a personal responsibility instead of a citizenship-based right. Dr. Parekh indicates, "Our system is different in that we only have about 90 percent of Americans with health insurance. Most of our peer countries have 99 to 100 percent." Acknowledging the dichotomy between personal responsibility and the "nanny state," Dr. Parekh explains, "In our neoliberal environment, it's your fault you are obese. It's a culture focused on personal responsibility, but it ignores the fact that you can't be personally responsible in a toxic environment." Pointing to the example of impoverished residents who have to take two buses to get to a produce store, Dr. Parekh asserts, "Zip code really determines obesity." Dr. Hyman responds, "If you don't actually provide the environment that allows people to make easy, healthy choices, it's hard to do the right thing." The two doctors agree that the environment in which one lives is the largest health determinant.

Likewise, instead of characterizing health as a meritocracy and potentially blaming the victim, I signal how social justice in health care access facilitates improved community-wide health outcomes. As a social epidemiologist, I argue that health is related to how society is organized. I agree with Marmot, who reframes health inequalities as *the* major health problem and indicates that, despite increasingly technical medical interventions, health inequalities are on the rise due to socially unjust values. Marmot writes, "My simple proposal is that health and health inequity are good measures of how we are doing as a society. They are outcomes and they are indicators. By that I mean that health and health equity are valued in themselves" (2015, 42). As a medical anthropologist, I write in the same vein as Farmer, who asks how far the nation is willing to go for people living on society's fringes. How we deal with diseases, especially among the poor, is a standard for measuring not only our medical and scientific skill but also our society's capacity for justice and compassion.

The United States government espouses the principle of equality. At the same time, the World Health Organization identifies health as a "fundamental human right" and calls for universal health coverage (Ghebreyesus 2017). So why are the principle of equality and a commitment to the right to health not reflected in our health care policy?[16] According to Farmer, differential valuation of life explains both the biosocial origins of disease and disparate health outcomes. In contrast, Dr. Parekh's bipartisan perspective is less incriminating: "We all agree that prevention is important. So why haven't policymakers . . . elevated this issue to the top?" Answering his own question, Dr. Parekh explains that policymakers tend to react to problems, whereas prevention requires a proactive approach. In describing policymakers in this way, Dr. Parekh is not highlighting "reactivity" as a personal character flaw of the policymakers; instead, he notes how the political system discourages policymakers from investing resources in prevention and public health.

The Congressional Budget Office evaluates the effectiveness of public spending over ten-year periods. While prevention may prove beneficial over a twenty-year period, in the short term it tends to look like a "cost sink" instead of money well spent. Clinical nutritionist Dr. Peter Osborne, identifying himself as a businessman, describes his resistance to using public funds for conventional health care that has proven to be astronomically expensive in the long run. He furthermore asserts, "I think that taxpayer dollars should not be spent on a system that doesn't work." From a functional medicine perspective, the government's disincentivization of disease prevention leads to systemic problems in health care delivery and, ultimately, to financial mismanagement. What is the solution to these systemic problems?

As an ethnographic observer, I noticed over the course of my research period that functional medicine interlocutors' expressions of hope regarding individual recovery shifted to affirmations of the need for politicized action at the community level. For example, Maskell asserts in one email newsletter that instead of waiting for politicians or commercial development to lead the way, communities should take charge of their own health (see also Maskell 2020).[17] In so doing, Maskell echoes Marmot, who suggests that in the United States, if the central government is unwilling to make health equity a goal, a pathway forward may be action at the local level (Marmot 2015). While their message can be critiqued for deemphasizing the role of the state, Maskell argues in the November 2020 Functional Forum, on the eve of the presidential election, "If we really want to make progress over the next four years, we need to have a political action wing. We do need to be focusing on what we can be doing politically." He stresses that functional medicine proponents will have to be nimble in their efforts to bring functional medicine to the masses and that this may mean "getting on the back of other movements" like direct primary care and Medicare for All.

Similarly, Dr. Parekh indicates that advocacy for preventive health care is important since the only way to scale up preventive health is through government action. He explains, "The reason why the government is so important is, the private sector is critical, but there is only so much from a scale perspective that philanthropy or nonprofit organizations can do." Dr. Parekh asserts that while individual nongovernmental organizations are able to meet the needs of thousands of individuals, only the government is able to meet the needs of millions of Americans.

According to Dr. Parekh, a grassroots movement that galvanizes the public can, in turn, prompt a deeper commitment to "evidence-based policymaking." His argument echoes that of Maskell, who quotes anthropologist Margaret Mead: "Never doubt that a small group of thoughtful, committed citizens can change the world. Indeed, it is the only thing that ever has" (Maskell 2020, 28). Dr. Parekh explains that the American public needs to indicate to their political representatives, "I'm doing everything I can, but if there is not community support, policy systems, and environmental change helping my family, it is going to be very difficult to do." I agree that while the state is responsible for ensuring the health of its citizens, grassroots movements can help spur the state to fulfill its obligation.

Fortunately, functional medicine interlocutors are beginning to vocalize that, as part of their role as healers, they must advocate for policies that would improve conditions for their patients. Former Idaho state representative Paulette Jordan, who ran for the US Senate in 2020, opined in the November 2020 Functional Forum that the health care crisis would be elevated to the level of top priority during the 2021–2025 presidential term due to the COVID-19 pandemic. Jordan argued that the current medical system must be dismantled and a new system, based on universal access to functional medicine as primary care, should be built in its place. She advocated for reengineering health care so that functional medicine services are reimbursed through insurance, rendering preventive and restorative services accessible to the population at large.

Thus far, preventive medicine for bioconsumers has too often been allowed to stand in for what Maskell calls "precision public health." True, universal access to precision public health is needed. I argue that—since the adjective "precision" suggests a narrow focus—meeting the unique needs of bioindividuals requires *expanding* the notion of public health. In making this argument, I engage Marmot's, Dr. Parekh's, and health economist Irene Papanicolas's emphasis on the importance of cross-sector collaborations for preventive health. Reflecting on how 60 percent of American adults have one or more chronic diseases (CDC 2022), Dr. Parekh asserts that addressing social determinants of health requires a package of policy changes. He explains, "Whether it is affordable housing, whether it is education or prekindergarten education, paid family leave—there are a series of interventions that go beyond the four walls of the clinical setting." In the same vein, Papanicolas indicates, "Personally, I support robust social spending on things like education, housing, and family care. They improve health outcomes and indeed social outcomes." All the examples Dr. Parekh and Papanicolas mention are examples of health justice in action.

Health justice is not merely about access to health care but about access to the necessary resources for creating and sustaining health. Dr. Parekh provides one specific example: even if a patient receives excellent nutrition counseling, they will not be able to implement the advice they receive if they do not have access to nutritious food. He reiterates that clinical interventions must be reinforced through clinical-community linkages. In essence, increasing access to health care will not be successful without also increasing individuals' access to health-sustaining resources.

There are rare examples of clinical-community linkages already unfolding. For example, Dr. Hyman shares on his podcast *The Doctor's Farmacy* how Community Rx uses a new e-prescribing system to connect patients to community resources on the south side of Chicago that can help them with their specific diagnoses. Furthermore, the Cleveland Clinic created a community program to deliver whole-food meals to a nearby African American neighborhood. During the program, the impoverished residents received nutrition coaching, were taken grocery shopping, and were taught to cook the healthful foods they had learned about. These interventions produced extraordinary improvements in the participants' health—Dr. Hyman points out that the effect of meal provisioning was approximately four times stronger than the effect of diabetes drugs that are considered "a raging success." In response to Dr. Hyman, Dr. Parekh shares that when Geisinger Health provided ten meals per week to diabetes patients through their "Fresh Food Farmacy," the results were dramatic decreases in hemoglobin A1C. Agreeing with Dr. Parekh and Dr. Hyman, a number of functional medicine interlocutors consider meal provisioning a public health intervention and an effective form of disease prevention.[18]

Investments in social programs not only bolster equity and justice, they may also lower health care costs. Dr. Parekh specifically emphasizes the importance of the *ratio* of social services to health care when analyzing chronic-disease outcomes. The United States has a one-to-one ratio of social services to health care spending. That is, the United States spends 18 percent of its gross domestic product—nearly one in five dollars of the entire economy—on health care and approximately the same amount on social services. In contrast, peer countries make double the investment in social services as compared to health care spending—a two-to-one ratio. Dr. Parekh explains, "That ratio matters because there's been research even domestically that looks at the fifty states in our country, and those states that have a higher social service to health care services ratio, they have better outcomes." According to the data, states that spend more on social services have fewer chronic-disease risk factors and lower rates of chronic disease and mortality.

In contrast, states that have a low ratio of social spending are the ones with the highest levels of obesity and other leading causes of preventable deaths. Dr. Parekh specifies, "The CDC estimates that every year there are 250,000 potentially preventable deaths in the United States. That's just taking five leading causes of death: heart disease, stroke, cancer, chronic lower respiratory disease, and unintentional injury." Listening to Dr. Parekh, Dr. Hyman observes that social services are vital since adequate social services can often prevent disease, whereas the health care system is set up to treat disease after it occurs. Seen from this perspective, social services speak to two core goals of functional medicine: to identify the root cause of disease and to prevent disease.

In making this observation, I build upon Timothy Frie's proposal that functional medicine proponents apply systems-biology thinking to policy, thus promoting cross-agency initiatives, programs, research, and education. Frie is the founder and executive director of Reform Health Caucus, a not-for-profit, nonpartisan political action committee that aims to educate down-ballot officeholders and candidates about functional medicine principles, practices, and advantages. During the November 2020 Functional Forum, Frie argued for community wellness programs and framed nutrition, food, and health literacy as critical public health issues. He hopes to spark conversations about proactive prevention to increase both lifespan and healthspan in lieu of costly, reactive interventions to eliminate symptoms. I urge other functional medicine proponents to follow his lead by engaging in a politicized struggle for health equity. At stake is health care as a basic human right—not a privilege reserved for those who can afford it.

ACKNOWLEDGMENTS

In the spring of 2019, I applied for a Faculty Development Leave from the University of Texas Rio Grande Valley (UTRGV). My plan for the proposed leave was to write a book on medical migration across the US-Mexico border. My application was approved for spring 2020. However, as the spring 2019 semester came to a close, I began toying with another book idea—something much more personal. I confided in my two "writing buddies"—Andrés Amado and Marisa Palacios Knox—both of whom emboldened me to seek permission to change the book project for my upcoming leave.

My first step was to reach out to Casey Kittrell, editor in chief at the University of Texas Press. Casey had nurtured and guided my first book, *No Alternative: Childbirth, Citizenship, and Indigenous Culture in Mexico*, beginning when I was a doctoral candidate. In many ways, he helped me become the author I am today. I was incredibly inspired by this new idea, but what I was proposing felt so far off the beaten path that I was unsure if others would recognize its value as a scholarly monograph. It felt like a risk. We spoke on the phone and he wholeheartedly supported my idea. If not for his support in that moment, I would not have had the confidence to pursue my passion project.

While in lockdown during the COVID-19 pandemic, I wrote a mega-manuscript at my dining room table that, with Casey's guidance, was later transformed into two books—*Nested Ecologies: A Multilayered Ethnography of Functional Medicine* and this book. When my husband, Rikin, would come into the kitchen to heat his meals, I would carry my laptop into the bathroom, where I would continue writing. I am sure he found my behavior somewhat strange, but he has always respected how important my writing is to me. (And if there was ever any doubt, certainly none remains after being each other's sole companion for over a year in lockdown!) I am grateful to Rikin for his support and encouragement after witnessing me turn our home into a "writing café." Also, more than anything else in our marriage so far, I am thankful for his partnership in my healing journey. By facilitating my health and well-being, and loving me in sickness and in health, he supports all my efforts as a wife, mother, daughter, professor, and author.

Although I was by myself, I was not alone. I was accompanied by Andrés and Marisa in the dining room "writing café." Before the pandemic, we had met in person, taking turns picking the café of the day or visiting each other's homes. During the pandemic, we met every weekday afternoon via Zoom. We took breaks every forty-five minutes or so to catch up, exchange ideas, and insert a few moments of levity into our otherwise focused sessions. Using technology to adapt to the circumstances of lockdown, it was almost as if they were at my kitchen table with me—like "old times," when I had occasionally hosted our writing meetups and invited them to explore my fairly extensive tea collection. (However, they might say it was as if they were hosting me in their homes!) Although we are in different fields, these two colleagues provided me with ongoing feedback throughout the writing process. I deeply value their insights and I cherish their friendship.

During my initial writing of the mega-manuscript, I wrote about one chapter per week. My close friend from graduate school James Battle invited me to join his virtual writing group on Friday mornings. At the beginning of each week, two writing group members submitted a chapter or article draft to the entire group via email, allowing the others to read the submitted work and provide comments and suggestions at the Friday meeting. Over the course of several months, I submitted most of the chapters in this book to the group and I benefited greatly from their generative comments. In addition to James, I am indebted to Sandra Harvey, Victoria Massie, and Dennis Browe for their close reading of my work. Sandra encouraged me to write in an experimental style, Victoria asked thought-provoking questions, Dennis pushed me to hone my critique of the phenomena I was observing, and James shared his honest opinions about when a chapter was still lacking versus when I had "found my stride."

One of the questions James asked me was whether the 347 practitioners included in my ethnography indeed formed a social network. Is there a functional medicine community? Or are the practitioners included in my ethnography random individuals that I happened to have come across? Having conducted the ethnography, I knew I was observing a cohesive functional medicine community; however, James's question pointed to the need for graphic visualizations of the cohesion I had observed. I enlisted the help of my favorite "computer whiz"—my younger brother, Jason Vega. He was completing his bachelor's degree in computer science at UC San Diego and is now pursuing a PhD in computer science at the University of Illinois Urbana-Champaign, where he is researching artificial intelligence, trustworthy machine learning, and fairness in federated learning. I sent Jason the data table in the appendix and he produced the people- and source-centric social networks depicted in figures 0.1 and 0.2. The job was more than he bargained for, and I am very appreciative of his hard work.

As I continued writing the first draft, it quickly became clear that the manuscript was too long for publication. I had written well over three hundred thousand words. Even after untangling the two manuscripts, my writing still needed serious tightening. Each week, I emailed a new chapter draft to my mother, Tuen Wong. My mom is a former English major. While I was producing words, she was eliminating them. We did not see each other for sixteen months during the pandemic, but, in some way, her involvement in my writing process helped me to feel her presence. Moreover, my mom has always been supportive of all my decisions, including my chosen paths for career, child-rearing, health, and healing. She never questions my judgment or doubts the "alternative" methods I pursue. She repeatedly tells me I know what is best for my body. Her faith gives me faith.

After this pruning process, I shared drafts of my work with a trusted colleague at UTRGV, Bill Yaworsky. Since I joined the anthropology department, Bill and I had developed a habit of exchanging manuscripts and offering each other feedback. Bill is a social and cultural anthropologist with research interests in Latin America, politics, and social psychology. He is humble to a fault. Every time he reads my work, he reminds me that he is not a medical anthropologist, so his opinion is simply that of an educated lay reader—then he delivers feedback that is invariably useful and constructive. I often needed the perspective of an anthropologist who is not positioned squarely within my own subdiscipline, and Bill's comments helped me to gauge how my work would be perceived by the wider audience I was hoping to write for.

This manuscript greatly benefited from the generous and insightful comments of three reviewers. An anonymous reviewer urged me to organize the chapters in a way that is readily navigable to readers. Carlos Novas challenged me to critically explore whether functional medicine is a pseudoscience, how functional medicine practitioners engage in boundary work, the role of wearable devices and the quantified Self in functional medicine, and whether functional medicine online communities advance capitalist agendas or are contributing to an alternative media. Furthermore, his generative comments pushed me to engage more deeply with the existing medical anthropology literature on illness narratives, bioeconomy, biocapital, biosociality, and the US health care system. Finally, Carole Browner identified specific places where I had provided excessive detail and alerted me to issues with the US health care system of which I had not previously been aware. Each of these reviewers shaped this book in a unique and valuable way.

As I was in the process of revising this book, my daughter, Madelena, transformed (seemingly overnight!) from a baby to a toddler. My mom cared for Madelena on weekday afternoons, thus allowing me precious time for focused work. I am so grateful for how she contributed to my finishing this book. Madelena is blessed to have her as a grandma, and I cherish her as my mom.

APPENDIX

PERSONS DESCRIBED IN THIS BOOK

This section includes individuals I have cited because of their positionality vis-à-vis functional medicine and public discourse, the sources of their statements that are quoted or referenced in the text, and their roles and credentials. It does not include the social scientists I have referenced throughout the book or the functional medicine patients I have anonymized using pseudonyms.

Person	**Source**	**Role**
Matthew Accurso	*The Human Longevity Project* docuseries	Entrepreneur; health consultant
Ted Achacoso	*The Human Longevity Project* docuseries	MD
Lara Adler	*The Human Longevity Project* docuseries	Environmental toxins expert; certified holistic health coach
Dave Asprey	*Super Human: The Bulletproof Plan to Age Backward and Maybe Even Live Forever*; *Bulletproof Radio* podcast; *Bulletproof* YouTube channel; Bulletproof email; *The Doctor's Farmacy* podcast; Eat4Earth online event; *Evelyn Lambrecht* podcast; Biohack Your DNA Summit; email by Williams	Entrepreneur; founder, Bulletproof
Josh Axe	*Dr. Josh Axe* YouTube channel	DNM; DC; CNS

Sarah Ballantyne	The Paleo Mom website; her "BONUS gift" for the Overcoming Hashimoto's Summit is included in Misty Williams's email newsletter *Healing Rosie*	PhD, medical biophysics; functional health educator
Josiah Bartz	"Enhancing Patient Care with Virtual Group Visits" webinar; September 2017 Functional Forum	Business development manager, Lifestyle Matrix Resource Center
Razi Berry	*The Human Longevity Project* docuseries; NaturalPath website	Publisher, *International Journal of Naturopathic Medicine* and *Naturopathic Doctor News & Review*; founder and publisher, NaturalPath website
Tom Bilyeu	*Impact Theory* podcast	Cofounder and president, Quest Nutrition; cofounder, CEO, and host, *Impact Theory* podcast
Jeffrey Bland	*FxMed* podcast; *The Human Longevity Project* docuseries; September 2017 Functional Forum; Interpreting Your Genetics Summit; "Simplexity Medicine: Health Care Reimagined" webinar; 2020 Institute for Functional Medicine Annual International Conference	PhD, biochemistry; FACN; CNS
Tom Blue	*The Human Longevity Project* docuseries	Strategic advisor (industry), Institute for Functional Medicine; former executive director and chief strategy officer, American Academy of Private Physicians
Elizabeth Boham	*The Doctor's Farmacy* podcast	MD; MS; RD
David Brady	*Betrayal* docuseries	ND
Dale Bredesen	*Autoimmune Secrets* docuseries	MD
Kelly Brogan	*The Human Longevity Project* docuseries; *Betrayal* docuseries; "Tantalizing Evidence of a Brain Microbiome" blog post on Kelly Brogan, MD website	MD

Marena Burnett	September 2019 Functional Forum	Senior director of health care engagement and innovation, Centering Health Institute
Krista Burns	American Posture Institute email	DC
Lloyd Burrell	EMF Health Summit email	Host, EMF Health Summit; founder, ElectricSense
Zach Bush	Food Revolution Network interview; EMF Health Summit; *Autoimmune Secrets* docuseries; "Intrinsic Health Coaching Program" web page; "The Virome: A Template for a Regenerative Future" webinar; Eat4Earth online event	MD
Benjamin Chan	*FxMed* podcast	PhD, biology; associate research scientist, Paul Turner lab
Rangan Chatterjee	*The Human Longevity Project* docuseries	MD
John Chen	*FxMed* podcast; *The Community Cure*, by Maskell	PharmD; DOM; LAc; medical consultant, Evergreen Herbs
Nalini Chilkov	*The Human Longevity Project* docuseries	DOM
Titus Chiu	*The Human Longevity Project* docuseries	MD
Jon Cohen	TEDMED talk	MD
Taylor Conroy	Described by Maskell	Founder, The Idea Collective; TEDx speaker
Alauna Curry	"Functional Medicine, COVID-19 and Racial Disparities, Bridging the Gap" webinar	MD
Bridgit Danner	DIY Detox Summit email	Functional health coach; detoxification expert
Jay Davidson	Mitochondrial Summit; Viral and Retroviral Summit; Microbe Formulas advertisement on Facebook; *Autoimmune Secrets* docuseries	DC; PScD; cofounder, Microbe Formulas and CellCore Biosciences

Reed Davis	*The Human Longevity Project* docuseries	Functional diagnostic nutritionist
René Dubos (1901–1982)	His contribution is described by Servan-Schreiber in *Anticancer* and by Prescott and Logan in *The Secret Life of Your Microbiome*	PhD, microbiology; microbiologist, Rockefeller University
Mette Dyhrberg	*Autoimmune Secrets* docuseries	Digital health innovator; CEO, Mymee
Marvin Edeas	*The Human Longevity Project* docuseries	MD; PhD; microbiome researcher
Darryl Edwards	*The Human Longevity Project* docuseries	Founder, Primal Play
Ryan Eliason	Social Entrepreneur Empowerment email	Founder, Visionary Business School
Stephen Ezell	MyGreenFills email; he promoted Sarah Otto and Matt Potts's *Gut Solution* docuseries	CEO, MyGreenFills
Cindy Fallon	"The Innate Immune System" webinar	PhD, organic chemistry
Paul Farmer (1959–2022)	Described by Hyman in presentation "Application of Functional Medicine in a Large Medical System (Cleveland Clinic)"; *Food Fix*, by Hyman	MD; PhD, medical anthropology; Kolokotrones University Professor; chair, Department of Global Health and Social Medicine, Harvard Medical School
Kara Fitzgerald	*FxMed* podcast; *FxMed* email newsletter; "Functional Medicine, COVID-19 and Racial Disparities, Bridging the Gap" webinar; Doctor Kara Fitzgerald website	ND; host, *FxMed* podcast
Bill Frist	*The Doctor's Farmacy* podcast	MD; former senator and US Senate majority leader
Joel Fuhrman	*Autoimmune Secrets* docuseries	MD; president, Nutritional Research Foundation; faculty, Health Sciences Division, North Arizona University
Jason Fung	*The Human Longevity Project* docuseries	MD

Jerry Fusilier	September 2019 Functional Forum	Open Source Wellness patient
Christopher Gardner	2020 Institute for Functional Medicine Annual International Conference	PhD, nutrition science; Rehnborg Farquhar Professor of Medicine at Stanford University
Donna Gates	Body Ecology website; Body Ecology email; Interpreting Your Genetics Summit	MEd; ABAAHP; nutritional consultant
Tracy Gaudet	2020 Institute for Functional Medicine Annual International Conference; "Visionary Tracy Gaudet, MD, Explains Whole Health Care within the VA" on ifm.org; 2018 End Well Symposium	MD
Jeffrey Geller	September 2019 Functional Forum; *Evolution of Medicine* podcast	MD
Niki Gratrix	*Autoimmune Secrets* docuseries; her role is described by Howard	Nutritionist; health coach; cofounder, Optimum Health Clinic
Patrick Hanaway	2020 Institute for Functional Medicine Annual International Conference	MD; past president, American Board of Integrative Holistic Medicine; chief medical education officer, Institute for Functional Medicine; founding medical director, Cleveland Clinic
Heidi Hanna	Fatigue Super Conference	PhD, holistic nutrition; MS, mental health counseling
Michelle Hauser	2020 Institute for Functional Medicine Annual International Conference	MD; MS, epidemiology and clinical research; MPA; FACP; FACLM; DipABLM; chef; clinical associate professor of medicine, Stanford University; obesity medicine director, Medical Weight Loss Program at Stanford Lifestyle and Weight Management Center
Rick Henriksen	Healing Rosie email	MD; MPP

Andrew Heyman	*George Washington University School of Medicine and Health Sciences Integrative Medicine* podcast; Advances in Mitochondrial Medicine Symposium	MD; MHSA
Andrew Hill	*The Human Longevity Project* docuseries	PhD, cognitive neuroscience; cognitive neuroscientist and founder, Peak Brain Institute
Leroy Hood	His contribution is described by Bland	MD; PhD; biologist, California Institute of Technology and University of Washington
Alex Howard	Fatigue Super Conference; Fatigue Super Conference email	CEO, Optimum Health Clinic
Mark Hyman	*The Doctor's Farmacy* podcast; *The Human Longevity Project* docuseries; "Application of Functional Medicine in a Large Medical System (Cleveland Clinic)" presentation; *Food Fix*; *The Conscious-ish Show*; his contribution to *Betrayal* is described by Nandi; 2020 Institute for Functional Medicine Annual International Conference	MD; host, *The Doctor's Farmacy* podcast
Janet (pseudonym)	Member of my functional medicine team	MS; CNS; CKNS; CN
Sayer Ji	GreenMedInfo email; Interpreting Your Genetics Summit; "How Raw Honey Could Save Your Microbiome (and Travel Back in Time)" article; *The Human Longevity Project* docuseries; Ji's PDF "gift" was included in a promotional email from O'Bryan for *Betrayal*	Founder, GreenMedInfo
Angel Jockers	Dr. Jockers email; *Autoimmune Secrets* docuseries	"Lead happiness manager," DrJockers.com

David Jockers	*Dr. Jockers* email newsletter; *The Human Longevity Project* docuseries	DNM; DC; MS
Jolene (pseudonym)	Member of my functional medicine team	Nutrition resident
Tawny Jones	*The Community Cure*, by Maskell; *Evolution of Medicine* podcast; *The Doctor's Farmacy* podcast	Chief administrator, Cleveland Clinic Center for Functional Medicine
Paulette Jordan	November 2020 Functional Forum	Idaho state representative (2014–2018)
Anup Kanodia	2017 Functional Forum	MD
Datis Kharrazian	*The Human Longevity Project* docuseries; *FxMed* newsletter	PhD; DHSc; DC; MS; MMSc; FACN
Katie Kimball	Kitchen Stewardship email	Creator, Kitchen Stewardship website
Chris Kresser	*FxMed* podcast; *The Human Longevity Project* docuseries; *Unconventional Medicine*	LAc; functional health coach; author; ancestral nutritionist
Vishen Lakhiani	*The Doctor's Farmacy* podcast; *The Human Longevity Project* docuseries	Entrepreneur; founder and CEO, Mindvalley
Beth Lambert	*The Human Longevity Project* docuseries	Executive director, Parents Ending America's Childhood Epidemic (PEACE)
Jonathan Landsman	EMF Health Summit; NaturalHealth365 email; Landsman's PDF "gift" was included in a promotional email from O'Bryan for *Betrayal*	Personal health consultant; author; radio talk show host
Carolyn Ledowsky	MTHFR Support Australia website, email	Naturopath; founder, MTHFR Fertility and MTHFR Support Australia
Anna Lembke	TEDx talk	MD; professor, medical director of addiction medicine, Stanford University School of Medicine; chief, Stanford Addiction Medicine Dual Diagnosis Clinic
Todd LePine	*The Doctor's Farmacy* podcast; "The Gut and Skin Microbes" HealthMeans interview	MD

Cynthia Li	*The Doctor's Farmacy* podcast	MD
William Li	TED talks; *The Doctor's Farmacy* podcast; *Eat to Beat Disease*	MD
Grace Liu	*The Human Longevity Project* docuseries	PharmD; CEO, the Gut Institute
Tieraona Low Dog	*Remedy: Ancient Medicine for Modern Illness* docuseries; Tieraona Low Dog, M.D. website; "Meet the Real Medicine Woman" article by Janet Ungless; "Telehealth: Navigating the Changing Landscape of Medicine" Fullscript webinar	MD
Robert Luby	*FxMed* email newsletter	MD; director of medical education initiatives, Institute for Functional Medicine
Max Lugavere	*The Human Longevity Project* docuseries	Health and science journalist; filmmaker
Amy R. Mack	"Expanding Access to Functional Medicine in Vulnerable Communities" article on Institute for Functional Medicine website	MD; CEO, Institute for Functional Medicine
Molly Maloof	October 2017 Functional Forum	MD; lecturer, Stanford University
James Maskell	Fatigue Super Conference; *The Energy Blueprint* podcast; October 2017 and September 2019 Functional Forums; email newsletter; "Enhancing Patient Care with Virtual Group Visits" webinar; *The Human Longevity Project* docuseries; *The Evolution of Medicine*; *The Community Cure*; *The Rogue Health Economist* daily livecast; "Building Healthcare from Scratch" TEDMED talk; Morgan Health; Advances in Mitochondrial Medicine Symposium	BSc, economics; entrepreneur; author; founder, Evolution of Medicine; cofounder, Functional Forum; functional medicine advocate

Steven Masley	*Betrayal* docuseries	MD; FAHA; FACN; CNS; CCD
Wayne Matson	His contribution is described by Bland	PhD, analytical chemistry; metabolomics researcher
Safiya McCarter	"Functional Medicine, COVID-19 and Racial Disparities, Bridging the Gap" webinar	ND; LAc
Celeste McGovern	*Betrayal* docuseries	Health and science journalist, columnist
Joseph Mercola	His contribution to *Betrayal* is described by Nandi; Eat4Earth online event	DO
Deanna Minich	*The Human Longevity Project* docuseries	PhD, nutrition; certified nutritionist, trained by the Institute for Functional Medicine
Charles Modlin	*The Community Cure*, by Maskell; *The Doctor's Farmacy* podcast	MD; MBA; physician lead for public health, executive director of minority health, and founder and director of the Minority Men's Health Center, Cleveland Clinic
Christopher Mote	"Enhancing Patient Care with Virtual Group Visits" webinar	DO; DC
Rodger Murphree	*The Gut Solution* docuseries; *Autoimmune Secrets* docuseries	DC
Mike Mutzel	*The Human Longevity Project* docuseries	MS, clinical nutrition; graduate, Institute for Functional Medicine's AFMCP program; creator, *High Intensity Health* YouTube channel and podcast
Amy Myers	*The Autoimmune Solution*; *The Thyroid Connection*; Amy Myers MD® website; *Myers Way® Guide to Candida* eBook; The Myers Way® Community Facebook group	MD
Sarah Myhill	Fatigue Super Conference	MD

Andrea Nakayama	*The Human Longevity Project* docuseries; *FxNutrition* email newsletter; Fatigue Super Conference; Interpreting Your Genetics Summit; *Betrayal* docuseries; *Evelyn Lambrecht* podcast	Functional medicine nutritionist
Partha Nandi	*Ask Dr. Nandi* email; Dr. Nandi website	MD; FACP; author; talk show host
Robert Naviaux	Advances in Mitochondrial Medicine Symposium	MD
Mary Newport	*Autoimmune Secrets* docuseries	MD
Michele Nickels	*High Intensity Health* YouTube channel	ND; LAc
Edward Noffsinger	*The Community Cure*, by Maskell; his DIGMA model is described as an inspiration for Dr. Saxena's group visits	MD
Christiane Northrup	*The Energy Blueprint* podcast; Christiane Northrup M.D. website	MD
Tom O'Bryan	*Autoimmune Secrets* docuseries; *The Human Longevity Project* docuseries; *Betrayal* docuseries; his *Betrayal* docuseries was advertised in emails from Wohlfert, Wahls, Sarna, Ballantyne, Shojai, Maskell, Nandi, and Ji	DC; CCN; DACBN
Dean Ornish	*Voices of the Food Revolution*, by John Robbins and Ocean Robbins	MD
Peter Osborne	*Betrayal* docuseries	PScD; nutritionist
Sarah Otto	*The Gut Solution* docuseries	Filmmaker; health researcher
Irene Papanicolas	"Why Your Health Care Costs So Much" TEDMED talk	PhD, economics; assistant professor of health economics, Department of Social Policy, London School of Economics

Dan Pardi	*The Human Longevity Project* docuseries	PhD, cognitive neuroscience; MS, exercise physiology; CEO, humanOS.me
Anand Parekh	*The Doctor's Farmacy* podcast	MD; chief medical advisor, Bipartisan Policy Center; former deputy assistant secretary for health, US Department of Health and Human Services
Kirk Robert Parsley	*The Human Longevity Project* docuseries	MD
Sachin Patel	*The Human Longevity Project* docuseries	Functional health coach; founder, Living Proof Institute
Vincent Pedre	*FxMed* podcast; FxMed email; *The Gut Solution* docuseries	MD
David Perlmutter	His contribution to *Betrayal* is described by Nandi; email by Williams	MD; FACN; ABIHM
Martin Picard	*The Energy Blueprint* podcast	PhD, mitochondrial biology of aging; neurology researcher, Columbia University
Mark Pimentel	His collaborative relationship with Sarna is described by Sarna	MD
Joseph Pizzorno	2020 Institute for Functional Medicine Annual International Conference; Eat4Earth online event	ND
Nick Polizzi	Described by Vaszily	Executive producer, *Remedy: Ancient Medicine for Modern Illness* docuseries; author, *The Sacred Science*; creator, The Sacred Science website
Matt Potts	*The Gut Solution* docuseries	Filmmaker; health researcher
Jason Prall	Mitochondrial Summit; Fatigue Super Conference; *The Human Longevity Project* docuseries	Filmmaker; functional health coach

Susan Prescott	*The Secret Life of Your Microbiome* (coauthored with Alan C. Logan); 2020 Institute for Functional Medicine Annual International Conference	MD
Mary Purdy	September 2019 Functional Forum	RN; RDN
Kaya Purohit	*The Doctor's Farmacy* podcast	Chief content officer, Hyman Digital
Harpreet Rai	*The Human Longevity Project* docuseries	CEO and board member, Oura Health
Matt Riemann	*The Human Longevity Project* docuseries	Founder and CEO, Ultimate Human Foundation
John Robbins	*Voices of the Food Revolution*	Cofounder and president, Food Revolution Network
Ocean Robbins	*Food Revolution Network* email; *Voices of the Food Revolution*	Cofounder and CEO, Food Revolution Network
Marwan Sabbagh	*The Doctor's Farmacy* podcast	MD
Steven Sandberg-Lewis	His collaborative relationship with Sarna is described by Sarna	ND; DHANP
Shivan Sarna	*SIBO* email newsletter	SIBO expert, recovery coach
Shilpa Saxena	Advances in Mitochondrial Medicine Symposium; 2013 Heal Thy Practice Conference	MD; creator, Group Visit Toolkit
David Servan-Schreiber (1961–2011)	*Anticancer: A New Way of Life*	MD; PhD, cognitive neuroscience
Christopher Shade	Quicksilver Scientific advertisement on Facebook; *Autoimmune Secrets* docuseries	PhD, environmental science/aquatic chemistry; CEO, Quicksilver Scientific
Ayesha Sherzai	Your Best Years Start Now online event	MD
Dean Sherzai	Your Best Years Start Now online event	MD; PhD, health care leadership with a focus on community health
Pedram Shojai	*Interconnected* docuseries email	DOM; LAc; wellness consultant

Allison Siebecker	Her collaborative relationship with Sarna is described by Sarna	ND; MSOM; LAc
David Sinclair	*Impact Theory* YouTube channel; *The Doctor's Farmacy* podcast	PhD, biochemistry and molecular biology; professor of genetics, Harvard Medical School
Marvin Singh	*FxMed* email newsletter	MD
Karta Purkh Singh Khalsa	*Remedy: Ancient Medicine for Modern Illness* docuseries	AD; D.N.-C; RH
Rhonda Smith	September 2019 Functional Forum	Director, Integrative Medicine for the Underserved (IM4US)
Ryan Sternagel	Stern Method website; Stern Method email	Co-creator, the Stern Method
Teddy Sternagel	Stern Method website	Co-creator, the Stern Method
Inna Topiler	Overcoming Hashimoto's Summit emails	MS; CNS
Paul Turner	*FxMed* podcast	PhD, microbial ecology and evolution; Rachel Carson Professor of Ecology and Evolutionary Biology, Yale School of Medicine
Brian Vaszily	The Art of Antiaging email	Host, Your Best Years Start Now online event
Rob Verkerk	"What Happened to 'Do No Harm'?" article	PhD, multitrophic interactions in agricultural systems; executive and scientific director, Alliance for Natural Health International
Elena Villanueva	Mitochondrial Summit; *Autoimmune Secrets* docuseries	DC; integrative health coach; founder, Modern Holistic Health
JJ Virgin	Her contribution to *Betrayal* is described by Nandi; email by Williams	Holistic nutritionist; fitness instructor; personal trainer

Terry Wahls	*Betrayal* docuseries; Toxic Mold Summit; Mitochondrial Summit; *FxMed* podcast; Terry Wahls M.D. website; email newsletter; Wahls Protocol Facebook group; *The Community Cure*, by Maskell; Reverse Alzheimer's Summit 2.0; *Health Theory* YouTube channel	MD
Chris Wark	*The Human Longevity Project* docuseries	Cancer survivor; health coach
Rick Warren	*The Community Cure*, by Maskell; *The Doctor's Farmacy* podcast	Founding pastor, Saddleback Church
Todd Watts	Microbe Formulas advertisement on Facebook; *Autoimmune Secrets* docuseries	DC; PScD; cofounder, Microbe Formulas and CellCore Biosciences
Volkmar Weissig	*The Human Longevity Project* docuseries	PhD; professor of pharmaceutical sciences at Midwestern University
Ari Whitten	*The Energy Blueprint* podcast	PhD candidate, clinical psychology; health coach; fatigue specialist
Misty Williams	*Healing Rosie* email newsletter; Healing Rosie website	Functional medicine advocate; creator, Healing Rosie
Ryan Wohlfert	*Upgraded Parents* email newsletter	DC; co-owner, Total Health Spine and Nutrition
Lara Zakaria	*FxMed* podcast; "Functional Medicine, COVID-19 and Racial Disparities, Bridging the Gap" webinar	PharmD; Institute for Functional Medicine certified practitioner; nutritionist; public health professional
Sherry Zhang	*GenoPalate* email newsletter	PhD, molecular biology; founder and CEO, GenoPalate

NOTES

Prelude

1. According to Water Resources Mission Area (2019) data on arsenic contamination in US water supplies—published online by the United States Geological Survey (USGS)—the arsenic level in Sacramento, California, where I grew up, 5 μg/L, can also contribute to cancer over time.

2. Here I am extending to health care the anthropologist Arjun Appadurai's 1996 proposal of different "scapes": mediascapes, technoscapes, ethnoscapes, financescapes, and ideoscapes (33).

Introduction

1. The Institute for Functional Medicine has been accredited since 2001, and the current accreditation term will be in effect through the end of July 2028.

2. Data from James Maskell's email newsletter, *Evolution of Medicine*, June 4, 2022.

3. I am placing "race" and "racial" in quotation marks to destabilize ready assumptions about the biological underpinnings of so-called "race." Along with other critical "race" studies scholars, I argue that "race" as a social category has implications for individuals' every experience of privilege or discrimination; however, "race" does not exist as a biological given (see Roberts 2012).

4. Practitioners are not impervious to the concern about stigma. For example, Dr. David Servan-Schreiber concealed his struggle with cancer for fourteen years before releasing his best-selling book, *Anticancer: A New Way of Life* (2009).

Chapter 1. Is Functional Medicine Pseudoscience?

1. In this chapter, I am responding to medical anthropologists Jennifer Jo Thompson and Mark Nichter (2016), who consider how engaged medical anthropologists might serve as brokers who facilitate interprofessional communities between conventional and functional medicine practitioners. They furthermore highlight opportunities for medical anthropologists to contribute to evaluations of preventive health services on patient well-being and behavior change.

2. While the term "P4 medicine" usually refers to "predictive, preventive, personalized, and participatory" medicine, I noticed over the course of my ethnographic research that many functional medicine interlocutors emphasized *precision* over *prevention*, thus underscoring methodological differences between functional medicine and conventional medicine. While conventional medicine aims to "prevent" through one-size-fits-all preventive measures, functional medicine aims to use precise diagnostics and interventions to create health. In this vein, Maskell argues that while providers can never know what they have "prevented," precision medicine uses a data-driven approach to diagnose, track progress, and determine outcomes.

3. Popper's deductive approach to the scientific method is opposed to Hilary Putnam's (1991) later notion of science as an inductive process.

4. Only licensed health care professionals are eligible for the IFM's Functional

Medicine Certification Program. According to the IFM's website, common eligible career paths among those seeking IFM certification are acupuncturist, certified nutrition specialist, dentist, doctor of chiropractic, doctor of optometry, doctor of osteopathy, doctor of podiatric medicine, medical doctor, mental health professional, naturopathic doctor, nurse practitioner, occupational therapist, pharmacist, physical therapist, physician assistant, registered dietician, and registered nurse (https://www.ifm.org/certification-membership/certification-program/eligibility/).

5. Functional medicine interlocutors also critique how research-funding structures determine "askable questions" and undermine research on holistic wellness. See section in chapter 7, "Troubling the Waters: 'Fundable' Research Questions and 'Reimbursable' Interventions."

6. I will explore this further in chapter 3.

7. 42 US Code § 300aa–22: Standards of responsibility.

8. Dr. Tracy Gaudet critiqued the "reactive disease care system" during her presentation for the IFM's 2020 Annual International Conference.

9. While lower-class Americans undoubtedly experience anxiety as well—likely more so than their wealthier counterparts—my analysis focuses on the anxieties of middle- and upper-class Americans since they are the potential clients of functional medicine. Some forms of anxiety are more pronounced among the wealthy. For example, anxieties among the wealthy were exacerbated by economic instability during the 2008 Great Recession (see Jetten, Mols, and Healy 2017).

10. I describe functional medicine's emphasis on a patient's life history and the practitioner's intentional attempts to listen instead of speaking during the initial intake (lasting an average of ninety minutes) in chap. 1 of *Nested Ecologies*.

11. See my *Nested Ecologies*, chap. 1, regarding how functional medicine practices may represent an emerging paradigm shift in medicine.

12. This is the topic of chapter 3.

13. See my *Nested Ecologies*, chap. 2, for an in-depth explanation of systems biology.

14. In chapter 5, I problematize the nature of entrepreneurialism among functional medicine doctors.

15. In *Nested Ecologies*, chap. 1, I explore how, with respect to Popper's "demarcation problem," functional medicine may be what Pigliucci and Boudry (2013) refer to as a "paradigmatic case," and I observe how numerous functional medicine proponents use the language of "shifting the paradigm" to describe their work. Thomas Kuhn (1962), critiquing Popper, offered a "revolutionary approach" to science, arguing that facts, theories, and methods are normative behaviors within the "culture" of science and that normative science continues to operate under the existing paradigm until a scientific revolution spurs a paradigm shift. Seen through this lens, the question is, how might functional medicine practitioners act as "scientific revolutionaries" (see *Nested Ecologies*, 20, 36)?

16. See chapter 7.

Interlude. Mapping Out My Systems Biology

1. See my *Nested Ecologies*, chap. 2.

Chapter 2. Wounded Healers

1. This vignette is based on Dr. Terry Wahls's explanations of her personal healing

journey at the Toxic Mold Summit, at the Mitochondrial Summit, at the Reverse Alzheimer's Summit 2.0, on the docuseries *Betrayal*, in a *Health Theory* YouTube episode, and in an *FxMed* podcast interview with host Dr. Kara Fitzgerald in March 2020.

2. The Wahls Protocol diet includes lots of plants and sufficient protein. It is structured to make sure the cells and mitochondria are well nourished, the body is being supplied with building blocks for cell membranes, and the detox pathways are upregulated. The diet includes nine cups of fruits and vegetables per day: three cups of greens (measured raw), three cups of sulfur-family vegetables (broccoli, cauliflower, cabbage, Brussels sprouts, onions, garlic), and three cups of mushrooms and colorful fruits and vegetables (colored all the way through, not just the peel). Wahls recommends gluten-free grains, soaked overnight. She also recommends nutritional yeast as a good source of B vitamins.

3. I have written this narrative using information from Amy Myers's book *The Autoimmune Solution: Prevent and Reverse the Full Spectrum of Inflammatory Symptoms and Diseases*, 3–18.

4. Andrea's story here comes from her presentation at the Fatigue Super Conference and from a mass email to me.

5. Dr. Todd LePine is an exception to the rule in functional medicine since his entry into the field was not shaped by experiences he or a family member had as a chronic-disease sufferer. Dr. LePine explains, "I personally fell into functional medicine because I started hitting my head against the wall using pharmaceutical approaches. . . . What I ended up really needing were more tools in my tool box." He described his transformative experience while attending a seminar with Dr. Jeffrey Bland, saying, "It was really through Jeff Bland, his being able to connect the dots between the biochemistry, the physiology, and the pathophysiology, [that] really showed [me] that our bodies have this innate capacity to heal [themselves]." Dr. LePine explains that, given the right conditions, people do not need drugs or doctors to return to the body's natural homeostasis, which is health. Having transitioned to functional medicine, he indicates, "My job is to keep you away from surgeons and off of drugs as best as possible."

6. See my *Nested Ecologies*, chap. 3, for a detailed analysis of functional medicine discourse on epigenetics.

7. See chapter 7 for my critique of how Big Pharma funding structures determine askable questions and discoverable results, thus shaping the knowledge base of researchers like Sarah.

8. This paves the way for those without medical degrees to position themselves as functional medicine experts alongside MD counterparts (see chapter 1). At the IFM's 2020 Annual International Conference, Dr. Gaudet critiqued the term "nonclinicians," arguing that it evinces the hierarchical and hegemonic nature of biomedicine. She suggested that these individuals instead be called "wellness experts," thus conveying the value of their expert knowledge.

9. The emergence of illness-narrative analysis among anthropologists and sociologists can be traced back to public debates about the effectiveness of medicine and critiques of medical hegemony in the 1970s (Bury 2001).

10. The personal stories of these wounded healers are the central topic of chapter 7.

11. Anup's words point to how hope—an integral facet of the healing process—is intersubjectively constituted by functional medicine providers and patients (Mattingly 2010).

12. Mike Bury (2001) categorizes "heroic" narratives as a subform of "core narrative." Core narratives reveal connections between illness experiences and deeper cultural meanings attached to suffering.

13. See chapter 5 for a more in-depth discussion of branding practices in functional medicine.

14. See chapters 4 and 8.

Interlude. Taking the Reins

1. As mentioned in the introduction, the names of my personal providers are pseudonyms.

2. As noted in chapter 1, Dr. Kelly Brogan describes how, after many years of conventional medicine protocols involving multiple medications, her patients not only improve but also "achieve states of being that they never even knew were possible."

Chapter 3. Relational Shifts

1. See chapter 1 for a discussion of how functional medicine aims to create data matrices on individual patients ($n = 1$) instead of relying on randomized control trials that consider patients to be interchangeable units.

2. The Oura Ring is a sleep and activity tracker. Promotional materials suggest that the ring can help users "sleep better than ever before."

3. Social science scholars have argued that in this age of biotechnology, when biological materials and substances such as stem cells and genomes increasingly figure into product-making and profit-seeking ventures, a new type of capital has emerged: biocapital. Stefan Helmreich (2008) creates a cartography of how the term "biocapital" has been articulated in academia, tracing the varying degrees to which scholars have focused on biotic substance versus economic speculation and sentiment. He ultimately identifies two distinct "species" of biocapital. The first, which he describes as "Marxist feminist," emphasizes the role of sex/gender and "race" in the binary of production versus reproduction. The second, a "Weberian Marxist" approach, closely analyzes questions of information management and speculation, juxtaposing relations of production with ethical subjectivity, while somewhat neglecting biomatter. I will return to the "Marxist feminist" approach in chapter 6. In this chapter, I refer to the "Weberian Marxist" approach.

4. In suggesting this, Birch and Tyfield (2012, 299, 301–302, 309, 320) critique the fetishization among science and technology studies (STS) scholars of everything "bio" and the production of numerous "bio-concepts." They argue that STS scholars, focusing on the technoscientific, have theorized about the bioeconomy without paying adequate attention to the financial and economic restructuring of the economy.

5. Although his analysis is also Weberian Marxist, Rose, a sociologist, places greater emphasis on biomatter. He argues that contemporary biopolitics operate on a molecular level (2007a). Rose rescales what Michel Foucault called "life itself," rendering it microscopic, fungible, and multiple. When describing the "spirit of biocapital," he notes that vitality can be stabilized, frozen, stored, commoditized, exchanged, and traded in the service of both health and wealth (2007b).

6. I will expand on these arguments in chapter 8 and the conclusion.

7. I describe Dr. Wahls's story of being a wounded healer in chapter 2.

8. I discuss Dr. Wahls's group medicine approach in greater detail in chapter 8.

9. I endeavor to go deeper into patients' perspectives in the next chapter.

10. See my *Nested Ecologies*, chap. 3, for an in-depth analysis of functional medicine discourse regarding epigenetics.

Interlude. The Three Cs

1. Their stories are featured in chapters 2 and 4.

Chapter 4. Digitized Patient Communities

1. These four themes clearly overlap with the four themes identified by Natasja Kingod et al. (2017) in a qualitative systematic review of how online peer-to-peer support shaped the daily lives of individuals with chronic illness (i.e., illness-associated identity work, social support and connectivity, experiential knowledge sharing, and collective voice and mobilization). However, my ethnographic observations deviate significantly from their work with regard to patient criticism of, and group-wide strategizing to sidestep, the high costs of functional medicine.

2. See the Autoimmune Association's website for information on autoimmune conditions: https://www.aarda.org/diseaselist/.

3. See chapter 3 for my analysis of how "biohacking" is primarily accessible to privileged bioconsumers.

4. I caution readers against attributing the higher incidence of chronic disease and autoimmunity among women to female physiologies that are somehow "wrong" or to female hormones that are "out of balance." Instead, I argue that differences between men's and women's health outcomes can often be traced to gendered inequalities.

5. Assumptions regarding a universal womanhood can be critiqued from the perspective of social inequalities such as "race" and class, among others.

6. In the latter context, Yolo Akili's quote evokes functional medicine discourse regarding epigenetics and transgenerational trauma, although this may not have been his original intent. See my *Nested Ecologies*, chap. 3, for a discussion of the role trauma plays in intergenerational epigenetics.

7. A small subset of providers offer what can be described as concierge medicine for the masses. Examples include Dr. Angela Bymaster and Brett Bymaster at the Healing Grove Health Center in San Jose, CA, and membership-based services like Wild Health and Parsley Health. While the Healing Grove Health Center offers services to low-income patients, 2022 memberships at Wild Health start at approximately $100 per month, while memberships at Parsley Health cost approximately $175 per month.

8. I should also signal that some functional medicine providers offer "group-delivered care." I briefly mention how Dr. Wahls has implemented group-delivered care in chapter 3 and again later in this chapter. I describe group visits in depth in chapter 8.

9. In chapters 1 and 3, I critique "empowerment"—a critique I continue in this section.

10. Per his website, at jonathanotto.tv. While not all of his work falls squarely within the realm of functional medicine, many functional medicine interlocutors have appeared in his docuseries.

11. I paid this registration fee, booked my hotel, and purchased my flight to Phoenix to attend this conference, but it was deferred and switched to an online format due to the COVID-19 pandemic. I later completed 13.75 continuing medical education credits through my online participation in three of the five modules.

12. Individuals who check out functional medicine books from the library and implement lifestyle changes without advanced diagnostics or one-to-one care, as Dr. Wahls described in chapter 3, are exceptions to the rule.

13. For an ethnography of communalism and collectivist life that offers critical hope for a less individualist and more socially just world, see Smith-Morris (2019).

14. Per his website, at www.mindvalley.com.

15. Mindvalley accomplishes this goal by creating programs that "give people instant community." For example, the company hosts a one-to-three-week event called "Mindvalley University." The event's web page reads, "Imagine—one of the most iconic cities becoming both your home and your playground for twenty-one magical days with a tribe of people who become your new best friends. . . . From scheduled learning sessions to spontaneous gatherings, you share a deep connection." To join the event, individuals must purchase an All Access subscription for $599/year along with a ticket to the event, starting at $695 for one week. The FAQ page for the event indicates, "This ticket also gives you access to our exclusive Facebook group so you can connect with other attendees and share important information before, during, and after the event." However, the ticket price does not include travel, accommodations, meals, or "additional tribe activities." For another event, A-Fest, the website explains, "To attend A-Fest, you will first need to become a Global Campus Member for $995/year. Membership unlocks a range of benefits, including discounted access to A-Fest, starting at $3,595 to $5,595 USD." The cost of the ticket includes "bonding, networking, and connecting with some of the most interesting and inspirational people you'll ever meet." As with Mindvalley University, the ticket does not include transportation or accommodations. It is important to note that Mindvalley does not claim to provide functional medicine care. However, Lakhiani is a frequent interlocutor in the media spaces I explored for my ethnographic research on functional medicine. He was interviewed by Dr. Mark Hyman on his podcast *The Doctor's Farmacy*, by Jason Prall on the docuseries *The Human Longevity Project*, by Tom Bilyeu on his podcast *Impact Theory*, and by Dave Asprey on his podcast *Bulletproof Radio* and his YouTube channel *Bulletproof*. Furthermore, functional medicine interlocutors are frequent speakers at Mindvalley events. Dr. Hyman, Prall, Bilyeu, and Asprey have all spoken at past A-Fest events. Thus, my critique of the commodification of community is not aimed at Lakhiani's work at Mindvalley. Instead, my goal is to demonstrate how the commodification of community unfolds within functional medicine and how this relates to a larger context of emerging entrepreneurship around community-as-commodity.

16. I describe Dr. Wahls's recovery from multiple sclerosis in chapter 2.

17. At the same time, as certain groups accumulate thousands, and even tens of thousands, of members, the distinctions between "patient," "client," and "follower" are increasingly blurred. See chapter 5, "Doctor-Influencers."

18. For a discussion of how functional medicine is remaking traditional medicine, please see chapter 6.

19. During my digital ethnography, I heard a woman who subscribed to *The Gut Solution* platinum package describe the benefit of the docuseries' online Facebook community in as positive terms as the ones the individuals in the patient-organized Facebook groups use. She described the impact the community had had on her healing process, saying, "What really kept [my progress] going was the Facebook forum. In numbers we are powerful. If it were just me left to my own devices . . . I would not

have figured this out." Thus, I do not mean to dismiss the benefit these groups confer; rather, I aim to critique the commodification of "community" that occurs when access to these Facebook groups is sold as part of a "packaged deal."

20. Schermuly, Petersen, and Anderson (2019) argue that in the digital age, instead of struggling for rights, patients strive to achieve a public profile and attract funding. In 2021, they extended their argument regarding how the agency and hopes of citizens are central to the workings of political rule by applying a governmentality lens.

21. It can also be argued that some of these hosts sought out care from functional medicine providers while on their own healing journeys and filmed master classes with the providers so they could monetize the content later through a docuseries, thus recouping their costs and even turning a profit. Jonathan Otto explains that when his wife's father struggled with kidney failure, Jonathan asked one functional medicine practitioner to carve out two weeks of his time. Jonathan flew a film crew out to film "the entire process" of his father-in-law receiving in-depth functional medicine consultations. While this cost him over $10,000, he notes, those who purchase the platinum package get this content "totally free." Similarly, Sarah Otto and Matt Potts describe their struggles with autoimmunity and mental health, respectively. In some clips, Dr. Rodger Murphree is shown at a whiteboard giving an explanatory lecture to Sarah. Matt explains that because of "the financial risks they took flying around the world and creating the video and printed materials," they are not able to give away the packaged materials for free.

22. In addition to the purposes outlined in this chapter, Deborah Lupton (2014) signals that these forums ostensibly contribute to large aggregated data collections that are used to conduct medical research, develop medical treatments, and improve services.

Chapter 5. Doctor-Influencers

1. My comments about the intentional strategies employed by functional medicine entrepreneurs are not meant to devalue their desire to help and heal consumers.

2. Williams's online Ask-Me-Anything event featured one functional medicine practitioner, but her partnership is with the SteadyMD company. I discuss corporate sponsorships later in this chapter.

3. I discuss Dr. Wahls's June and July 2019 email newsletters in chapter 3.

4. It is important to note that students of the Visionary Business School are not exclusively, or even primarily, involved in functional medicine. However, as Robbins points out in the email, "home-based health coach[ing]" and "global natural foods enterprises" are among the types of "socially conscious businesses" that business school alumni launch.

5. On the same day, I also received three promotional emails for Jonathan Landsman's "Indoor Air Pollution"—a webinar that ultimately advertised specific air filters that Landsman asserts are superior to HEPA filters. In a follow-up email, Landsman wrote, "Just a quick note that the very special 50% off deal on the Air Doctor filtration units ($329 instead of $629!) ends at MIDNIGHT on TUESDAY, JULY 9th! The first 300 to purchase get their next set of filters, a $60 value, FREE, as a bonus! And you get a FIVE-YEAR warranty (rather than a one-year warranty) if you order by TUESDAY, JULY 9th!"

6. Community-based marketing also unfolds independently of online platforms

such as HealthMeans. Virtually all the digital content I analyzed while conducting research for this book—including podcasts and YouTube videos—was created by functional medicine practitioners and educators recording interviews with each other. As a result, the individual functional medicine practitioners I observed were interviewed by multiple other practitioners and educators in the functional medicine community. For example, Dr. William Li was a guest on Mark Hyman's podcast *The Doctor's Farmacy*, Chris Wark's podcast *Chris Beat Cancer*, and Dave Asprey's podcast *Bulletproof Radio*. Elsewhere in this book, I describe Dr. Hyman's, Wark's, and Asprey's various contributions as interviewees. By toggling between the roles of interviewer and interviewee, functional medicine practitioners and health educators are able to interview each other multiple times and on diverse platforms, thereby garnering greater visibility and ultimately bolstering their individual income.

7. In a literature review of 154 peer-reviewed academic publications on influencer marketing, Liselot Hudders, Steffi De Jans, and Marijke De Veirman (2021) reveal that the majority of studies focus on the use of influencers as a covert commercial marketing tactic, with the aim of evaluating the efficacy of influencers' sponsored recommendations.

8. This is also similar to the way affiliates cull from HealthMeans email scripts when promoting online events.

9. See the following text section, "Doctor-Influencers: When People Become Brands," for a deeper analysis of how doctor-influencers become brands.

10. Dr. Pedre is also a medical advisor for Fullscript. In essence, functional medicine practitioners market the products and services of corporate sponsors in ways that are strikingly similar to how they promote docuseries (thus underscoring how docuseries are self-knowledge products).

11. In the conclusion of *Nested Ecologies*, I apply the concept of nested ecologies—a heuristic tool I use to describe how individuals' internal ecologies (e.g., the trillions of microbes that inhabit each human body) are nested within an external ecology that is shaped by physical, environmental, political, economic, and cultural factors—to the US food system and describe functional medicine interlocutors' role in advocating for food justice.

12. See my comments above about how Dr. Wahls leverages the Wahls brand when promoting sponsors. I will further explore how doctor-influencers become brands in the following section, "Doctor-Influencers: When People Become Brands."

13. See chapter 3.

14. The Functional Forum offers in-person practitioner education through mixed-media "medutainment" (i.e., the union of "medicine," "education," and "entertainment"), by combining TED-style talks, videos, and audience interaction, which is later archived as "episodes" on YouTube. This monthly conference is paired with local events among dozens of functional medicine "communities" across the United States.

15. See chapter 4.

16. In chapter 3, I explore how functional medicine patients are positioned as "clients."

17. See chapter 2.

18. Hendry, Hartung, and Welch's aim is not to qualify influencer pedagogy as "good" or "appropriate," nor do they examine whether health and wellness influencers are (un)qualified sources of health education.

19. Since the functional medicine influencers I followed while conducting research for this book infrequently identified themselves as affiliates, in many cases I could not be certain an affiliate structure was in place.

20. See chapter 4. In making this argument, I am building on Lupton's (2014) notion of the "digital patient experience economy."

21. I will expand on this theme in chapter 7.

Chapter 6. Ancient Healing Traditions

1. When describing economic and power inequality in the contemporary world system, I prefer the terms "Global North" and "Global South." However, I am using the terms "Western" and "non-Western" since these are the terms used by the subjects in my study.

2. Mutzel asserts that "a lot of people" decide to buy organic, gluten-free, grain-free food at Whole Foods, but this statement belies the socioeconomic limitations that many bioconsumers face. Embedded in his comment is an assumption of middle- to upper-class standing, which in turn signals how functional medicine approaches are primarily consumed by privileged individuals. Mutzel's assertion may be correct for the audience he is addressing; however, it is out of touch with society at large.

3. Dr. Heyman clarifies that he cannot describe all ancient healing traditions with the same expertise, but he asserts, "I can speak a bit more authentically from the model of Traditional Chinese Medicine, which is where my original training was." Before earning an MD and a master's degree in health services administration, Dr. Heyman received formal training in Five-Element Shiatsu and Traditional Chinese Medicine.

4. See my comments at the end of this section, in chapter 1, and in Vega (2018, 190–192).

5. See chapter 1. Also see my *Nested Ecologies*, chap. 2.

6. See my *Nested Ecologies*, chap. 3, where I describe prominent studies in epigenetics and analyze how these have shaped functional medicine.

7. For a comparison of cancer frequency in an Asian context across time (i.e., Japan), see Yatani, Shiraishi, and Nakakuki 1988.

8. See Stewart and Kleihues (2003).

9. Functional medicine interlocutors suggest that, in contrast to conventional medicine, functional medicine teaches practitioners to resist binary thinking. The romanticization of "Others" is one example of how functional medicine practitioners fail to resist binary thinking. See my *Nested Ecologies*, chap. 1.

10. Consider how this relates to moral foundations theory and the idea that innate intuitions guide culture-specific virtues (see Haidt and Joseph 2007).

11. I will explore functional medicine's emphasis on community in chapter 8.

12. Dr. Northrup's website, Christiane Northrup M.D., is at https://www.drnorthrup.com/.

13. What is characterized as "vitality" in the literature on biocapital is often called "wellness" in functional medicine discourse.

14. Sarah Franklin (2006) uses the term "biocapital" to describe the translation of embryology into stem cell derivation and redirection and discusses how this extraction, isolation, and mobilization of reproductive agency provokes novel ethical articulations. Vora (2015) extends Franklin's approach to biocapital when she explores how biological commodities such as human organs for transplant, medical therapeutic

devices engineered from human biological materials, and the temporary use of human bodies through gestational surrogacy or clinical trial participation are understood in terms of surplus and thus potentiated for outsourcing.

15. See the New Thought Walden Awards web page on the Unity Worldwide Ministries website at https://www.unityworldwideministries.org/association-global-new-thought-agnt.

16. See chapter 5.

17. In this chapter, I refer to both Dr. Cynthia Li and Dr. William Li. For the sake of clarity, I refer to them using their full names throughout the remainder of the chapter.

18. My mother is Chinese. My father is of mixed Mexican, Nahua, and Blackfoot descent.

19. This Confucian phrase is elsewhere written "Hara hachi bun me" (腹八分目).

20. However, I also observed one example of a functional medicine interlocutor who is a person of color positioning himself as an expert in an ethnomedicine that is unrelated to his personal heritage. In a mass email, Dr. Pedram Shojai invited *Interconnected* docuseries viewers to join him in an exclusive retreat. The retreat's online description read, "Surrounded by nature, Pedram will lead the training and teach you specific Tai Chi, Qi Gong, and meditation exercises focusing on the alignment of your mind, body and spirit." Dr. Shojai, an Iranian American, has carved out a unique space in functional medicine as someone trained in Chinese martial arts and Oriental medicine—not the traditional medicine or martial arts of his native Iran. As a person of color who practices traditional medicine, Dr. Shojai is unusual within functional medicine circles. The majority of the ethnomedical healers I encountered during my ethnographic research are phenotypically White.

21. Consider how, in the absence of biological Blackness, Rachel Dolezal self-identified as Black based upon her affinity for Blackness. Dolezal, the former president of the National Association for the Advancement of Colored People (NAACP) in Spokane, Washington, was scrutinized for passing as Black and accused of cultural appropriation. Dolezal's critics argued that her NAACP presidency reinscribed historic power inequalities between Whites and Blacks and suggested that if Dolezal truly considered herself an ally to Black people, she would have understood why the presidents of NAACP chapters must be Black.

22. See the "about" page on Khalsa's website, International Integrative Educational Institute, https://internationalintegrative.com/about/kp-khalsa/.

23. For example, an article titled "Meet the Real Medicine Woman" appeared in *Prevention* (Ungless 2013). In this article, Dr. Low Dog explains that she is one-sixteenth Comanche and also part Lakota, but she does not indicate what portion of her heritage is Lakota.

24. Dr. Low Dog's website, Tieraona Low Dog, M.D., is at https://drlowdog.com/.

25. A year later, CNN reported on the use of TCM for COVID-19 (see Gan and Yeung 2021).

26. See Dr. Chen's biographies on the Evergreen Herbs website at https://www.evherbs.com/about-us/meet-our-family and on the Llasa OMS site at https://app.livestorm.co/lhasa-oms/how-coronavirus-covid-19-is-currently-treated-in-china-with-tcm-featuring-john-chen.

27. See the introduction to *Nested Ecologies*.

28. April 1, 2020, https://www.washingtonpost.com/opinions/2020/04/01/andrew-yang-coronavirus-discrimination/.

29. See figures 0.1 and 0.2 in the introduction depicting social networks among functional medicine interlocutors.

Chapter 7. Big Pharma and Health Insurance

1. Furthermore, as Dr. Lembke indicates, doctors may prescribe medications because they are afraid of receiving bad ratings from patient-consumers.

2. See my *Nested Ecologies*, chap. 1, for functional medicine interlocutors' arguments regarding the need for a paradigm shift in medicine.

3. Please see the "Protection from high medical costs" section of the "Why health insurance is important" web page of HealthCare.gov at https://www.healthcare.gov/why-coverage-is-important/protection-from-high-medical-costs/.

4. Please see the graph "National per capita health expenditure in the United States from 1960 to 2021 (in U.S. dollars)," located in the "Health, Pharma & Medtech (Health System)" section of Statista's website at https://www.statista.com/statistics/184955/us-national-health-expenditures-per-capita-since-1960/.

5. See Castañeda et al. (2011) for an assessment of the ACA based on the perspectives of future health care professionals. See Henry (2015) for a discussion of how the ACA has affected physician assistants, nurse practitioners, and community health centers.

6. Amy Dao and Jessica Mulligan (2016) ask if health insurance will become a vehicle for the provision of social protections. See Dr. Lembke's comments in the conclusion of this book regarding how, in the absence of adequate social programs and services, the health care system is used in the United States as a social safety net.

7. According to Dao and Mulligan (2016), health insurance in the era of the ACA accentuates tensions between social solidarity and individual responsibility, private markets and public goods, and granting universal access and rationing limited resources.

8. Maskell's statement foreshadows my discussion in the next section about how health insurance creates financial conflicts of interest.

9. I describe this program in further depth in chapter 8.

10. See the "Autoimmune Disease List" web page of the Global Autoimmune Institute website for a complete list of all autoimmune diseases: https://www.autoimmuneinstitute.org/resources/autoimmune-disease-list/.

11. Beidelschies et al. (2019) cite C. Buttorff, T. Ruder, and M. Bauman, *Multiple Chronic Conditions in the United States* (Santa Monica, CA: RAND Corporation, 2014), 15.

12. To support their argument, Beidelschies et al. (2019) cite G. A. Cuckler, A. M. Sisko, J. A. Poisal, et al., "National Health Expenditure Projections, 2017–2026: Despite Uncertainty, Fundamentals Primarily Drive Spending Growth," *Health Affairs* 37, no. 3 (2018): 482–492, https://doi.org/10.1377/hlthaff.2017.1655. Cuckler, Sisko, and Poisal's study documents how health spending is projected to grow 5.5 percent annually—representing 19.7 percent of the economy by 2026—because of income growth, increases in prices for medical goods and services, and enrollment shifts from private health insurance to Medicare due to the aging population (482).

13. The *JAMA* study tested the outcomes of Dr. Hyman's Cleveland Clinic Center for Functional Medicine.

14. See chapters 2 and 3 for in-depth exploration of how functional medicine reconfigures the patient-provider relationship.

15. See my discussion in chapter 1 regarding how functional medicine challenges current assumptions regarding study design.

16. Dr. Bush acknowledges that there is a "tiny fraction" of the NIH budget dedicated to "prevention," but he clarifies that these funds are aimed at public health education initiatives, not the basic science of how to create health.

17. I will further develop my argument regarding the state's responsibility for the health of citizens in the conclusion.

18. See the Medicare Payment Advisory Commission's *Report to the Congress: Medicare Payment Policy*, March 2022, chap. 12, at https://www.medpac.gov/wp-content/uploads/2022/03/Mar22_MedPAC_ReportToCongress_Ch12_SEC.pdf.

19. While Maskell made this comment well before the COVID-19 pandemic began, his point became even more significant when both patients and providers were sheltered in place.

Chapter 8. Group Visits

1. This story is derived from Maskell's book *The Community Cure*, 70–73; from Group Visit Toolkit materials; and from Dr. Saxena's description of these experiences at the Heal Thy Practice Conference in 2013.

2. During her culinary medicine demonstration at the IFM's 2020 Annual International Conference, Dr. Michelle Hauser—the obesity medicine director of the Medical Weight Loss Program at the Stanford Lifestyle and Weight Management Center—indicated that shared medical appointments could be used as a "portal" for nutrition and culinary education in primary care.

3. This story is derived from Maskell's book *The Community Cure*, 101–102; the *Evolution of Medicine* podcast; Dr. Wahls's website; and Dr. Wahls's email newsletters.

4. This story is derived from Maskell's book *The Community Cure*, 54–58; the *Evolution of Medicine* podcast; the *Doctor's Farmacy* podcast; and Dr. Hyman's presentation "Application of Functional Medicine in a Large Medical System (Cleveland Clinic)."

5. See chapter 7.

6. According to Maskell at the Fatigue Super Conference, "The data shows that 66 percent of people—two-thirds of people—are doing so much better after that group that they don't need to see the doctor." According to Josiah Bartz, business development manager of the Lifestyle Matrix Resource Center, "By the end, 60-80% don't need to see the doctor."

7. See chapter 4 regarding digitized patient communities.

8. At the time of his presentation, CCCFM had already established collaborations with the Cleveland Clinic's Orthopaedic & Rheumatologic Institute; Digestive Disease & Surgery Institute; Respiratory Institute; Neurological Institute; Endocrinology & Metabolism Institute; Miller Family Heart, Vascular & Thoracic Institute; Glickman Urological & Kidney Institute; Ob/Gyn & Women's Health Institute; Genomic Medicine Institute; Pediatric Institute; Sports Medicine Center; and Wellness & Preventive Medicine.

9. See chapter 6 regarding the health-promoting effects of human connection and how, from a functional medicine perspective, humans enjoyed more social connection in the past than we do in the present day.

10. See chapter 5 for an in-depth exploration of how functional medicine entrepreneurs use gated content and other strategies to attract patient-clients.

11. The practitioner "breaks even" at three patients in the group visit; however, group visits tend to involve multiple times the number of patients needed to break even.

12. I will problematize notions of "self-care" later in this chapter and in the conclusion by pointing to the state's role in ensuring health as a citizenship-based right.

13. The page with the pricing of this seminar was at https://terrywahls.com/seminar/; it has since been removed from the site.

14. The page with the pricing of this program was at https://terrywahls.com/thewahlsinstitute/; it has since been removed from the site.

15. Dr. Terry Wahls, "Getting Started on the Wahls Protocol," https://terrywahls.com/start/; Dr. Wahls, July 2019 email newsletter (see chapters 3 and 5).

16. Jonathan Otto and Sarah Otto's "platinum packages" are sold at a fraction of the price of nonbrokered programs comprised of online materials and group tele-education (e.g., the Wahls Protocol Seminar and the Health Optimization Program). The price difference may be attributed to the fact that the brokered model requires significantly less time commitment from individual providers since they are not responsible for recruiting patients, nor do they provide "continuity of care" through consecutive group visits. These packages may provide patients with some access to functional medicine providers; however, they are not an adequate replacement for one-on-one care.

17. I discuss this concept in the next section.

18. See chapter 5.

19. See chapter 5.

20. Maskell rendered this discursive tendency even more obvious when he described his admiration for Joseph Campbell's work. See Joseph Campbell, 2018, *The Hero's Journey: Joseph Campbell on His Life and Work* (Novato, CA: New World Library).

21. See the page at https://zachbushmd.com/services/.

22. See my *Nested Ecologies*, chap. 2.

23. See chapter 1 and my *Nested Ecologies*, chap. 3.

24. Consider Rebecca Adkins Fletcher's (2014) argument that blaming patients erases the responsibility of providers toward their patients.

25. See my argument in *Nested Ecologies*, 147–150, 243, about functional medicine proponents' structural myopia.

26. See chapter 2.

27. See the conclusion.

28. For an anthropological perspective, see Cheal (1988).

29. See Christakis and Fowler (2007).

30. See my *Nested Ecologies*, chap. 4.

31. For more about Frome, see the article "How a Small British Town Used Social Connections to Make Residents Happier and Healthier" (Anderson 2019).

Conclusion

1. See Vega (2018, 5) regarding how very particular racialized individuals are invited to professional conferences to substantiate preexisting narratives and legitimize the interests of nonracialized others.

2. Referring to Kuehn 2019.

3. Dr. Prescott and Dr. Bland were co-presenters in the module "Global Conversations: Sustainable Solutions for Population Health Systems." They are also co-authors of the 2020 article "Spaceship Earth Revisited: The Co-Benefits of Overcoming Biological Extinction of Experience at the Level of Person, Place and Planet."

4. Dr. Safiya McCarter asserted that functional medicine is actually behind conventional medicine in having conversations about "racial" equity.

5. For an in-depth explanation of the relationship between the medical anthropology concept of a "syndemic" and functional medicine's "systems biology" approach, see my *Nested Ecologies*, chap. 2.

6. I will expand on the valuable role engaged medical anthropologists can play in the delivery of functional medicine later in this conclusion.

7. See, for example, my comments regarding acts of violence against Asian Americans during the COVID pandemic in chapter 6. Also see my comments in *Nested Ecologies* (220, 251) regarding the toxic environmental exposures faced by Hispanic farm workers.

8. Dr. Bland cited Brandt and Botelho (2020).

9. See Dr. Heyman's and Dr. Brogan's similar comments in my *Nested Ecologies*, chap. 1.

10. See chapter 8.

11. Dr. Modlin clarified that both Blacks and women are negatively affected when they are not included in pharmaceutical development.

12. See chapters 2 and 4.

13. See chapter 7.

14. See my *Nested Ecologies.*

15. See my *Nested Ecologies.*

16. See Michel Foucault's 1976 lecture "Society Must Be Defended" on biopower as the power to "'make' live or 'let' die" (2003, 241).

17. See chapter 8.

18. In chapter 8, I noted that Dr. Hanaway has argued for providing nutritious food as a strategy for preventing chronic disease.

WORKS CITED

Abadía-Barrero, C. 2016. "Neoliberal Justice and the Transformation of the Moral: The Privatization of the Right to Health Care in Colombia." *Medical Anthropology Quarterly* 30, no. 1, 62–79.

Abidin, Crystal. 2016. *Please Subscribe! Influencers, Social Media, and the Commodification of Everyday Life*. PhD diss., University of Western Australia.

Adkins Fletcher, Rebecca. 2014. "Keeping up with the Cadillacs: What Health Insurance Disparities, Moral Hazard, and the Cadillac Tax Mean to the Patient Protection and Affordable Care Act." *Medical Anthropology Quarterly* 30, no. 1, 18–36.

Alarcón-Herrera, Maria T., Daniel A. Martin-Alarcon, Mélida Gutiérrez, Liliana Reynoso-Cuevas, Alejandra Martín-Domínguez, Mario A. Olmos-Márquez, Jochen Bundschuh. 2020. "Co-occurrence, Possible Origin, and Health Risk Assessment of Arsenic and Fluoride in Drinking Water Sources in Mexico: Geographical Data Visualization." *Science of the Total Environment* 689:134168.

Allen, Davina. 2000. "Doing Occupational Demarcation: The 'Boundary-Work' of Nurse Managers in a District General Hospital." *Journal of Contemporary Ethnography* 29, no. 3, 326–356.

Altheide, David L. 1997. "The News Media, the Problem Frame, and the Production of Fear." *The Sociological Quarterly* 38, no. 4, 647–668.

American Cancer Society. 2020. "Risk Factors for Cervical Cancer." Cervical Cancer. Last revised January 3, 2020. https://www.cancer.org/cancer/types/cervical-cancer/causes-risks-prevention/risk-factors.html.

Anderson, Jenny. 2019. "How a Small British Town Used Social Connections to Make Residents Happier and Healthier." Quartz, December 3. https://www.yahoo.com//video/small-british-town-used-social-150031829.html.

Appadurai, Arjun. 1996. *Modernity at Large: Cultural Dimensions of Globalization*. Minneapolis: University of Minnesota Press.

Asprey, Dave. 2019. *Super Human: The Bulletproof Plan to Age Backward and Maybe Even Live Forever*. New York: Harper Wave.

Aten, Jason. 2020. "The FTC Is About to Crack Down on Influencer Ads on Instagram, TikTok, and YouTube." Inc., February 13. https://www.inc.com/jason-aten/the-ftc-is-about-to-crack-down-on-influencer-ads-on-instagram-tiktok-youtube.html.

Atkinson, P. 1997. "Narrative Turn or a Blind Alley?" *Qualitative Health Research* 7:325–344.

Austin, J. L. 1962. *How to Do Things with Words*. Oxford, UK: Clarendon.

Barassi, Veronica. 2015. *Activism on the Web: Everyday Struggles against Digital Capitalism*. New York: Routledge.

Barber, Sharrelle. 2020. "Death by Racism." *The Lancet Infectious Diseases* 20, no. 8, 903.

Barg, Frances K., Shimrit Keddem, Wendy Shiekman Cohen, and Rebecca Henderson. 2013. "An Anthropology of Caregiving." In *Multidisciplinary Coordinated Caregiving: Research, Practice, Policy*, edited by Ronda C. Talley and Shirley S. Travis, 177–194. New York: Springer.

Baruah, Anali Ambani. 2017. *Travel Imagery in the Age of Instagram: An Ethnography of Travel Influencers and the "Online Tourist Gaze."* Master's thesis, University of London.

Beer, David, and Roger Burrows. 2013. "Popular Culture, Digital Archives and the New Social Life of Data." *Theory, Culture, & Society* 30, no. 4, 47–71.

Beidelschies, Michelle, Marilyn Alejandro-Rodriguez, Xinge Ji, Brittany Lapin, Patrick Hanaway, and Michael Rothberg. 2019. "Association of the Functional Medicine Model of Care with Patient-Reported Health-Related Quality-of-Life Outcomes." *Journal of the American Medical Association* 2, no. 10, e1914017.

Berchick, Edward, Jessica Barnett, and Rachel Upton. 2019. "Health Insurance Coverage in the United States: 2018." United States Census Bureau, report no. P60-267 (RV).

Betancourt, Joseph R. 2004. "Cultural Competence—Marginal or Mainstream Movement?" *New England Journal of Medicine* 351:953–954.

Beyerstein, Barry L. 1996. "Distinguishing Science from Pseudoscience." Department of Psychology, Simon Fraser University. Prepared for the Centre for Curriculum and Professional Development.

Birch, Kean, and David Tyfield. 2012. "Theorizing the Bioeconomy: Biovalue, Biocapital, Bioeconomics or . . . What?" *Science, Technology, & Human Values* 38, no. 3, 299–327.

Bisht, Babita, Warren G. Darling, Ruth E. Grossmann, E. Torage Shivapour, Susan K. Lutgendorf, Linda G. Snetselaar, Michael J. Hall, M. Bridget Zimmerman, and Terry L. Wahls. 2014. "A Multimodal Intervention for Patients with Secondary Progressive Multiple Sclerosis: Feasibility and Effect on Fatigue." *Alternative and Complementary Medicine* 20, no. 5, 347–355.

Bochner, Arthur Paul. 2001. "Narrative's Virtues." *Qualitative Inquiry* 7, no. 2, 131–157.

Boon, Sarah. 2017. "21st Century Science Overload." Canadian Science Publishing, January 7. http://blog.cdnsciencepub.com/21st-century-science-overload/.

Borba, Vânia Vieira, Gisele Zandman-Goddard, and Yehuda Shoenfeld. 2018. "Prolactin and Autoimmunity." *Frontiers in Immunology* 9:73.

Boston, P. Qasimah, M. Miaisha Mitchell, Kourtney Collum, and Clarence C. Gravlee. 2015. "Community Engagement and Health Equity." *Practicing Anthropology* 37, no. 4, 28–32.

Bourdieu, Pierre. 1984. *Distinction: A Social Critique of the Judgement of Taste.* Cambridge, MA: Harvard University Press.

Bourgois, Philippe. 1998. "The Moral Economies of Homeless Heroin Addicts: Confronting Ethnography, HIV Risk, and Everyday Violence in San Francisco Shooting Encampments." *Substance Use & Misuse* 33, no. 11, 2323–2351.

Bourgois, Philippe, Bridget Prince, and Andrew Moss. 2004. "The Everyday Violence of Hepatitis C among Young Women Who Inject Drugs in San Francisco." *Human Organization* 63, no. 3, 253–264.

Brandt, Allan, and Alyssa Botelho. 2020. "Not a Perfect Storm—Covid-19 and the Importance of Language." *New England Journal of Medicine* 382, no. 16, 1493–1495.

Bredesen, Dale E. 2014. "Reversal of Cognitive Decline: A Novel Therapeutic Program." *Aging* 6, no. 9, 707–717.

Briggs, Charles, and Clara Mantini-Briggs. 1986. *Learning How to Ask: A Sociolinguistic Appraisal of the Role of the Interview in Social Science Research.* Cambridge: Cambridge University Press.

Briggs, Charles, and Clara Mantini-Briggs. 2008. *Poéticas de vida en espacios de muerte: Género, poder y estado en la cotidianeidad warao*. Quito, Ecuador: Abya Yala.

Brons, Lajos. 2015. "Othering, an Analysis." *Transcience: A Journal of Global Studies* 6, no. 1, 69–90.

Browner, Carole H., and Nancy Press. 1996. "The Production of Authoritative Knowledge in American Prenatal Care." *Medical Anthropology Quarterly* 10, no. 2, 141–156.

Bruner, Jerome. 1986. *Actual Minds, Possible Worlds*. Cambridge, MA: Harvard University Press.

Burk, Robert D., Zigui Chen, Charles Saller, Katherine Tarvin, Andre L. Carvalho, Cristovam Scapulatempo-Neto, Henrique C. Silveira, et al. 2017. "Integrated Genomic and Molecular Characterization of Cervical Cancer." *Nature* 543:378–384.

Burri, Regula Valérie. 2008. "Doing Distinctions: Boundary-Work and Symbolic Capital in Radiology." *Social Studies of Science* 38, no. 1, 35–62.

Bury, Mike. 2001. "Illness Narratives: Fact or Fiction?" *Sociology of Health & Illness* 23, no. 3, 263–285.

Bush, Corinne, Jeffrey Blumberg, Ahmed El-Sohemy, Deanna Minich, Jóse Ordavás, Dana Reed, and Victoria Yunez Behm. 2019. "Toward the Definition of Personalized Nutrition: A Proposal by the American Nutrition Association." *Journal of the American College of Nutrition* 39, no. 1, 5–15.

Carlson, Robert. 1996. "The Political Economy of AIDS among Drug Users in the United States: Beyond Blaming the Victim or Powerful Others." *American Anthropologist* 98, no. 2, 266–278.

Castañeda, H., N. Kline, M. Rapp, N. Demetriou, N. Ahmed, I. Chan, T. Crocker, et al. 2011. "Assessing the 2010 Affordable Care Act: Perspectives of Future Health Care Professionals." *Practicing Anthropology* 33:44–48.

CBS News. 2015. "Herbal Supplements Filled with Fake Ingredients, Investigators Find." Health. Updated February 3, 2015. https://www.cbsnews.com/news/herbal-supplements-targeted-by-new-york-attorney-general/.

CDC (Centers for Disease Control and Prevention). 2022. "Chronic Diseases in America." National Center for Chronic Disease Prevention and Health Promotion. Last modified December 13, 2022. https://www.cdc.gov/chronicdisease/resources/infographic/chronic-diseases.htm.

Cheal, David. 1988. *The Gift Economy*. New York: Routledge.

Christakis, Nicholas A., and James H. Fowler. 2007. "The Spread of Obesity in a Large Social Network over 32 Years." *New England Journal of Medicine* 357:370–379.

Clark, Jack A., and Elliot G. Mishler. 1992. "Attending Patients' Stories: Reframing the Clinical Task." *Sociology of Health & Illness* 14, no. 3, 344–371.

Cleary, Ekaterina Galkina, Jennifer M. Beierlein, Navleen Surjit Khanuja, Laura M. McNamee, and Fred D. Ledley. 2018. "Contribution of NIH Funding to New Drug Approvals 2010–2016." *Proceedings of the National Academy of Sciences* 115, no. 10, 2329–2334.

Cleveland Clinic. 2022. "HPV (Human Papillomavirus)." https://my.clevelandclinic.org/health/diseases/11901-hpv-human-papilloma-virus.

Cohen, Lawrence. 2000. *No Aging in India: Alzheimer's, the Bad Family, and Other Modern Things*. Berkeley: University of California Press.

Costanza Torri, Maria. 2010. "Increasing Knowledge and Traditional Use of Medicinal Plants by Local Communities in Tamil Nadu: Promoting Self-Reliance at the Grassroots Level through a Community-Based Entrepreneurship Initiative." *Complementary Health Practice Review* 15, no. 1, 40–51.

Crenshaw, Kimberlé. 2014. "The Structural and Political Dimensions of Intersectional Oppression." In *Intersectionality: A Foundations and Frontiers Reader*, edited by Patrick R. Granzka, 16–21. Boulder, CO: Westview.

Dan, Laura. 2022. "The Blue Zones: Lifestyle Habits of the World's Longest-Living Populations." *Diet and Lifestyle* (blog), Fullscript, September 15. https://fullscript.com/blog/blue-zones.

Dana, Leo Paul, and Jan Åge Riseth. 2011. "Reindeer Herders in Finland: Pulled to Community-Based Entrepreneurship and Pushed to Individualistic Firms." *The Polar Journal* 1, no. 1, 108–123.

Dao, Amy, and Jessica Mulligan. 2016. "Toward an Anthropology of Insurance and Health Reform: An Introduction to the Special Issue." *Medical Anthropology Quarterly* 30, no. 1, 5–17.

Dao, Amy, and Mark Nichter. 2016. "The Social Life of Health Insurance in Low- to Middle-Income Countries: An Anthropological Research Agenda." *Medical Anthropology Quarterly* 30, no. 1, 122–143.

DasGupta, Sayantani, and Rita Charon. 2004. "Personal Illness Narratives: Using Reflective Writing to Teach Empathy." *Academic Medicine* 79, no. 4, 351–356.

de Botton, Alain. 2004. *Status Anxiety*. New York: Vintage Books.

De Courville Nicol, Valérie. 2021. *Anxiety in Middle-Class America: Sociology of Emotional Insecurity in Late Modernity*. New York: Routledge.

Degli-Esposti, Sara. 2014. "When Big Data Meets Dataveillance: The Hidden Side of Analytics." *Surveillance and Society* 12, no. 2, 209–225.

d'Hérelle, F. 1917. "Sur un microbe invisible antagoniste des bacilles dysentérique." *Academie des Sciences Paris* 165:373–375.

Dimitri, Carolyn, and Lydia Oberholtzer. 2009. "Marketing U.S. Organic Foods: Recent Trends from Farms to Consumers." United States Department of Agriculture Economic Research Service.

DuBois, W. E. B. 2007. *Dusk of Dawn: An Essay towards an Autobiography of a Race Concept*. New York: Oxford University Press.

DuFault, Beth Leavenworth, and John W. Schouten. 2020. "Self-Quantification and the Datapreneurial Consumer Identity." *Consumption Markets & Culture* 23, no. 3, 290–316.

Dyer, Owen. 2002. "WHO Links Long-Term Pill Use to Cervical Cancer." *BMJ* 324, no. 7341, 808.

Eisenstein, Charles. 2011. *Sacred Economics: Money, Gift and Society in the Age of Transition*. Berkeley, CA: North Atlantic Books.

Ellis, Carolyn, and Arthur P. Bochner. 2000. "Autoethnography, Personal Narrative, Reflexivity: Researcher as Subject." In Norman K. Denzin and Yvonna S. Lincoln, eds., *Handbook of Qualitative Research*, 733–768. Thousand Oaks, CA: Sage.

Epstein, Steven. 2007. *Inclusion: The Politics of Difference in Medical Research*. Chicago: University of Chicago Press.

Ericson, Richard, Dean Barry, and Aaron Doyle. 2000. "The Moral Hazards of Neoliberalism: Lessons from the Private Insurance Industry." *Economy and Society* 29, no. 4, 532–558.

Ettorre, Elizabeth. 2005. "Gender, Older Female Bodies and Autoethnography: Finding My Feminist Voice by Telling My Illness Story." *Women's Studies International Forum* 28, no. 6, 535–546.

Ettorre, Elizabeth. 2006. "Making Sense of My Illness Journey from Thyrotoxicosis to Health: An Autoethnography." *Auto/Biography* 14:153–175.

Farmer, Paul. 2001. *Infections and Inequalities: The Modern Plagues*. Berkeley: University of California Press.

Farmer, Paul, Bruce Nizeye, Sara Stulac, and Salmaan Keshavjee. 2006. "Structural Violence and Clinical Medicine." *PLOS Medicine* 3, no. 10, 1686–1691.

FDA (Food and Drug Administration). 2016. "Arsenic in Rice and Rice Products Risk Assessment Report." Center for Food Safety and Applied Nutrition. https://www.fda.gov/files/food/published/Arsenic-in-Rice-and-Rice-Products-Risk-Assessment-Report-PDF.pdf.

Fisher, Andrew T., Lizbeth López-Carrillo, Brenda Gamboa-Loira, and Mariano E. Cebrián. 2017. "Standards for Arsenic in Drinking Water: Implications for Policy in Mexico." *Journal of Public Health Policy* 38, no. 4, 395–406.

Fisher, Eran. 2015. "How Less Alienation Creates More Exploitation? Audience Labour on Social Network Sites." In *Marx in the Age of Digital Capitalism*, edited by Christian Fuchs and Vincent Mosco, 171–183. Leiden, Netherlands: Brill.

Fitzgerald, Kara N., Romilly Hodges, Douglas Hanes, Emily Stack, David Cheishvili, Moshe Szyf, Janine Henkel, et al. 2021. "Potential Reversal of Epigenetic Age Using a Diet and Lifestyle Intervention: A Pilot Randomized Clinical Trial." *Aging* 13, no. 7, 9419–9432.

Flesch, Hannah. 2013. "A Foot in Both Worlds: Education and the Transformation of Chinese Medicine in the United States." *Medical Anthropology* 32, no. 1, 8–24.

Foucault, Michel. 2003. *"Society Must Be Defended." Lectures at the Collège de France, 1975–1976*. London: Picador.

Franklin, Sarah. 2003. "Ethical Biocapital: New Strategies of Cell Culture." In *Remaking Life and Death: Toward an Anthropology of the Biosciences*, edited by Margaret M. Lock and Sarah Franklin, 97–128. Santa Fe, NM: School of American Research Press.

Franklin, Sarah. 2006. "Mapping Biocapital: New Frontiers in Bioprospecting." *Cultural Geographies* 13:301–304.

Freccero, J. 1986. "Autobiography and Narrative." In *Reconstructing Individualism: Autonomy, Individuality, and the Self in Western Thought*, edited by Thomas C. Heller, Morton Sosna, and David E. Wellbery, 16–29. Stanford, CA: Stanford University Press.

Fuchs, Christian. 2019. *Rereading Marx in the Age of Digital Capitalism*. London: Pluto.

Fuchs, Christian, and Vincent Mosco, eds. 2015. *Marx in the Age of Digital Capitalism*. Leiden, Netherlands: Brill.

Gaberšček, Simona, and Katja Zaletel. 2011. "Thyroid Physiology and Autoimmunity in Pregnancy and after Delivery." *Expert Review in Clinical Immunology* 7, no. 5, 697–706.

Galdas, Paul M., Francine Cheater, and Paul Marshall. 2005. "Men and Health Help-Seeking Behavior: Literature Review." *Journal of Advanced Nursing* 49, no. 6, 616–623.

Galetovic Carabantes, Alexandra, and Nilda A. G. G. de Fernicola. 2003. "Arsénico en el agua de bebida: Un problema de salud pública." *Revista Brasileira de Ciências Farmacêuticas* 39, no. 4, 365–372.

Gálvez, Alyshia. 2018. *Eating NAFTA: Trade, Food Policies, and the Destruction of Mexico.* Berkeley: University of California Press.

Gan, Nectar, and Jessie Yeung. 2021. "China Approves Sale of Traditional Medicine Products to Treat Covid-19." CNN. https://www.cnn.com/2021/03/04/asia/china-tcm-approved-covid-intl-hnk-scli/index.html.

García Canclini, Néstor. (1990) 2009. *Culturas híbridas: Estrategias para entrar y salir de la modernidad.* Mexico City: Grijalbo.

Garro, Linda. 1992. "Chronic Illness and the Construction of Narratives." In *Pain as Human Experience: An Anthropological Perspective*, edited by Mary-Jo DelVecchio Good, Paul E. Brodwin, Byron J. Good, and Arthur Kleinman, 100–137. Berkeley: University of California Press.

Gawande, Atul. 2009. "The Cost Conundrum." *New Yorker*, June 1. https://www.newyorker.com/magazine/2009/06/01/the-cost-conundrum.

Gawande, Atul. 2011. "The Hot Spotters: Can We Lower Medical Costs by Giving the Neediest Patients Better Care?" *New Yorker*, January 24. https://www.newyorker.com/magazine/2011/01/24/the-hot-spotters.

Gazella, Karolyn A. 2005. "Tieraona Low Dog, MD, Educator, Scientist, and Herbal Medicine Expert." *Alternative Therapies in Health and Medicine* 11, no. 1, 84–91.

Getrich, Christina M., Jacqueline M. García, Angélica Solares, and Miria Sano. 2018. "Buffering the Uneven Impact of the Affordable Care Act: Immigrant-Serving Safety-Net Providers in New Mexico." *Medical Anthropology Quarterly* 32, no. 2, 233–253.

Ghebreyesus, Tedros Adhanom. 2017. "Health Is a Fundamental Human Right." World Health Organization, December 10. https://www.who.int/news-room/commentaries/detail/health-is-a-fundamental-human-right.

Gibbon, Sahra, and Carlos Novas. 2007. *Biosocialities, Genetics, and the Social Sciences: Making Biologies and Identities.* New York: Routledge.

Gieryn, Thomas F. 1983. "Boundary-Work and the Demarcation of Science from Non-Science: Strains and Interests in Professional Ideologies of Scientists." *American Sociological Review* 48, no. 6, 781–795.

Golam Mostafa, Mohammad, Zarat Jahin Queen, and Nicola Cherry. 2017. "Histopathology of Cervical Cancer and Arsenic Concentration in Well Water: An Ecological Analysis." *International Journal of Environmental Research and Public Health* 14:1185.

Good, Byron J. 1994. *Medicine, Rationality, and Experience: An Anthropological Perspective.* Cambridge: Cambridge University Press.

Guthman, Julie. 2008a. "Bringing Good Food to Others: Investigating the Subjects of Alternative Food Practice." *Cultural Geographies* 15:431–447.

Guthman, Julie. 2008b. "'If They Only Knew': Color Blindness and Universalism in California Alternative Food Institutions." *The Professional Geographer* 60:387–397.

Guthman, Julie. 2008c. "Neoliberalism and the Making of Food Politics in California." *Geoforum* 39:1171–1183.

Hadley, Craig, and Deborah Crooks. 2012. "Coping and the Biosocial Consequences of Food Insecurity in the 21st Century." *American Journal of Biological Anthropology* 149, no. S55, 72–94.

Hadley, Craig, and Crystal Patil. 2008. "Seasonal Changes in Household Food Insecurity and Symptoms of Anxiety and Depression." *American Journal of Biological Anthropology* 135, no. 2, 225–232.

Haidt, Jonathan. 2007. *The Happiness Hypothesis: Putting Ancient Wisdom and Philosophy to the Test of Modern Science*. New York: Arrow Books.

Haidt, Jonathan, and Craig Joseph. 2007. "The Moral Mind: How Five Sets of Innate Intuitions Guide the Development of Many Culture-Specific Virtues, and Perhaps Even Modules." In *The Innate Mind*, vol. 3, *Foundations and the Future*, edited by Peter Carruthers, Stephen Laurence, and Stephen Stich, 367–392. New York: Oxford University Press.

Hansson, Sven Ove. 2013. "Defining Pseudoscience and Science." In *Philosophy of Pseudoscience: Reconsidering the Demarcation Problem*, edited by Massimo Pigliucci and Maarten Boudry, 61–78. Chicago: University of Chicago Press.

Hansson, Sven Ove. 2017. "Science Denial as a Form of Pseudoscience." *Studies in History and Philosophy of Science* 63:39–47.

Haraway, Donna. 1988. "Situated Knowledges: The Science Question in Feminism and the Privilege of Partial Perspective." *Feminist Studies* 14, no. 3, 575–599.

Haraway, Donna. 1997. *Modest_Witness@Second_Millennium. FemaleMan©_Meets_OncoMouse.*™ New York: Routledge.

Haraway, Donna. 2007. *When Species Meet*. Minneapolis: University of Minnesota Press.

Hård, Mikael, and Andrew Jamison. 2005. *Hubris and Hybrids: A Cultural History of Technology and Science*. New York: Routledge.

Harvard News Office. 2011. "Paul Farmer: 'Accompaniment' as Policy." *Harvard Magazine*, May 25. https://www.harvardmagazine.com/2011/05/paul-farmer-accompaniment-as-policy.

Harvey, David. 1990. *The Condition of Postmodernity: An Enquiry into the Origins of Cultural Change*. Cambridge, MA: Blackwell.

Harvey, David. 2005. *A Brief History of Neoliberalism*. New York: Oxford University Press.

Harvey, David. 2010. "The Enigma of Capital and the Crisis This Time." Paper presented at the American Sociological Association Meetings, Atlanta, August 16, 2010. https://davidharvey.org/2010/08/the-enigma-of-capital-and-the-crisis-this-time/.

Hayden, Cori. 2003. *When Nature Goes Public: The Making and Unmaking of Bioprospecting in Mexico*. Princeton, NJ: Princeton University Press.

Helmreich, Stefan. 2008. "Species of Biocapital." *Science as Culture* 17, no. 4, 463–478.

Hendry, Natalie Ann. 2022. "'Hey Lovely! Don't Miss This Opportunity!': Digital Temporalities of Wellness Culture, Email Marketing, and the Promise of Abundance." *Journal of Sociology*, published online May 17. https://doi.org/10.1177/14407833221101397.

Hendry, Natalie Ann, Catherine Hartung, and Rosie Welch. 2021. "Health Education,

Social Media, and Tensions of Authenticity in the 'Influencer Pedagogy' of Health Influencer Ashy Bines." *Learning, Media and Technology* 47, no. 4, 427–439.

Henry, Lisa. 2015. "Physician Assistants, Nurse Practitioners, and Community Health Centers under the Affordable Care Act." *Human Organization* 74:42–51.

Henry, Lisa. 2017. "Understanding Food Insecurity among College Students: Experience, Motivation, and Local Solutions." *Annals of Anthropological Practice* 41, no. 1, 6–19.

Hertz, Rosanna. 2006. "Stories as Evidence." *Qualitative Sociology* 29:539–543.

Hobsbawm, Eric, and Terence Ranger. 1983. *The Invention of Tradition*. Cambridge: Cambridge University Press.

Horn, Susan D., and Julie Gassaway. 2007. "Practice-Based Evidence Study Design for Comparative Effectiveness Research." *Medical Care* 45, no. 10 (supp. 2), S50–S57.

Hsueh, Ming-Feng, Patrik Önnerfjord, Michael P. Bolognesi, Mark E. Easley, and Virginia B. Kraus. 2019. "Analysis of 'Old' Proteins Unmasks Dynamic Gradient of Cartilage Turnover in Human Limbs." *Science Advances* 5, no. 10, eaax3203.

Hudders, Liselot, Steffi De Jans, and Marijke De Veirman. 2021. "The Commercialization of Social Media Stars: A Literature Review and the Conceptual Framework on the Strategic Use of Social Media Influencers." In *Social Media Influencers in Strategic Communication*, edited by Nils S. Borchers, 327–375. New York: Routledge.

Hunsaker Hawkins, Anne. 1990. "A Change of Heart: The Paradigm of Regeneration in Medical and Religious Narrative." *Perspectives in Biology and Medicine* 33, no. 4, 547–559.

Hydén, Lars-Christer. 1997. "Illness and Narrative." *Sociology of Health & Illness* 19, no. 1, 48–69.

Hyman, Mark. 2020. *Food Fix: How to Save Our Health, Our Economy, Our Communities, and Our Planet—One Bite at a Time*. Boston: Little Brown Spark.

Inhorn, Marcia, and Kimberly A. Buss. 1995. "Medical Anthropology and Epidemiology: Divergences or Convergences?" *Social Science & Medicine* 40, no. 3, 285–290.

Jarrett, Kylie. 2016. *Feminism, Labour and Digital Media: The Digital Housewife*. New York: Routledge.

Jetten, Jolanda, Frank Mols, and Nikita Healy. 2017. "'Fear of Falling': Economic Instability Enhances Collective Angst among Societies' Wealthy Class." *Journal of Social Issues* 73, no. 1, 61–79.

Johansson, Victoria, Anna Sigridur Islind, Tomas Lindroth, Eva Angenete, and Martin Gellerstedt. 2021. "Online Communities as a Driver for Patient Empowerment: Systematic Review." *Journal of Medical Internet Research* 23, no. 2, 1–18.

Jordan, Brigitte. 1992. *Birth in Four Cultures*. Long Grove, IL: Waveland.

Kandil, Caitlin Yoshiko. 2020. "Asian Americans Report over 650 Racist Acts over Last Week, New Data Says." NBC News. https://www.nbcnews.com/news/asian-america/asian-americans-report-nearly-500-racist-acts-over-last-week-n1169821.

Kapoor, Ilan. 2004. "Hyper-Self-Reflexive Development? Spivak on Representing the Third World 'Other.'" *Third World Quarterly* 4:627–647.

Kent, Rachael. 2018. "Social Media and Self-Tracking: Representing the 'Health Self.'" In *Self-Tracking: Empirical and Philosophical Investigations*, edited by Btihaj Ajana, 61–76. London: Palgrave Macmillan.

Kent, Rachael. 2020. "Self-Tracking and Digital Food Cultures: Surveillance and

Representation of the Moral 'Healthy Body.'" In *Digital Food Cultures*, edited by Deborah Lupton and Zeena Feldman, 19–34. London: Routledge.
Kent, Rachael. 2021. "Digital Food Tracking: Combining Traditional and Digital Ethnographic Methods to Identify the Influence of Social Media Sharing of Health and Foods Upon Users' Everyday Lives." In *Research Methods in Digital Food Studies*, edited by Jonatan Leer and Stinne G. S. Krogager, chap. 11. New York: Routledge.
Kim, Tae. 2018. "Goldman Sachs Asks in Biotech Research Report: 'Is Curing Patients a Sustainable Business Model?'" CNBC, April 11. https://www.cnbc.com/2018/04/11/goldman-asks-is-curing-patients-a-sustainable-business-model.html.
Kingod, Natasja, Bryan Cleal, Ayo Wahlberg, and Gitte R. Husted. 2017. "Online Peer-to-Peer Communities in the Daily Lives of People with Chronic Illness: A Qualitative Systematic Review." *Qualitative Health Research* 27, no. 1, 89–99.
Kleinman, Arthur. (1988) 2020. *The Illness Narratives: Suffering, Healing, and the Human Condition*. New York: Basic Books.
Kleinman, Arthur. 1992. "Pain and Resistance: The Delegitimation and Relegitimation of Local Worlds." In *Pain as Human Experience: An Anthropological Perspective*, edited by Mary-Jo DelVecchio Good, Paul E. Brodwin, Byron J. Good, and Arthur Kleinman, 169–197. Berkeley: University of California Press.
Kleinman, Arthur, and Peter Benson. 2006. "Anthropology in the Clinic: The Problem with Cultural Competency and How to Fix It." *PLOS Medicine* 3, no. 10, e294.
Kortright, Kaitlyn E., Benjamin K. Chan, Jonathan L. Koff, and Paul E. Turner. 2019. "Phage Therapy: A Renewed Approach to Combat Antibiotic-Resistant Bacteria." *Cell Host & Microbe* 25, no. 2, 219–232.
Kresser, Chris. 2017. *Unconventional Medicine: Join the Revolution to Reinvent Healthcare, Reverse Chronic Disease, and Create a Practice You Love*. Austin, TX: Lioncrest.
Kuehn, Bridget M. 2019. "Heritage Diets and Culturally Appropriate Dietary Advice May Help Combat Chronic Diseases." *Journal of the American Medical Association* 322, no. 23, 2271–2273. https://doi.org/10.1001/jama.2019.18431.
Kuhn, Thomas. 1962. *The Structure of Scientific Revolutions*. Chicago: University of Chicago Press.
Lakoff, Andrew. 2008. "The Generic Biothreat, or, How We Became Unprepared." *Cultural Anthropology* 23, no. 3, 399–428.
Lamas, Eugenia, Rodrigo Salinas, Carla Coquedano, Marie-Pierre Simon, Cedric Bousquet, Marcela Ferrer, and Sergio Zorrilla. 2017. "The Meaning of Patient Empowerment in the Digital Age: The Role of Online Patient-Communities." In *The Practice of Patient Centered Care: Empowering and Engaging Patients in the Digital Era*, edited by Rolf Engelbrecht, Ran Balicer, and Mira Hercigonja-Szekeres, 43–47. Amsterdam, Netherlands: IOS.
Lee, S. Agnes, and Michelle Farrell. 2006. "Is Cultural Competency a Backdoor to Racism?" *Anthropology News*, February and March special eds.
Lehtonen, Turo-Kimmo, and Ine Van Hoyweghen. 2014. "Editorial: Insurance and the Economization of Uncertainty." *Journal of Cultural Economy* 7, no. 4, 532–540.
Lester, Rebecca. 2019. *Famished: Eating Disorders and Failed Care in America*. Berkeley: University of California Press.
Li, William. 2019. *Eat to Beat Disease*. New York: Hachette.

Lock, Margaret. 1990. "Rationalization of Japanese Herbal Medication: The Hegemony of Orchestrated Pluralism." *Human Organization* 49, no. 1, 41.

Lock, Margaret. 2001. "The Alienation of Body Tissue and the Biopolitics of Immortalized Cell Lines." *Body & Society* 7, nos. 2–3, 63–91.

Lock, Margaret. 2002. *Twice Dead: Organ Transplants and the Reinvention of Death.* Berkeley: University of California Press.

Lock, Margaret, Patricia Alice Kaufert, and Alan Harwood. 1998. *Pragmatic Women and Body Politics.* Cambridge: Cambridge University Press.

López, Leslie. 2005. "De Facto Disentitlement in an Information Economy: Enrollment Issues in Medicaid Managed Care." *Medical Anthropology Quarterly* 19, no. 1, 26–46.

Luhmann, Niklas. 1998. *Observations on Modernity.* Translated by William Whobrey. Stanford, CA: Stanford University Press.

Lundh, Andreas, Joel Lexchin, Barbara Mintzes, Jeppe Schroll, and Lisa Bero. 2017. "Industry Sponsorship and Research Outcome." *Cochrane Database of Systematic Reviews* 16, no. 2, https://doi.org/10.1002/14651858.mr000033.pub3.

Luo, Erdan, Daiyan Zhang, Hua Luo, Bowen Liu, Keming Zhao, Yonghua Zhao, Ying Bian, and Yitao Wang. 2020. "Treatment Efficacy Analysis of Traditional Chinese Medicine for Novel Coronavirus Pneumonia (COVID-19): An Empirical Study from Wuhan, Hubei Province, China." *Chinese Medicine* 15:34.

Lupton, Deborah. 2014. "The Commodification of Patient Opinion: The Digital Patient Experience Economy in the Age of Big Data." *Sociology of Health & Illness* 36, no. 6, 856–869.

Lupton, Deborah. 2016. *The Quantified Self.* Cambridge, UK: Polity.

Maboloc, Christopher Ryan. 2017. "On the Scientific Method of Kuhn and Popper: Implications of Paradigm-Shifts to Development Models." *Philosophia* 46:387–399.

Makary, Martin A., and Michael Daniel. 2016. "Medical Error: The Third Leading Cause of Death in the U.S." *BMJ* 353:i2139.

Mann, Michael. 2013. "Globalizations." In *The Sources of Social Power*, vol. 4, *Globalizations, 1945–2011*, 1–12. Cambridge: Cambridge University Press.

Mannix, Liam. 2019. "'Cannot Be Trusted . . . Causing Harm': Top Medical Journal Takes on Big Pharma." The Age, December 4. https://www.theage.com.au/national/cannot-be-trusted-causing-harm-top-medical-journal-takes-on-big-pharma-20191203-p53ggj.html.

Manzerolle, Vincent, and Atle Mikkola Kjøsen. 2015. "Digital Media and Capital's Logic of Acceleration." In *Marx in the Age of Digital Capitalism*, edited by Christian Fuchs and Vincent Mosco, 151–179. Leiden, Netherlands: Brill.

Marcus, George E. 1995. "Ethnography in/of the World System: The Emergence of Multi-Sited Ethnography." *Annual Review of Anthropology* 24, no. 1, 5–117.

Margolin, Josh. 2020. "FBI Warns of Potential Surge in Hate Crimes against Asian Americans amid Coronavirus: Critics Say Rhetoric Has Fueled Ill Will." ABC News, March 27. https://abcnews.go.com/US/fbi-warns-potential-surge-hate-crimes-asian-americans/story?id=69831920.

Marks, Deborah. 1999. *Disability: Controversial Debates and Psychosocial Perspectives.* New York: Routledge.

Marmot, Michael. 2015. *The Health Gap: The Challenge of an Unequal World.* London: Bloomsbury.

Martyn, Amy. 2018. "Goldman Sachs Warns Biotech Clients that Curing Patients May Not Be 'Sustainable.'" ConsumerAffairs, April 13. https://www.consumeraffairs.com/news/goldman-sachs-warns-biotech-clients-that-curing-patients-may-not-be-sustainable-041318.html.

Marx, Karl. (1867) 1992. *Capital*, vol. 1. London: Penguin.

Maskell, James. 2016. *The Evolution of Medicine: Join the Movement to Solve Chronic Disease and Fall Back in Love with Medicine*. n.p.: Knew.

Maskell, James. 2020. *The Community Cure: Transforming Health Outcomes Together*. Austin, TX: Lioncrest.

Mattingly, Cheryl. 1994. "The Concept of the Therapeutic 'Emplotment.'" *Social Science & Medicine* 38, no. 6, 811–822.

Mattingly, Cheryl. 2010. *The Paradox of Hope: Journeys through a Clinical Borderland*. Berkeley: University of California Press.

Mayer, Emeran. 2018. *The Mind-Gut Connection: How the Hidden Conversation within Our Bodies Impacts Our Mood, Our Choices, and Our Overall Health*. New York: Harper Wave.

McGregor, Sue. 2001. "Neoliberalism and Health Care." *International Journal of Consumer Studies* 25, no. 2, 82–89.

Menéndez, Eduardo. 1996. *De algunos alcoholismos y algunos saberes: Atención primaria y proceso de alcoholización*. Mexico City: CIESAS.

Menéndez, Eduardo. (2002) 2010. *La parte negada de la cultura: Relativismo, diferencias y racismo*. Argentina: Prohistoria Ediciones.

Miner, Horace. 1956. "Body Ritual among the Nacirema." *American Anthropologist* 58:503–507.

Minocha, Aneeta. 1980. "Medical Pluralism and Health Services in India." *Social Science & Medicine*. Part B: Medical Anthropology 14, no. 4:217–223.

Mishler, Elliot G. 1984. *The Discourse of Medicine: Dialectics of Medical Interviews*. Norwood, NJ: Ablex.

Mishler, Elliot G., Jack A. Clark, Joseph Ingelfinger, and Michael P. Simon. 1989. "The Language of Attentive Patient Care: A Comparison of Two Medical Interviews." *Journal of General Internal Medicine* 4, no. 4, 325–335.

Molina, Natalia. 2013. *How Race Is Made in America: Immigration, Citizenship, and the Historical Power of Racial Scripts*. Berkeley: University of California Press.

Morini, Cristina, and Andrea Fumagalli. 2010. "Life Put to Work: Towards a Life Theory of Value." *ephemera: theory and politics in organization* 10, nos. 3/4, 234–252.

Morris, Zoë Slote, Steven Wooding, and Jonathan Grant. 2011. "The Answer Is 17 Years, What Is the Question: Understanding Time Lags in Translational Research." *Journal of the Royal Society of Medicine* 104, no. 12, 510–520.

Mount Sinai Tisch Cancer Center. n.d. "HPV and Cervical Cancer Myths vs. Facts." https://www.mountsinai.org/care/cancer/services/gynecologic/conditions/cervical/myths-facts.

Moynihan, Ray, Lisa Bero, Sue Hill, Minna Johansson, Joel Lexchin, Helen Macdonald, Barbara Mintzes, et al. 2019. "Pathways to Independence: Towards Producing and Using Trustworthy Evidence." *BMJ* 367:l6576.

Mulligan, Jessica. 2016. "Insurance Accounts: The Cultural Logics of Health Care Financing." *Medical Anthropology Quarterly* 30, no. 1, 37–61.

Mulligan, Jessica. 2017. "The Problem of Choice: From the Voluntary Way to Affordable Care Act Health Insurance Exchanges." *Social Science & Medicine* 181:34–42.

Mulligan, Jessica, and Heide Castañeda. 2018. *Unequal Coverage: The Experience of Health Care Reform in the United States*. New York: New York University Press.

Myers, Amy. 2015. *The Autoimmune Solution: Prevent and Reverse the Full Spectrum of Inflammatory Symptoms and Diseases*. San Francisco: HarperOne.

Myers, Amy. 2021. *The Thyroid Connection: Why You Feel Tired, Brain-Fogged, and Overweight—and How to Get Your Life Back*. Boston: Little Brown Spark.

Naftulin, Julia. 2016. "Here's How Many Times We Touch Our Phones Every day." Insider, July 13. https://www.businessinsider.com/dscout-research-people-touch-cell-phones-2617-times-a-day-2016-7.

Nelson, Nancy L. 2005. "Ideologies of Aid, Practices of Power: Lessons for Medicaid Managed Care." *Medical Anthropology Quarterly* 19, no. 1, 103–122.

Office of the Press Secretary. 2015. "Remarks by the President on Precision Medicine." The White House. https://obamawhitehouse.archives.gov/the-press-office/2015/01/30/remarks-president-precision-medicine.

Onomake, Umoloyouwe Ejiro. 2021. "Social Media Relationships." Oxford Research Encyclopedias (website), Oxford University Press. https://doi.org/10.1093/acrefore/9780190854584.013.114.

Otero, Gerardo. 2018. *The Neoliberal Diet: Healthy Profits, Unhealthy People*. Austin: University of Texas Press.

Parekh, Anand K. 2019. *Prevention First: Policymaking for a Healthier America*. Baltimore: Johns Hopkins University Press.

Parry, Bronwyn. 2004. *Trading the Genome: Investigating the Commodification of Bio-Information*. New York: Columbia University Press.

Pauling, Linus, Harvey Itano, S. J. Singer, and Ibert Wells. 1949. "Sickle Cell Anemia, A Molecular Disease." *Science* 110, no. 2865, 543–548.

Petersen, Alan, Allegra Clare Schermuly, and Alison Anderson. 2019. "The Shifting Politics of Patient Activism: From Bio-Sociality to Bio-Digital Citizenship." *Health* 23, no. 4, 478–494.

Pigliucci, Massimo, and Maarten Boudry, eds. 2013. *Philosophy of Pseudoscience: Reconsidering the Demarcation Problem*. Chicago: University of Chicago Press.

Pizzorno, Joseph. 2017. "Toxin Exposure Reduction." *Integrative Medicine* 16, no. 6, 8–10.

Polanyi, Karl. 2001. *The Great Transformation: The Political and Economic Origins of Our Time*. 2nd ed. Boston: Beacon Press.

Pols, Jeannette, Dick Willems, and Margunn Aanestad. 2019. "Making Sense with Numbers: Unravelling Ethico-Psychological Subjects in Practices of Self-Quantification." *Sociology of Health & Illness* 41, no. S1, 98–115.

Pon, Gordon. 2009. "Cultural Competency as New Racism: An Ontology of Forgetting." *Journal of Progressive Human Services* 20:59–71.

Popper, Karl. (1934) 1959. *The Logic of Scientific Discovery*. Translated from German by Julius Freed. London: Hutchinson.

Prescott, Susan L., and Jeffrey S. Bland. 2020. "Spaceship Earth Revisited: The Co-Benefits of Overcoming Biological Extinction of Experience at the Level of Person, Place and Planet." *International Journal of Environmental Research and Public Health* 17, no. 4, 1407.

Prescott, Susan L., and Alan C. Logan. 2017. *The Secret Life of Your Microbiome: Why Nature and Biodiversity are Essential to Health and Happiness.* Gabriola Island, BC: New Society.

Price, Nathan, Andrew Magis, John Earls, Gustavo Glusman, Roie Levy, Christopher Lausted, Daniel McDonald, Ulrike Kusebauch, Christopher Moss, Yong Zhou, Shizhen Qin, Robert Moritz, Kristin Brogaard, Gilbert Omenn, Jennifer Lovejoy, and Leroy Hood. 2017. "A Wellness Study of 108 Individuals Using Personal, Dense, Dynamic Data Clouds." *Nature Biotechnology* 35:747–756.

Putnam, Hilary. 1991. "The Corroboration of Theories." In *Philosophy of Science*, edited by Richard Boyd, Philip Gasper, and J. D. Trout, 121–138. Cambridge: Massachusetts Institute of Technology Press.

Putnam, Robert D. 2000. *Bowling Alone: The Collapse and Revival of American Community.* New York: Simon & Schuster.

Rabinow, Paul. 1992. "Artificiality and Enlightenment: From Sociobiology to Biosociality." In *Incorporations*, edited by Jonathan Crary and Sanford Kwinter, 521–566. New York: Zone.

Rabinow, Paul. 1996. *Essays on the Anthropology of Reason.* Princeton, NJ: Princeton University Press.

Ragin, Charles. (1987) 2014. *The Comparative Method: Moving beyond Qualitative and Quantitative Strategies.* Berkeley: University of California Press.

Rajan, Kaushik Sunder. 2006. *Biocapital: The Constitution of Postgenomic Life.* Durham, NC: Duke University Press.

Rajan, Kaushik Sunder. 2007. "Biocapital as an Emergent Form of Life: Speculations on the Figure of the Experimental Subject." In *Biosocialities, Genetics, and the Social Sciences.* Abingdon, UK: Routledge.

Rapp, Rayna. 2000. *Testing Women, Testing the Fetus: The Social Impact of Amniocentesis in America.* New York: Routledge.

Reed-Danahay, Deborah. 1997. Introduction to *Auto/ethnography: Rewriting the Self and the Social*, 1–17. Oxford, UK: Berg.

Rees, Tobias. 2016. *Plastic Reason: An Anthropology of Brain Science in Embryogenetic Terms.* Berkeley: University of California Press.

Richards, Rose. 2008. "Writing the Othered Self: Autoethnography and the Problem of Objectification in Writing about Illness and Disability." *Qualitative Health Research* 18, no. 12, 1717–1728.

Robbins, John, and Ocean Robbins. 2013. *Voices of the Food Revolution: You Can Heal Your Body and Your World—With Food!* Newburyport, MA: Conari.

Roberts, Dorothy. 2012. *Fatal Invention: How Science, Politics, and Big Business Re-create Race in the Twenty-first Century.* New York: New Press.

Rose, Nikolas. 2007a. "Molecular Biopolitics, Somatic Ethics and the Spirit of Biocapital." *Social Theory and Health* 5:3–29.

Rose, Nikolas. 2007b. *The Politics of Life Itself: Biomedicine, Power, and Subjectivity in the Twenty-First Century.* Princeton, NJ: Princeton University Press.

Rose, Nikolas. 2008. "The Value of Life: Somatic Ethics and the Spirit of Biocapital." *Dædalus* 137, no. 1, 36–48.

Ruckenstein, Minna, and Mika Pantzar. 2017. "Beyond the Quantified Self: Thematic Exploration of a Dataistic Paradigm." *New Media & Society* 19, no. 3, 401–418.

Rylko-Bauer, Barbara, and Paul Farmer. 2002. "Managed Care or Managed Inequality?

A Call for Critiques of Market-Based Medicine." *Medical Anthropology Quarterly* 16, no. 4, 476–502.

Sadowski, Jathan. 2020. *Too Smart: How Digital Capitalism Is Extracting Data, Controlling Our Lives, and Taking Over the World.* Cambridge: Massachusetts Institute of Technology Press.

Savage, Mike. 2013. "The 'Social Life of Methods': A Critical Introduction." *Theory, Culture & Society* 30, no. 4, 3–21.

Scheper-Hughes, Nancy, and Philippe Bourgois. 2004. *Violence in War and Peace: An Anthology.* Hoboken, NJ: Wiley.

Scheper-Hughes, Nancy, and Margaret Lock. 1987. "The Mindful Body: A Prolegomenon to Future Work in Medical Anthropology." *Medical Anthropology Quarterly* 1, no. 1, 6–41.

Schermuly, Allegra Clare, Alan Petersen, and Alison Anderson. 2021. "'I Am Not an Activist!': Digital Self-Advocacy in Online Patient Communities." *Critical Public Health* 31, no. 2, 204–213.

Servan-Schreiber, David. 2009. *Anticancer: A New Way of Life.* New York: Viking.

Sforzo, Gary A., Miranda P. Kaye, Irina Todorova, Sebastian Harenberg, Kyle Costello, Laura Cobus-Kuo, Aubrey Faber, Elizabeth Frates, and Margaret Moore. 2017. "Compendium of the Health and Wellness Coaching Literature." *American Journal of Lifestyle Medicine* 20, no. 10, 1–12.

Singer, Merrill. 1994. "AIDS and the Health Crisis of the U.S. Urban Poor: The Perspective of Critical Medical Anthropology." *Social Science & Medicine* 39, no. 7, 931–948.

Singer, Merrill. 2009. *Introduction to Syndemics: A Critical Systems Approach to Public and Community Health.* San Francisco: Jossey-Bass.

Singer, Merrill, David Himmelgreen, Margaret R. Weeks, Kim E. Radda, and Rolando Martinez. 1997. "Changing the Environment of AIDS Risk: Findings on Syringe Exchange and Pharmacy Sales of Syringes in Hartford, CT." *Medical Anthropology* 18, no. 1, 107–130.

Smith-Morris, Carolyn. 2019. *Indigenous Communalism: Belonging, Healthy Communities, and Decolonizing the Collective.* New Brunswick, NJ: Rutgers University Press.

Spivak, Gayatri Chakravorty. 1988. "Can the Subaltern Speak?" In *Marxism and Interpretation of Culture*, edited by Cary Nelson and Lawrence Grossbery, 66–111. Champaign: University of Illinois Press.

Stearns, Peter N. 2006. *American Fear: The Causes and Consequences of High Anxiety.* New York: Routledge.

Stewart, B. W., and P. Kleihues. 2003. *World Cancer Report 2003.* Lyon, France: IARC.

Stingone, Jeanette A., Germaine M. Buck Louis, Shoji F. Nakayama, Roel C. H. Vermeulen, Richard K. Kwok, Yuxia Cui, David M. Balshaw, and Susan L. Teitelbaum. 2017. "Toward Greater Implementation of the Exposome Research Paradigm within Environmental Epidemiology." *Annual Review of Public Health* 38:315–327.

Stoner, Bradley. 1986. "Understanding Medical Systems: Traditional, Modern, and Syncretic Health Care Alternatives in Medically Pluralistic Societies." *Medical Anthropology Quarterly* 17, no. 2, 44–48.

Strathern, Marilyn. 1992a. *After Nature: English Kinship in the Late Twentieth Century.* Cambridge: Cambridge University Press.

Strathern, Marilyn. 1992b. *Reproducing the Future: Essays on Anthropology, Kinship, and the New Reproductive Technologies*. New York: Routledge.

Strathern, Marilyn. 1994. "Displacing Knowledge: Technology and the Consequences for Kinship." In *Life and Death under High Technology Medicine*, edited by Ian Robinson. Manchester, UK: Manchester University Press..

Sullivan, Mark. 1986. "In What Sense Is Contemporary Medicine Dualistic?" *Culture, Medicine, and Psychiatry* 10:331–350.

Terzic, Andre, and Scott Waldman. 2011. "Chronic Diseases: The Emerging Pandemic." *Clinical and Translational Science* 4, no. 3, 225–226.

Thompson, Charis. 2005. *Making Parents: The Ontological Choreography of Reproductive Technologies*. Cambridge: Massachusetts Institute of Technology Press.

Thompson, Jennifer Jo, and Mark Nichter. 2016. "Is There a Role for Complementary and Alternative Medicine in Preventive and Promotive Health? An Anthropological Assessment in the Context of U.S. Health Reform." *Medical Anthropology Quarterly* 30, no. 1, 80–99.

Tuhiwai Smith, Linda. 2012. *Decolonizing Methodologies: Research and Indigenous Peoples*. London: Zed Books.

Twort, Frederick William. 1915. "An Investigation on the Nature of Ultra-microscopic Viruses." *The Lancet* 186:4814.

Ungless, Janet. 2013. "Meet the Real Medicine Woman." *Prevention*, November 24. https://www.prevention.com/life/a20452157/meet-the-medicine-woman-tieraona-low-dog/.

Vega, Rosalynn A. 2017a. "Childbirth and Medical Pluralism in Multiethnic Mexico." *L'Uomo Societá tradizione sviluppo* 1:125–156.

Vega, Rosalynn A. 2017b. "Racial I(nter)dentification: The Racialization of Maternal Health through the Oportunidades Program and in Government Clinics in Mexico." *Salud à Colectiva* 13, no. 3, 489–505.

Vega, Rosalynn A. 2018. *No Alternative: Childbirth, Citizenship, and Indigenous Culture in Mexico*. Austin: University of Texas Press.

Vega, Rosalynn A. 2023. *Nested Ecologies: A Multilayered Ethnography of Functional Medicine*. Austin: University of Texas Press.

Verkerk, Rob. 2019. "What Happened to 'Do No Harm'?" *What Doctors Don't Tell You*, October.

Vora, Kalindi. 2015. *Life Support: Biocapital and the New History of Outsourced Labor*. Minneapolis: University of Minnesota Press.

Wagner, William G. 2005. "Confronting Utilization Review in New Mexico's Medicaid Mental Health System: The Critical Role of 'Medical Necessity.'" *Medical Anthropology Quarterly* 19, no. 1, 64–83.

Wahls, Terry. 2014. *The Wahls Protocol: A Radical New Way to Treat All Chronic Autoimmune Conditions Using Paleo Principles*. New York: Penguin.

Wahls, Terry L., Catherine A. Chenard, and Linda G. Snetselaar. 2019. "Review of Two Popular Eating Plans within the Multiple Sclerosis Community: Low Saturated Fat and Modified Paleolithic." *Nutrients* 11, no. 2, 352.

Wainwright, Steven P., Clare Williams, Mike Michael, Bobbie Farsides, and Alan Cribb. 2006. "Ethical Boundary-Work in the Embryonic Stem Cell Laboratory." *Sociology of Health & Illness* 28, no. 6, 732–748. https://doi.org/10.1111/j.1467-9566.2006.00539.x.

Warren, Carol A. B., Dane Archer, Carlfred B. Broderick, S. Collas, Debra Dobbs, and Glena Flores. 2000. "Writing the Other, Inscribing the Self." *Qualitative Sociology* 23, no. 2, 183–198.

Water Resources Mission Area. 2019. "Arsenic and Drinking Water." United States Geological Survey. https://www.usgs.gov/mission-areas/water-resources/science/arsenic-and-drinking-water#:~:text=In%20a%20national%20study%20of,1%20%C2%B5g%2FL%20or%20greater.

Weeks, John. 2019. "Cleveland Clinic's Functional Medicine Outcomes in *JAMA*: Six Perspectives." *Today's Practitioner*, November 8. https://todayspractitioner.com/uncategorized/cleveland-clinics-functional-medicine-outcomes-in-jama-six-perspectives/.

Whitson, Jennifer R. 2013. "Gaming the Quantified Self." *Surveillance & Society* 11, nos. 1/2, 163–176.

Wiley, Sarah. 1992. "Adaptation and the Biocultural Paradigm in Medical Anthropology: A Critical Review." *Medical Anthropology Quarterly* 6, no. 3, 216–236.

Willging, Cathleen E. 2005. "Power, Blame, and Accountability: Medicaid Managed Care for Mental Health Services in New Mexico." *Medical Anthropology Quarterly* 19, no. 1, 84–102.

Williams, Roger. 1998. *Biochemical Individuality: Basis for the Genetotrophic Concept.* New York: McGraw Hill.

Wilson, Ara. 2004. *The Intimate Economies of Bangkok: Tomboys, Tycoons, and Avon Ladies in the Global City.* Berkeley: University of California Press.

Wiltshire, J. 1994. "Beyond the Ouija Board: Dialogue and Heteroglossia in the Medical Narrative." *Literature and Medicine* 13, no. 2, 211–228.

Wittel, Andreas. 2015. "Digital Marx: Toward a Political Economy of Distributed Media." In *Marx in the Age of Digital Capitalism*, edited by Christian Fuchs and Vincent Mosco, 68–104. Leiden, Netherlands: Brill.

Wolever, Ruth Q., Leigh Ann Simmons, Gary A. Sforzo, Diana Dill, Miranda Kaye, Elizabeth M. Bechard, Mary Elaine Southard, Mary Kennedy, Justine Vosloo, and Nancy Yang. 2013. "A Systematic Review of the Literature on Health and Wellness Coaching: Defining a Key Behavioral Intervention in Healthcare." *Global Advances in Health and Medicine* 2, no. 4, 38–57.

Yatani, R., T. Shiraishi, and K. Nakakuki. 1988. "Trends in Frequency of Latent Prostate Carcinoma in Japan from 1965–1979 to 1982–1986." *Journal of the National Cancer Institute* 80, no. 9, 683–687.

Yeung, Jessie. 2019. "Humans Have a 'Salamander-like' Ability to Regrow Cartilage, Study Finds." CNN, October 10. https://www.cnn.com/2019/10/10/health/humans-salamander-regenerate-intl-hnk-scli-scn/index.html.

INDEX

Photos and illustrations are indicated by italicized page numbers.

FSC
www.fsc.org
MIX
Papier | Fördert
gute Waldnutzung
FSC® C083411

Kolibri 360 GmbH
Ferdinand-Jühlke-Straße 7
99095 Erfurt, Deutschland
produktsicherheit@kolibri360.de